Evidence-based Management of

EPILEPSY

Steven C. Schachter

tfm Publishing Limited, Castle Hill Barns, Harley, Nr Shrewsbury, SY5 6LX, UK.
Tel: +44 (0)1952 510061; Fax: +44 (0)1952 510192
E-mail: nikki@tfmpublishing.com; Web site: www.tfmpublishing.com

Design & Typesetting: Nikki Bramhill BSc Hons Dip Law
First Edition: © September 2011
ISBN: 978 1 903378 77 9

Cover image: © 2011 3d4medical, www.3d4medical.com

Printed by Gutenberg Press Ltd., Gudja Road, Tarxien, PLA 19, Malta.
Tel: +356 21897037; Fax: +356 21800069.

Contents

Foreword

In assessing, treating and advising their patients, physicians make numerous decisions based on various types of information and evidence. Some of this information comes directly from an individual patient in the form of the medical history, physical findings and laboratory studies. Ideally, much of the evidence to support diagnostic and treatment strategies is attained from high-quality published clinical studies that are particularly relevant to the physician's pending decisions. Unfortunately, such evidence is not often available, leaving physicians to rely entirely on consensus statements, uncontrolled case reports or case series, or anecdotal experience.

The purpose of this book is to provide physicians caring for patients with epilepsy with the available evidence to support the diagnostic and treatment decisions that are frequently made in clinical practice together with an assessment of the strength of the supporting published evidence, using levels and grades as explained further on page ix. Chapter 1 focuses on the decisions to start, select, monitor and stop antiepileptic drugs (AEDs), Chapter 2 further elaborates on monitoring seizure frequency and severity, and Chapter 6 addresses an aspect of seizures that is often overlooked – the postictal state. Chapters 3 and 7 address a range of non-pharmacological treatments that become options when AEDs do not achieve the treatment objective of freedom from seizures and significant side effects, and Chapter 8 proposes the basis for evaluating a new class of devices – seizure prediction and detection systems – which are currently under development. Chapters 4, 5 and 12 discuss diagnostic and treatment issues specific to women of child-bearing potential, patients with concomitant depressive and anxiety disorders, and those with intellectual disabilities, respectively. The diagnosis and treatment of psychogenic non-epileptic seizures, a problem that vexes patients and physicians alike, is covered in Chapter 13.

Patients with epilepsy often ask their physicians about topics such as whether they could die from a seizure and how this could be prevented, what behavioral treatments may be of benefit to them, and if herbal remedies could help. The available evidence for these topics is presented in Chapters 7, 9, 10 and 11.

One of the informative and sobering outcomes of assessing the evidence-based management of epilepsy is the recognition that evidence simply does not currently exist to inform and support many of the potentially life-altering decisions that clinicians must make on a daily basis. Hence the authors suggest many areas where further clinical research is urgently needed.

To use the published evidence most effectively in their daily work, physicians should evaluate its strengths and weaknesses, as well as its relevance to a specific patient. Even the best evidence is not "one size fits all" but rather should be applied in the context of the clinical insights that emerge from the doctor-patient relationship, which still remains the most vitally important, irreplaceable cornerstone of the practice of medicine.

Steven C. Schachter MD

Contributors

Stefan Beyenburg MD Neurologist, Senior Clinical Lecturer in Neurology and Chef de Service, Department of Neurology, Centre Hospitalier de Luxembourg, Luxembourg

Ingo Borggräfe MD Pediatrician, Attending Physician and Head of the Pediatric Epilepsy Unit, Department of Pediatric Neurology and Developmental Medicine, University of Munich, Munich, Germany

Ivana Dojcinov MRCPsych Specialist Trainee in Psychiatry of Learning Disability, ABMU NHS Trust, Cardiff, UK

Dana Ekstein MD Senior Neurologist, Head, Epilepsy Center, Department of Neurology, Hadassah University Medical Center, Jerusalem, Israel

Lizbeth Hernandez-Ronquillo MD MSc Research Co-ordinator, Epilepsy Program, University of Saskatchewan, Division of Neurology, Department of Medicine, Royal University Hospital, Saskatoon, Canada

Andres M. Kanner MD Professor of Neurological Sciences and Psychiatry, Rush Medical College at Rush University; Director, Laboratory of EEG and Video-EEG-Telemetry; Associate Director, Section of Epilepsy and Rush Epilepsy Center, Rush University Medical Center, Chicago, Illinois, USA

Mike Kerr FRCPsych Professor, Learning Disability Psychiatry, Cardiff University, Cardiff, UK

Autumn M. Klein MD PhD Director, Program in Women's Neurology, Brigham and Women's Hospital; Instructor in Neurology, Harvard Medical School, Boston, Massachusetts, USA

Danielle G. Koby PhD Staff Psychologist, Department of Psychiatry, Division of Behavioral Medicine, The Miriam Hospital, Providence, Rhode Island, USA

Kimford Meador MD Professor of Neurology and Director of Epilepsy, Department of Neurology, Emory University, Atlanta, Georgia, USA

Joshua Mendelson MD Fellow in Neurology, Department of Neurology, Emory University, Atlanta, Georgia, USA

Soheyl Noachtar MD Neurologist and Psychiatrist, Associate Professor of Neurology and Head of the Epilepsy Center, Department of Neurology, University of Munich, Munich, Germany

Patricia Osborne Shafer RN MN Epilepsy Nurse Specialist, Beth Israel Deaconess Medical Center, Boston, Massachusetts, USA

Ivan Osorio MD Professor of Neurology, University of Kansas Medical Center, Kansas, USA

Mark Quigg MD MSc Professor of Neurology, Medical Director Clinical Neurophysiology: EEG, Neurological Sleep, Evoked Potentials, and Intensive Monitoring, University of Virginia, Charlottesville, Virginia, USA

Jan Rémi MD Epilepsy Fellow at the Epilepsy Center, Department of Neurology, University of Munich, Munich, Germany

Steven C. Schachter MD Professor of Neurology, Harvard Medical School, Beth Israel Deaconess Medical Center; Chief Academic Officer and Director of NeuroTechnology, Center for Integration of Medicine and Innovative Technology (CIMIT), Boston, Massachusetts, USA

Dieter Schmidt MD Formerly Professor of Neurology, Free University of Berlin, Currently Head of Epilepsy Research Group, Berlin, Germany

Joseph I. Sirven MD Professor of Neurology, Department of Neurology, Division of Epilepsy, Mayo Clinic Hospital, Phoenix, Arizona, USA

José F. Téllez Zenteno MD PhD Associate Professor, University of Saskatchewan, Division of Neurology, Department of Medicine, Royal University Hospital, Saskatoon, Canada

Acknowledgements

We are grateful to all of the contributors for taking on this important task and hope they will be proud to be part of a book which attempts to set out the evidence-based management of epilepsy.

We would also like to thank Nikki Bramhill and Jonathan Gregory from tfm Publishing Limited for their invaluable assistance.

Using evidence-based medicine

The process of gathering evidence is a time-consuming task. One of the main reasons for supporting the use of evidence-based medicine is the rate of change of new practices, and the increasing tendency for specialization. Medical information is widely available from a variety of sources for clinicians but keeping up-to-date with current literature remains an almost impossible task for many with a busy clinical workload. *Evidence-based Management of Epilepsy* has been written to aid this process. The chapters in this book have been written by internationally renowned experts who have applied the principles of evidence-based medicine and taken relevant clinical questions and examined the current evidence for the answers. The authors were asked to quote levels and grades of evidence for each major point, and to provide a summary of key points and their respective evidence levels at the end of each chapter. The levels of evidence and grades of evidence used in this book are shown in Tables 1 and 2 and are widely used in evidence-based medicine.

Table 1. Levels of evidence.

Level	Type of evidence
Ia	Evidence obtained from systematic review or meta-analysis of randomized controlled trials
Ib	Evidence obtained from at least one randomized controlled trial
IIa	Evidence obtained from at least one well-designed controlled study without randomization
IIb	Evidence obtained from at least one other type of well-designed quasi-experimental study
III	Evidence obtained from well-designed non-experimental descriptive studies, such as comparative studies, correlation studies and case studies
IV	Evidence obtained from expert committee reports or opinions and/or clinical experience of respected authorities

Table 2. Grades of evidence.

Grade of evidence	Evidence
A	At least one randomized controlled trial as part of a body of literature of overall good quality and consistency addressing the specific recommendation (evidence levels Ia and Ib)
B	Well-conducted clinical studies but no randomized clinical trials on the topic of recommendation (evidence levels IIa, IIb, III)
C	Expert committee reports or opinions and/or clinical experience of respected authorities. This grading indicates that directly applicable clinical studies of good quality are absent (evidence level IV)

Chapter 1

Starting, choosing, monitoring and stopping AEDs in epilepsy

Dieter Schmidt MD
Formerly Professor of Neurology, Free University of Berlin
Currently Head of Epilepsy Research Group, Berlin
Germany

Stefan Beyenburg MD
Neurologist, Senior Clinical Lecturer in Neurology
and Chef de Service, Department of Neurology
Centre Hospitalier de Luxembourg, Luxembourg

Introduction

Epilepsy is one of the most common neurological disorders and antiepileptic drugs (AEDs) are the mainstay of epilepsy treatment. Although there is an abundance of short-term regulatory randomized controlled trials to assess the efficacy and safety of individual experimental AEDs prior to marketing, surprisingly, few trials have addressed the management of epilepsy with marketed AEDs in clinical practice. Good management of epilepsy requires to know when to start AEDs, what AED to choose, how to monitor AED treatment and when to stop AEDs. The present chapter provides a brief criticial overview on the strength of the evidence for making these major management decisions in epilepsy.

Starting AEDs

The rationale for starting treatment is to have a lower risk of seizure recurrence and better well-being compared to no treatment or deferred treatment. In this section we discuss the effects of AED treatment versus no treatment on time to recurrence, long-term seizure outcome, as well as well-being in patients with a single seizure and in those with several seizures prior to treatment.

Patients presenting with a single seizure

Among patients with a single seizure, only about 25% will have a recurrence within 2 years in the absence of factors that predict a high probability of recurrence [1] (Ia/A). Risk factors for a higher seizure recurrence include primarily a known cause such as remote major head trauma or, in the case of generalized epilepsy, spike wave activity in the EEG [1] (Ia/A). Even in patients with one or more risk factors, the recurrence rate at 2 years is not above 40%. A number of randomized controlled trials have compared AED treatment versus deferred treatment in patients presenting with a first seizure [2-5] (Ib/A). Here we will discuss the largest trial [5] (Ib/A). For patients with a single seizure, the risk of relapse at 2 years of treatment was 32% for immediate treatment and 39% for deferred treatment. However, at 5 years, the risk was similar (42% for immediate and 51% for deferred treatment). The treatment effect between early and deterred treatment for 2-year remission was 12% at 2 years, 2% at 5 years and 1% at 8 years [5] (Ib/A). Regression analysis showed that the number of seizures before randomization, an abnormal EEG, and signs of a neurological or cognitive deficit increased the risk of seizure recurrence [6] (Ia/A). Low-risk patients were those with a single seizure, no neurological deficit, and a normal EEG. Medium-risk was seen in those with either 2-3 seizures or neurological signs or an abnormal EEG. All patients who had more seizures or more than one additional factor belonged to the high-risk group.

This is in agreement with randomized controlled trials showing that treatment reduces the risk of seizure recurrence on average by about 50% (range: 30-60%) and that those treated earlier have a better short-term seizure outcome versus those with no treatment or deferred treatment. However, the likelihood of being seizure-free at 3-5 years after a first or second seizure was similar whether treatment was started immediately or was deferred initially and started only if a further seizure occurred [5] (Ib/A). This is important evidence for two reasons: one, it shows for clinical practice that deferring treatment does not worsen prospects for becoming seizure-free, at least for those with low to medium risk for recurrence [6] (Ib/A); and, two, it provides clues for clinical science, that AEDs, even if they are actively blocking seizures, are not able to improve the course of the underlying disease, i.e. epilepsy. This finding is also in agreement with long-term studies of the natural history of treated epilepsy showing that early seizure remission may be followed by late relapse and thus does not guarantee permanent seizure freedom [7] (III/B).

Patients presenting with several recent seizures

Patients presenting with two or three seizures or even four or more seizures have a higher risk of seizure recurrence, which is further increased in those with neurological signs or an abnormal EEG [6] (Ib/A). High-risk patients, as defined above [6] (Ib/A), have a higher 5-year recurrence risk (73% vs. 50%) versus those with early treatment [6] (Ib/A). However, the risk following a second seizure has not been examined in a prospective population-based study of untreated patients [8] (Ib/A). The best available evidence for the risk of seizure recurrence comes from Hauser *et al* [9] (IIa/B) who prospectively followed 204 patients, 87% of which were treated with AEDs following their second seizure. The risk of a third seizure went up from 57% (95% CI, 45-70%) at 1 year and 73% (95% CI, 59-87%) at 4 years. The risk was higher in those with symptomatic epilepsy versus those with idiopathic or presumed symptomatic (cryptogenic) epilepsy. Shinnar et al [10] (Ia/A) reported similar findings in children followed up since their first seizure. A study reporting seizure recurrence in patients with several seizures who were randomized to treatment does not exist for ethical concerns, as it would deprive patients of needed proven treatment. The current recommendations on starting AEDs in patients with two or more seizures, particularly if they occurred within the last 6-12 months, are based on Hauser's data [9] (IIa/B). Given this finding, starting AEDs is almost always justified in those with two or more seizures within the last 6-12 months provided the seizures are disabling, and cannot be controlled by avoiding precipitants. However, there are exceptions, such as patients with benign syndromes of childhood or adolescence or seizures that can easily be controlled by avoiding precipitants.

Choosing the right AED

Choosing the right AED for the individual patient is the result of a complex decision process that involves a risk-benefit assessment of the drug versus other suitable AEDs for the individual patient. In addition, other factors, which may play in the decision to prefer a drug over another one, include personal preference and ease of use based on past experience, a feeling of comfort, and last not least, cost. Unfortunately the vast majority of trials dealing with efficacy and safety of AEDs are designed for regulatory agencies which are primarily focused on evidence for short-term efficacy and safety of the drug versus placebo in the case of add-on treatment or low-dose controls in active monotherapy trials.

Choosing the right AED for patients with newly diagnosed epilepsy

In this section we will limit the discussion to a brief critical review of four influential benchmark trials that examined the long-term, comparative risk-benefit balance of major individual AEDs given at a clinically adequate dosage for new-onset epilepsy in adults [8, 11, 12] (Ib/A).

What is the evidence to prefer carbamazepine over phenobarbital, phenytoin, primidone and valproate for newly diagnosed focal epilepsy in adults?

Mattson et al [11] (Ib/A) conducted a 10-center, double-blind trial to compare the efficacy and tolerability of four major antiepileptic drugs in the treatment of focal and focal-onset generalized tonic-clonic seizures in 622 adults. Patients were randomly assigned to treatment with carbamazepine, phenobarbital, phenytoin, or primidone and were followed for 2 years or until the drug failed to control seizures or caused unacceptable side effects. Overall treatment success, as measured by the proportion of patients remaining on treatment (retention rate), was highest with carbamazepine or phenytoin, intermediate with phenobarbital, and lowest with primidone (p<0.002). Differences in failure rates of the drugs were explained primarily by the fact that primidone caused more intolerable acute toxic effects, such as nausea, vomiting, dizziness, and sedation. Decreased libido and impotence were more common in patients given primidone. Phenytoin caused more dysmorphic effects and hypersensitivity. Control of tonic-clonic seizures did not differ significantly with the various drugs. Carbamazepine provided complete control of partial seizures more often than primidone or phenobarbital (p<0.03). The authors concluded that, overall, carbamazepine and phenytoin are recommended drugs of first choice for single-drug therapy of adults with focal partial or focal-onset generalized tonic-clonic seizures or with both.

The trial is an unsurpassed benchmark study, and the authors are congratulated for their work. In fact, the study could serve as a model to compare the utility of several modern AEDs in a long-term double-blind retention trial such as the one performed by Mattson *et al* [11] (Ib/A).

For the control of secondarily generalized tonic-clonic seizures, carbamazepine and valproic acid were comparably effective in a double-blind trial study of 136 patients and 138 patients, respectively [12] (Ib/A). For complex partial seizures, four of five outcome measures favored carbamazepine (100 patients) over valproic acid (106 patients): the total number of seizures (2.7 vs. 7.6, p=0.05), the number of seizures per month (0.9 vs. 2.2, p=0.01), the time to the first seizure (p<0.02), and the seizure-rating score (p<0.04). Carbamazepine was also superior according to a composite score that combined scores for the control of seizures and for adverse effects (p<0.001). Valproic acid was associated more frequently than carbamazepine with a weight gain of more than 5.5kg (12lb) (20% vs. 8%, p<0.001), with hair loss or change in texture (12% vs. 6%, p=0.02), and with tremor (45% vs. 22%, p<0.001). Rash was more often associated with carbamazepine (11% vs. 1%, p<0.001). The authors concluded that valproic acid is as effective as carbamazepine for the treatment of generalized tonic-clonic seizures, but carbamazepine provides better control of complex partial seizures and has fewer long-term adverse effects. Although the carbamazepine versus valproic acid trial is a benchmark study, and the authors are congratulated for their work, it has some limitations. The main limitation is that the teratogenicity of valproic acid versus carbamazepine could not be evaluated as this was a trial in male patients. It is also unfortunate that the trial did not assess the effects of enzyme-inducing carbamazepine versus non-enzyme-inducing valproic acid.

Do we have enough evidence which new AED to choose for newly diagnosed epilepsy?

A series of short-term, randomized double-blind trials have demonstrated that several of the newer generation AEDs are equal in effectivenmess to the standard old drug carbamazepine. This has been shown for lamotrigine [13] (Ib/A), levetiracetam [14] (Ia/A), and topiramate [15] (Ia/A), although the latter is in some dispute [8]. Oxcarbazepine has also shown similar efficacy compared to carbamazepine and phenytoin [8, 16, 17] (Ib/A). Recent guidelines found clear evidence for the effectiveness of a number of new generation AEDs in initial monotherapy in adults and children [18, 19] (Ia/A).

A recent evidence-based analysis of antiepileptic drug efficacy and effectiveness as initial monotherapy for epileptic seizures and syndromes came to sobering conclusions [20] (Ia/A). The authors concluded that the absence of rigorous comprehensive adverse effects data makes it impossible to develop an evidence-based guideline aimed at identifying the overall optimal recommended initial-monotherapy AED, old or new. There is an especially alarming lack of well-designed, properly conducted RCTs for patients with generalized seizures/epilepsies and for children in general. The majority of relevant existing RCTs have significant methodologic problems that limit their applicability to this guideline's clinically relevant main question. Multicenter, multinational efforts are needed to design, conduct and analyze future clinically relevant RCTs that can answer the many outstanding questions identified in this guideline.

The purpose of the review was to assess which AEDs have the best evidence for long-term efficacy or effectiveness as initial monotherapy for patients with newly diagnosed or untreated epilepsy. A 10-member subcommission of the Commission on Therapeutic Strategies of The International League Against Epilepsy (ILAE), evaluated available evidence found through a structured literature review including MEDLINE, Current Contents and the Cochrane Library for all applicable articles from 1940 until July 2005. Articles dealing with different seizure types (for different age groups) and two epilepsy syndromes were assessed for quality of evidence (four classes) based on predefined criteria. Criteria for class I classification were a double-blind randomized controlled trial (RCT) design, ≥48-week treatment duration without forced exit criteria, information on ≥24-week seizure freedom data (efficacy) or ≥48-week retention data (effectiveness), demonstration of superiority or 80% power to detect a ≤20% relative difference in efficacy/effectiveness versus an adequate comparator, and appropriate statistical analysis. Class II studies met all class I criteria except for having either treatment duration of 24 to 47 weeks or, for non-inferiority analysis, a power to only exclude a 21-30% relative difference. Class III studies included other randomized double-blind and open-label trials, and class IV included other forms of evidence (e.g. expert opinion, case reports). Quality of clinical trial evidence was used to determine the strength of the level of recommendation. A total of 50 RCTs and seven meta-analyses contributed to the analysis. Only four RCTs had class I evidence, whereas two had class II evidence; the remainder were evaluated as class III evidence. Three seizure types had AEDs with level A or level B efficacy and effectiveness evidence as initial monotherapy: adults with partial-onset seizures (level A, carbamazepine and phenytoin; level B, valproic acid), children with partial-onset seizures (level A, oxcarbazepine; level B, none), and elderly adults with partial-onset seizures (level A, gabapentin and lamotrigine; level B, none). One adult seizure type (adults with generalized-onset tonic-clonic [GTC] seizures), two pediatric seizure types (GTC seizures and absence seizures), and two epilepsy syndromes (benign epilepsy with centrotemporal spikes and juvenile myoclonic epilepsy) had no AEDs with level A or level B efficacy and effectiveness evidence as initial monotherapy.

The ultimate choice of an AED for any individual patient with newly diagnosed or untreated epilepsy should include consideration of the strength of the efficacy and effectiveness evidence for each AED along with other variables such as the AED safety and tolerability profile, pharmacokinetic properties, formulations, and expense [20] (Ia/A). In a nutshell, the ILAE treatment guidelines for initial monotherapy emphasize the poor quality of information available to inform everyday clinical practice.

When selecting a patient's AED, physicians and patients should consider all relevant variables and not just efficacy and effectiveness. Furthermore, the results of regulatory trials are difficult to translate into the clinical practice which always weighs the long-term effects and tolerability of one drug versus another suitable drug at clinically useful dosage. As a consequence, we will limit ourselves in this section to a brief critical review of long-term, randomized trials of comparative risk-benefit outcome with individual AEDs given at clinically adequate dosage [8, 11, 12] (Ib/A).

Should modern AEDs be preferred over older AEDs as first-line agents for newly diagnosed epilepsy?

Despite the introduction of many new AEDs over the last two decades, the older agents, carbamazepine, phenytoin and phenobarbital, remain the AEDs most commonly prescribed throughout the world. At the same time, there is growing concern regarding the possible adverse consequences of older AEDs such as CYP450 induction, such that it is appropriate to pose the question of whether the inducing drugs should still be considered first-line agents for the treatment of epilepsy. We review here the comparative evidence of new versus old AEDs stemming from several benchmark trials and evidence-based guidelines.

The SANAD trial

The SANAD trial is a randomized controlled trial that examined the longer-term outcomes of older versus newer antiepileptic drugs [8] (Ib/A). The aim was to compare clinicians' choice of one of the standard older epilepsy drug treatments (carbamazepine or valproate) versus appropriate comparator new drugs. It was a multicenter study recruiting patients with epilepsy from hospital outpatient clinics. Patients included had to have an adequately documented history of two or more clinically definite unprovoked epileptic seizures within the last year for whom treatment with a single antiepileptic drug represented the best therapeutic option. The clinical trial had two arms, one comparing new drugs with carbamazepine (Arm A) and the other with valproate (Arm B). Arm A was carbamazepine versus gabapentin versus lamotrigine versus oxcarbazepine versus topiramate. Arm B was valproate versus lamotrigine versus topiramate. The study measured time to treatment failure (withdrawal of the randomized drug for reasons of unacceptable adverse events or inadequate seizure control or both) and time to achieve a 12-month remission of seizures.

Time from randomization to first seizure, 24-month remission of seizures, incidence of clinically important adverse events, quality of life (QoL) outcomes and health economic outcomes were also considered.

The results of the SANAD trial were as follows. Arm A recruited 1721 patients (88% with symptomatic or cryptogenic partial epilepsy and 10% with unclassified epilepsy). Arm B recruited 716 patients (63% with idiopathic generalized epilepsy and 25% with unclassified epilepsy). In Arm A, lamotrigine had the lowest incidence of treatment failure and was statistically superior to all drugs for this outcome with the exception of oxcarbazepine. Some 12% and 8% fewer patients experienced treatment failure on lamotrigine than carbamazepine, the standard drug, at 1 and 2 years after randomization, respectively. The superiority of lamotrigine over carbamazepine was due to its better tolerability but there was satisfactory evidence indicating that lamotrigine is not clinically inferior to carbamazepine for measures of its efficacy. No consistent differences in QoL outcomes were found between treatment groups. Health economic analysis supported lamotrigine being preferred to carbamazepine for both cost per seizure avoided and cost per quality-adjusted life-year gained. In Arm B, for time to treatment failure, valproic acid was the standard drug. Valproic acid was preferred to both topiramate and lamotrigine, as it was the drug least likely to be associated with treatment failure for inadequate seizure control and was the preferred drug for time to achieving a 12-month remission. QoL assessments did not show any between-treatment differences. The health economic assessment supported the conclusion that valproate should remain the drug of first choice for idiopathic generalized or unclassified epilepsy, although there is a suggestion that topiramate is a cost-effective alternative to valproate. In the conclusions the authors suggested that lamotrigine may be a clinical and cost-effective alternative to the existing standard drug treatment, carbamazepine, for patients diagnosed as having partial seizures. For patients with idiopathic generalized epilepsy or difficult-to-classify epilepsy, the authors concluded that valproic acid remains the clinically most effective drug, although topiramate may be a cost-effective alternative for some patients. The authors noted that additional new antiepileptic drugs have been marketed since completion of the SANAD trial (levetiracetam, zonisamide and pregabalin) and suggested that these drugs should be compared in a similarly designed trial.

Although the SANAD trial is a benchmark study, and the authors are congratulated for their work, it has a few limitations. The main limitation is that it is an unblinded trial. The lack of a double-blind design introduces an assessment bias, particularly for measuring adverse events. It is also unfortunate that the SANAD trial did not assess the effects of enzyme-inducing carbamazepine versus non-enzyme-inducing newer AEDs. Finally, it would have been helpful to include only patients with definite idiopathic generalized epilepsy (IGE) into ARM A. The diagnostic heterogeneity was perhaps unavoidable but is unfortunate in view of the lack of RCT data for treatment outcome in patients with IGE.

A 23-member committee evaluated the available evidence up until 2003 [18, 19] **(Ib/A)**, demonstrating efficacy, tolerability, and safety of seven new antiepileptic drugs (AEDs) (gabapentin, lamotrigine, topiramate, tiagabine, oxcarbazepine, levetiracetam, and zonisamide) in the treatment of children and adults with newly diagnosed partial and generalized epilepsies. The committee reported that there is evidence either from comparative or dose-controlled trials that gabapentin, lamotrigine, topiramate, and oxcarbazepine have efficacy as monotherapy in newly diagnosed adolescents and adults with either partial or mixed seizure disorders. There is also evidence that lamotrigine is effective for newly diagnosed absence seizures in children. Evidence for effectiveness of the new AEDs in newly diagnosed patients with other generalized epilepsy syndromes is lacking. The authors concluded that the results of this evidence-based assessment provide guidelines for the prescription of AEDs for patients with newly diagnosed epilepsy and identify those seizure types and syndromes where more evidence is necessary. Although valuable, the guidelines could not provide evidence from comparative effectiveness research which AED to prefer over another suitable AED for treatment of new focal or generalized epilepsy.

Should non-enzyme-inducing new AEDs be preferred over enzyme-inducing AEDs as first-line agents?

Although many new AEDs including non-enzyme-inducing agents such as gabapentin or lamotrigine entered the market since the 1990s, the older agents, valproate, as well as carbamazepine, phenytoin and phenobarbital, which are potent inducers of the cytochrome P450 (CYP450) system, remain among the AEDs most commonly prescribed throughout the world. There is growing concern, however, regarding the possible adverse implications of CYP450 induction, raising the question whether enzyme-inducing AEDs should still be considered first-line agents for the treatment of focal epilepsy. A recent review of the evidence suggested that the older enzyme-inducing drugs are involved in sometimes deleterious drug-drug interactions and have many detrimental metabolic effects on vitamin D and bone metabolism, gonadal steroids, cholesterol and other markers of vascular risk [21] (IV/C) (see elsewhere in this book). Although there are data suggesting similar efficacy of the newer, non-inducing AEDs, longer and better-powered studies are needed to truly establish whether the newer AEDs are equivalent in efficacy to the older, inducing agents [21] (IV/C) (see above). Pending this, however, the existing data are sufficiently concerning to suggest that it may be prudent to start with non-inducing AEDs unless there is a clear indication for one of the inducing drugs.

Do we have enough evidence which new AED to choose for refractory epilepsy?

A 23-member committee evaluated the available evidence based on a structured literature review including MEDLINE, Current Contents, and the Cochrane Library for relevant articles from 1987 until March 2003 [18, 19] (Ia/A). The task was to assess the evidence demonstrating efficacy, tolerability, and safety of seven new antiepileptic drugs (AEDs) (gabapentin, lamotrigine, topiramate, tiagabine, oxcarbazepine, levetiracetam, and zonisamide) in the treatment of children and adults with refractory partial and generalized epilepsies. The authors found that all of the new AEDs were appropriate for adjunctive treatment of refractory focal seizures in adults. Gabapentin can be effective for the treatment of patients with mixed seizure disorders, and gabapentin, lamotrigine, oxcarbazepine, and topiramate for the treatment of refractory partial seizures in adults and children. Limited evidence suggests that lamotrigine and topiramate are also effective for adjunctive treatment of idiopathic generalized epilepsy in adults and children, as well as treatment of the Lennox-Gastaut syndrome. The authors of the guidelines concluded that the choice of AED depends upon seizure and/or syndrome type, patient age, concomitant medications, AED tolerability, safety, and efficacy. The results of this evidence-based assessment provide guidelines for the prescription of AEDs for patients with refractory epilepsy and identify those seizure types and syndromes where more evidence is necessary [18, 19] **(Ia/A)**. Although valuable, the guidelines could not provide evidence from comparative effectiveness research which AED to prefer over another suitable AED for treatment of refractory focal or generalized epilepsy. Unfortunately, we do not have (yet) suitable design strategies that allow us to compare two or more appropriate drugs for refractory epilepsy in a long-term double-blind retention trial.

How much better than placebo are new AEDs for treatment of refractory epilepsy?

Although adjunctive treatment with new AEDs is standard care in refractory epilepsy, as reviewed in the previous section, it is unclear how much of the effect can be directly attributed to the AEDs and how much to the beneficial changes seen with placebo. This prompted a systematic review and meta-analysis of the evidence to determine the placebo-corrected net efficacy of adjunctive treatment with modern AEDs on the market for refractory epilepsy [22] **(Ia/A)**. Of 317 potentially eligible articles reviewed in full text, 124 (39%) fulfilled eligibility criteria. After excluding 69 publications, 55 publications of 54 studies in a total of 11,106 adults and children with refractory epilepsy form the basis of evidence. The overall weighted pooled risk difference in favor of AEDs over placebo for seizure freedom in the total sample of adults and children was 6%, (95% CI, 4-8%; $z=6.47$; $p<0.001$) and 21% (95% CI, 19-24%; $z=17.13$; $p<0.001$) for 50% seizure reduction. Although the presence of moderate heterogeneity may reduce the validity of the results and limit generalizations from the findings, the authors concluded that the placebo-corrected efficacy of adjunctive treatment with modern AEDs is disappointingly small and suggest that better strategies of finding drugs are needed for refractory epilepsy, which is a major public health problem [22] **(Ia/A)**.

Monitoring AEDs

Most suggestions for monitoring AED levels routinely are not evidence-based [23-25] and there is still considerable debate on the clinical usefulness of therapeutic drug monitoring in epilepsy patients [24-27]. In other words, the impact of therapeutic drug monitoring on clinical outcome has not been evaluated systematically. For example, the authors of a recent Cochrane review [24] **(Ia/A)** found only one randomized controlled trial meeting their inclusion criteria to assess the usefulness of routine AED monitoring in patients with newly diagnosed epilepsy with AED monotherapy. In that open study, 180 epilepsy patients with newly diagnosed, untreated seizures were randomized to treatment with carbamazepine, valproate, phenytoin, phenobarbital or primidone either with or without therapeutic drug serum level monitoring. A 12-month remission from seizures was achieved by 60% of the patients randomized to therapeutic drug monitoring and by 61% in the control group. A total of 56% in the group with AED monitoring and 58% in the control group were seizure-free during the last 12 months of follow-up. Adverse effects were reported by 48% in the intervention group and 47% of the control group patients. Of those randomized to therapeutic drug monitoring, 62% completed the 2-year follow-up compared with 67% of the control group. Thus, there was no clear evidence to support routine AED serum level measurement for the optimization of treatment in these patients [28] **(Ib/A)**. In the only other available randomized trial, 127 patients with refractory epilepsy receiving mono- or polytherapy with different AEDs were randomly assigned to treatment with or without measuring AED serum levels. Blood sampling for determination of AED levels were done in all patients. However, the treating physician was not informed about the results. One hundred and five patients completed the 1-year follow-up. As a result, a substantial proportion of patients in both groups had AED concentrations either below or above the so called therapeutic range. Moreover, treatment outcome was not different in the two groups [29]. This early study provided no evidence to support routine monitoring of AED serum levels [29] **(Ib/A)**.

However, some evidence from non-randomized studies and everyday clinical practice points to the possible usefulness of therapeutic drug monitoring of specific AEDs during polytherapy, in selected patients (e.g. pregnant women with epilepsy) or in special circumstances [25, 30, 31] **(III/B & IV/C)**. Best practice guidelines for therapeutic drug monitoring by the ILAE Commission on Therapeutic Strategies [25] **(IV/C)** recently suggested that two separate terms should be used to define drug concentration ranges in relation to their clinical effects. The 'reference range' can be defined as a range of drug concentrations, which is quoted by a laboratory and specifies a lower limit below which a therapeutic response is relatively unlikely to occur, and an upper limit above which toxicity is relatively likely to occur. In contrast, the 'therapeutic range' can be regarded as the range of drug concentrations which is associated with the best achievable response in a given subject (Table 1). This range is representing the balance between antiseizure efficacy and dose-related side effects. Therefore, it represents a purely statistical standard of the AED serum level derived from population studies (mostly in medically refractory patients).

Table 1. Common doses and ranges of serum concentrations of major AEDs in adults. Modified from St. Louis EK [38] (IV/C).

AED	Usual dosages (adults)/day (mg)	Serum levels (µG/mL)
Carbamazepine	400-1600	4-12
Ethosuximide	500-1500	40-100
Felbamate	1800-4800	30-100
Gabapentin	900-3600	4-20
Lacosamide	200-600	?
Lamotrigine	300-600	1-20
Levetiracetam	1000-4000	5-40
Oxcarbazepine	600-3600	10-40
Phenobarbital	90-180	15-40
Phenytoin	200-400	8-20
Pregabalin	150-450	?
Primidone	500-1500	5-12
Rufinamide	400-3200	?
Tiagabine	16-64	100-300ng/mL
Topiramate	100-600	10-20
Valproate	600-2500	50-100
Vigabatrin	2000-3000	0.8-36
Zonisamide	100-600	10-40

? = 'therapeutic range' not yet established

Indications for monitoring AED serum levels

The primary indications for monitoring AED serum levels have been extensively discussed and may be summarized as follows [25] (IV/C):

* monitoring of AED serum concentrations is helpful after the initiation of treatment or after dose adjustment (to achieve a target concentration in the individual patient and to establish an individual therapeutic range);
* in patients treated with drugs showing dose-dependent pharmacokinetics (e.g. phenytoin);
* in the case of presumed AED toxicity;
* when seizures persist despite an adequate dosage;
* during treatment of special patient populations (e.g. children and the elderly, women with epilepsy becoming pregnant). The rationale for monitoring in these patients is to elucidate altered pharmacokinetics during physiological alterations due to aging, pregnancy, and comorbid conditions;
* in patients with presumed drug-drug interactions, to evaluate potential changes in steady state AED concentration;
* when a change in drug formulation is made, including switches involving generic formulations;
* when poor compliance is suspected or whenever there is an unexpected alteration in clinical response.

As indicated above, reference ranges are a statistical estimate of the concentration range at which the majority of patients can be expected to show an optimal response to AED treatment. Several other limitations should be kept in mind when analyzing the results of serum level measurements: Most of the studies for defining reference ranges have been conducted in medically refractory patients [32-34] (IIa/B & III/B). For most of the newer AEDs, reference ranges have not yet been clearly defined [35] (IV/C). Moreover, the upper limit of the range may vary from one patient to another. There are patients showing toxic symptoms even at low drug levels while others may tolerate and even need concentrations above the upper limit of the range to achieve seizure control without developing side effects [36, 37] (III/B). Thus, dose adjustments should never be made on the basis of serum level concentrations alone, but should always be made on the basis of a careful clinical evaluation of the individual patient ("treat the patient and not the serum concentration").

Stopping AEDs

Although approximately 70% of all newly diagnosed epilepsy patients become seizure-free with AEDs [39] (III/B), many seizure-free patients (and their physicians) prefer to continue medication, mainly for fear of a seizure recurrence. What is the evidence to assess the risk-benefit of AED discontinuation? Surprisingly, there is only one small randomized double-blind trial for AED withdrawal of adults becoming seizure-free on AEDs [40] (Ib/A). The best evidence from the earlier literature comes from a large unblinded randomized trial in patients who became seizure-free on AED treatment [41] (Ib/A), and several, but non-randomized observational studies [42-46] (III/B). In addition, a number of reviews offer valuable information [47-49] (Ia/A).

The risk of seizures

The decision to continue or to stop AED treatment in patients with prolonged seizure remission is a difficult one and requires a full assessment of the risk-benefit balance of drug discontinuation for the individual patient. In the Akershus study, the first double-blind, randomized trial [40] (Ib/A), 15% of patients randomized to treatment withdrawal and 7% of those randomized to remain on treatment had a recurrence at 12 months, a non-significant difference. However, compared to the latter, the former improved significantly in their neuropsychological performance. In this benchmark study, Lossius and colleagues [40] (Ib/A) randomized adult patients, seizure-free for more than 2 years on AED monotherapy, to AED withdrawal (n=79) and no withdrawal (n=81), and followed them up for 12 months, or until seizure recurrence. After withdrawal, recurrence rates were 27% after a median of 41 months off medication. Withdrawal did not affect quality of life and EEG. Predictors for remaining seizure-free after AED withdrawal over 1 year were normal neurological examination and use of carbamazepine prior to withdrawal. Although the Akershus study is first in class, it needs to be considered in the light of several limitations. Firstly, the study excluded patients with a high risk of seizure relapse after withdrawal, for example, patients with idiopathic generalized epilepsy with epileptiform discharges and patients with juvenile myoclonic epilepsy, patients seizure-free on polytherapy, and a history of two prior withdrawal attempts. This has introduced a bias towards lowering the risk of seizure relapses, in both arms. Secondly, as patients were not randomized on AED use, the better outcome of withdrawal in those withdrawn from carbamazepine, may, in part, reflect a selection bias when treatment was started, and should not be taken as evidence that withdrawing patients from carbamazepine is more successful than withdrawal from other AEDs. Thirdly, the AED treatment and prognosis of seizures occurring after relapse have not been included in the results. It would have been worthwhile to learn if most patients had one seizure and remained seizure-free after relapse or how often treatment was restarted and how successful it was. This would have been important for patient counselling.

What are the implications of this important study? Firstly, AED withdrawal in adults is associated with a considerable risk of seizure recurrence in one of six patients, more than double the risk in those who remain on drugs (though the difference was not significant in the small trial). Secondly, some patients have improved neuropsychological outcome, but quality of life is not better after withdrawal. This finding is in agreement with the MRC study, although Jacoby et al [50] (Ia/A) found a benefit in a subgroup of patients with low risk of recurrence. Thirdly, remaining on AEDs does not protect from seizure recurrence. In fact, 2 years after withdrawal, there is no difference in recurrence rate between the withdrawal and the no withdrawal group. The Akershus study provided robust class I evidence on the benefits and risks of withdrawing AEDs in low-risk seizure-free adults that we did not have before. Patients and physicians are now better equipped to make the difficult decision to withdraw AEDs, after taking into account other important factors, such as the preference of the patient and the sometimes grave social consequences of a seizure relapse.

A review of the impact of planned discontinuation of AEDs in seizure-free patients on seizure recurrence yielded 14 observational studies of seizure recurrence after discontinuation and its treatment outcome. Seizure recurrence rate after AED discontinuation ranged between 12 and 66% (mean 34%, 95% CI, 27-43) in the 13 reviewed studies involving over 2300 patients (no data in one study) [48] (Ia/A). According to a large review, the proportion of patients with relapses during or after treatment withdrawal ranges from 12 to 66% [51] (Ia/A). Using life-table analysis, the cumulative probability of remaining seizure-free in children was 66-96% at 1 year and 61-91% at 2 years (adults 39-74% and 35-57%, respectively). The relapse rate peaked in the first 12 months (especially in the first 6 months) and tended to diminish thereafter. In a meta-analysis of 25 studies, the pooled relapse risk was 25% (95% CI, 21-30%) at 12 months and 29% (95% CI, 24-34%) at 24 months [47] (Ia/A).

The risk of seizures compared to continued treatment

AED discontinuation doubles the risk of seizures for up to 2 years after stopping AEDs compared to continued treatment [52] (Ia/A). This was one of the results of a prospective, multicenter, unblinded randomized study of continued antiepileptic treatment versus slow withdrawal conducted in 1013 patients who had been free of seizures for at least 2 years [41] (Ib/A). By 2 years after randomization, 78% of patients in whom treatment was continued and 59% of those in whom it was withdrawn remained seizure-free, but thereafter the differences between the two groups diminished. This suggests that the long-term seizure outcome is not affected by drug discontinuation. Non-compliance with continued treatment accounted for only a small proportion of the risk to the group continuing with treatment. The most important factors determining outcome were longer seizure-free periods (reducing the risk) and more than one antiepileptic drug and a history of tonic-clonic seizures (increasing the risk). Other factors (e.g. history of neonatal seizures, specific electroencephalographic features) seemed to have smaller effects, but even in such a large study the confidence intervals for these observations were wide [41] (Ib/A). The failure to predict the risk of recurrence for the individual patient creates uncertainty and anguish, and is a matter of concern.

Outcome of relapse seizures

How long does it take to become seizure-free after restarting treatment in the case of recurrence? Although seizure control was regained within approximately 1 year in half of the cases becoming seizure-free, it took some patients as many as 5-12 years [48] (Ia/A). As discussed below, in 19% (mean of 14 studies, 95% CI, 15-24%), resuming medication did not control the epilepsy as before, and chronic drug-resistant epilepsy with many seizures over as many as 5 years was seen in up to 23% of patients with a recurrence [48] (Ia/A). In a longitudinal long-term study of childhood-onset epilepsy, it took 24 patients 8 years (mean, median 7.0 years, range: 5-20 years) to re-enter long-term remission after the last recurrence and it was more than 10 years in five of the 24 patients [46] (IIb/B). Delayed regaining of seizure control, defined as 1-year remission, was noted in an observational study from the Netherlands [42] (IIb/B). Among 41 patients, seizure control was regained within 6 months in only 40%. In addition, as will be discussed in detail below, three of the 41 patients never became seizure-free again during a follow-up of 5 years and their seizures could be considered to be drug-resistant [42] (IIb/B).

Seizures despite continued treatment

In fact, there is no evidence that continued treatment with AEDs guarantees permanent seizure freedom. In a prospective, long-term population-based study of 144 patients followed on average for 37 years, 67% were in terminal remission, with or without treatment [46] (IIb/B). However, 28 patients (19%) achieved terminal remission following a relapse after early or late remission, suggesting a remitting-relapsing pattern, and 20 patients (14%) had a relapse after prolonged remission and did not re-enter remission, indicating a worsening course of the disease. The continued use of AEDs in both children and adults may also be associated with adverse effects in a substantial fraction of the exposed population, including behavioral and cognitive side effects [53, 54] (IV/C) and are shown to improve after drug withdrawal [40] (Ib/A). Additional disadvantages of continuing treatment indefinitely include a higher risk of teratogenicity [30] (IV/C), drug interaction with concurrent medications [55] (IV/C), and, last not least, the concern that treatment may be unnecessary. Studies in untreated patients showed that almost half of individuals with chronic epilepsy are seizure-free for more than 5 years [56] (III/B).

Should physicians encourage seizure-free patients to discontinue AEDs?

Any physician who indiscriminately propagates AED discontinuation is in a difficult position in case of harmful seizure recurrence. Although continued treatment is no guarantee to remain seizure-free, patients tend to attribute any harm to the discontinuation of the treatment and may lose confidence and go elsewhere. Given these circumstances, patients at high risk for seizure recurrence should not be encouraged or even advised to discontinue AEDs. Seizure-free patients with juvenile myoclonic epilepsy, and seizure-free adults with symptomatic focal or generalized epilepsy belong to the high-risk group for seizure recurrence in whom discontinuation may in fact be dangerous. It is advisable to refrain from encouraging AED discontinuation. The decision process leading to discontinuation should be carefully documented and include the patient's preference.

Conclusions

Opinion remains divided about treating patients who have had only a single seizure, particularly in those with a low to medium risk of recurrence. However, even in those with a low risk who prefer treatment, treatment can be justified as it is for almost all with a much higher risk of recurrence, for example, those with two or more seizures within the preceding 6-12 months, and even those with the highest risk of recurrence after the first seizure. We need adequate, comparative double-blind trials for starting treatment with new versus old AEDs.

Based on the available evidence, carbamazepine is the preferred older drug for focal seizures based on efficacy and safety; however, it has disadvantages over non-enzyme-inducing newer drugs such as levetiracetam or lamotrigine which are equivalent in efficacy. Although there are no comparative double-blind retention trials among new AEDs, levetiracetam has the advantage over lamotrigine that it is not involved in drug interactions or hypersensitivity reactions. Although no adequate comparative trials are available for treatment of idiopathic generalized epilepsy, valproate is unsurpassed in efficacy compared to lamotrigine or topiramate. However, valproate has the highest risk of teratogenicity among all current AEDs requiring special precautions. We need adequate, comparative double-blind trials for drug treatment of idiopathic generalized epilepsy and for drug treatment of children.

AED monitoring should be only performed when there is a specific clinical question/reason. Blood samples should be taken at steady state (i.e. at a period greater than four to five times the AED half-life after any dosage change). In clinical practice this is immediately before the next oral dose, always (if possible) at a similar time. Situations that may influence AED serum levels in relation to clinical response should always be considered (e.g. polytherapy with other AED or concomitant drugs with possible pharmacodynamic interactions, comorbidity, conditions that may alter pharmacokinetics, seizure type and frequency). Patient education about limitations and overinterpretation of serum level measurements is important. The golden rule to "treat the patient and not the serum concentration" cannot be overemphasized.

AED discontinuation requires a careful risk-benefit assessment in view of the undeniable risks involved. These risks include difficulties to predict individual seizure outcome after discontinuation, frequent seizure recurrence, particularly in high-risk patients, and the often grave consequences of seizure recurrence. In addition, successful treatment of seizure recurrence is neither invariably immediate nor assured. Physicians should prudently refrain from encouraging AED discontinuation in high-risk patients.

Key points	Evidence level
◆ Based on a large unblinded randomized trial, the outcome of starting treatment in patients with a single seizure versus deferred treatment is that onset of remission is delayed but long-term outcome is not affected for those with a low-to-medium risk of relapse.	Ib/A
◆ Although no RCTs exist for immediate versus deferred treatment of patients with several recent seizures, the available evidence favors immediate treatment in those with several recent seizures.	IIb/B
◆ Unexpectedly, restarting AEDs after relapse does not invariably result in immediate or assured remission.	III/B
◆ Carbamazepine is unsurpassed in effectiveness for initial monotherapy of focal seizures versus phenobarbital and primidone, based on a benchmark comparative, long-term double-blind retention trial.	Ib/A
◆ Among newer AEDs, lamotrigine and levetiracetam are equivalent to carbamazepine in efficacy for initial monotherapy of focal seizures.	Ib/A
◆ The placebo-corrected efficacy of adjunctive treatment with modern AEDs is disappointingly small and suggests that better strategies of finding drugs are needed for refractory epilepsy.	Ia/A
◆ The existing data are sufficiently concerning to suggest that it may be prudent to start with non-inducing AEDs unless there is a clear indication for one of the inducing drugs.	IV/C
◆ There is no clear evidence to support routine AED serum level measurement for the optimization of treatment in patients treated with AED monotherapy.	Ib/A
◆ AED drug monitoring is indicated when altered pharmacokinetics or poor compliance is suspected, in the case of presumed neurotoxicity, to evaluate drug-drug interactions (e.g. during polytherapy).	III/B & IV/C
◆ AED discontinuation results in seizures in one of three previously seizure-free patients.	Ia/A
◆ Patients with juvenile myoclonic epilepsy and those with symptomatic partial epilepsy carry a higher risk of seizures upon AED discontinuation.	Ia/A
◆ One in five patients with seizures after stopping AEDs will not be seizure-free immediately after restarting AEDs.	III/B

References

1. Berg AT. Risk of recurrence after a first unprovoked seizure. *Epilepsia* 2008; 49: Suppl 1: 13-8.
2. Camfield P, Camfield C, Dooley J, Smith E, Garner B. A randomized study of carbamazepine versus no medication after a first unprovoked seizure in childhood. *Neurology* 1989; 39: 851-2.
3. First Seizure Trial Group (FIRST Group). Randomized clinical trial on the efficacy of antiepileptic drugs in reducing the risk of relapse after a first unprovoked tonic clonic seizure. *Neurology* 1993; 43: 478-83.
4. Gilad R, Lampl Y, Gabbay U, Eshel Y, Sarova-Pinhas I. Early treatment of a single generalized tonic-clonic seizure to prevent recurrence. *Arch Neurol* 1996; 53: 1149-52.
5. Marson A, Jacoby A, Johnson A, Kim L, Gamble C, Chadwick D. Immediate versus deferred antiepileptic drug treatment for early epilepsy and single seizures: a randomised controlled trial. *Lancet* 2005; 365: 2007-13.
6. Kim LG, Johnson TL, Marson AG, Chadwick DW, MRC MESS Study group. Prediction of risk of seizure recurrence after a single seizure and early epilepsy: further results from the MESS trial. *Lancet Neurol* 2006; 5: 317-22.
7. Sillanpää M, Schmidt D. Natural history of treated childhood-onset epilepsy: prospective, long-term population-based study. *Brain* 2006; 129: 617-24.
8. Marson AG, Appleton R, Baker GA, *et al.* A randomised controlled trial examining the longer-term outcomes of standard versus new antiepileptic drugs. The SANAD trial. *Health Technol Assess* 2007; 11: 1-134.
9. Hauser WA, Rich SS, Lee JR, Annegers JF, Anderson VE. Risk of recurrent seizures after two unprovoked seizures. *N Engl J Med* 1998; 338: 429-34.
10. Shinnar S, Berg AT, O'Dell C, *et al.* Predictors of multiple seizures in a cohort of children prospectively followed from the time of their first unprovoked seizure. *Ann Neurol* 2000; 48: 140-7.
11. Mattson RH, Cramer JA, Collins JF, *et al.* Comparison of carbamazepine, phenobarbital, phenytoin, and primidone in partial and secondarily generalized tonic-clonic seizures. *N Engl J Med* 1985; 313: 145-51.
12. Mattson RH, Cramer JA, Collins JF. Comparison of valproate with carbamazepine for focal epilepsy in adults. The Department of Veterans Affairs Epilepsy Cooperative Study No. 264 Group. A comparison of valproate with carbamazepine for the treatment of complex partial seizures and secondarily generalized tonic-clonic seizures in adults. *N Engl J Med* 1992; 327: 765-71.
13. Brodie MJ, Richens A, Yuen AW. Double-blind comparison of lamotrigine and carbamazepine in newly diagnosed epilepsy. UK Lamotrigine/Carbamazepine Monotherapy Trial Group. *Lancet* 1995; 345: 476-9.
14. Brodie MJ Perucca E, Ryvlin P, Ben-Menachem E, Meencke HJ, for the Levetiracetam Monotherapy Study Group. Comparison of levetiracetam and controlled-release carbamazepine in newly diagnosed epilepsy. *Neurology* 2007; 68: 402-8.
15. Privitera MD, Brodie MJ, Mattson RH, *et al.* Topiramate, carbamazepine and valproate monotherapy: double-blind comparison in newly diagnosed epilepsy. *Acta Neurol Scand* 2003; 107: 165-75.
16. Bill PA, Vigonius U, Pohlmann H, *et al.* A double-blind controlled clinical trial of oxcarbazepine versus phenytoin in adults with previously untreated epilepsy. *Epilepsy Res* 1997; 27: 195-204.
17. Guerreiro MM, Vigonius U, Pohlmann H, *et al.* A double-blind controlled clinical trial of oxcarbazepine versus phenytoin in children and adolescents with epilepsy. *Epilepsy Res* 1997; 27: 205-13.
18. French JA, Kanner AM, Bautista J, *et al.* Efficacy and tolerability of the new antiepileptic drugs I: treatment of new onset epilepsy: report of the Therapeutics and Technology Assessment Subcommittee and Quality Standards Subcommittee of the American Academy of Neurology and the American Epilepsy Society. *Neurology* 2004; 62: 1252-60.
19. French JA, Kanner AM, Bautista J, *et al.* Efficacy and tolerability of the new antiepileptic drugs II: treatment of refractory epilepsy: report of the Therapeutics and Technology Assessment Subcommittee and Quality Standards Subcommittee of the American Academy of Neurology and the American Epilepsy Society. *Neurology* 2004; 27: 1261-73.
20. Glauser T, Ben-Menachem E, Bourgeois B, *et al.* ILAE treatment guidelines: evidence-based analysis of antiepileptic drug efficacy and effectiveness as initial monotherapy for epileptic seizures and syndromes. *Epilepsia* 2006; 47: 1094-20.
21. Mintzer S, Mattson RT. Should non-enzyme-inducing AEDs be preferred over enzyme-inducing AEDs as first-line agents? *Epilepsia* 2009; 50. Suppl 8: 42-50.

22. Beyenburg S, Stavem K, Schmidt D. Placebo-corrected efficacy of modern antiepileptic drugs for refractory epilepsy: systematic review and meta-analysis. *Epilepsia* 2010; 51: 7-26.
23. Camfield P, Camfield C. Monitoring for adverse effects of antiepileptic drugs. *Epilepsia* 2006; 47(Suppl 1): 31-4.
24. Tomson T, Dahl ML, Kimland E. Therapeutic monitoring of antiepileptic drugs for epilepsy. *Cochrane Database Syst Rev* 2007; 1: CD002216.
25. Patsalos PN, Berry DJ, Bourgeois BFD, *et al.* Antiepileptic drugs - best practice guidelines for therapeutic drug monitoring: a position paper by the subcommission on therapeutic drug monitoring. ILAE Commission on Therapeutic Strategies. *Epilepsia* 2008; 49: 1239-76.
26. Chadwick DW. Overuse of monitoring of blood concentrations of antiepileptic drugs. *Br Med J (Clin Res Ed)* 1987; 294: 723-4.
27. Schoenenberger RA, Tanasijevic MJ, Jha A, Bates DW. Appropriateness of antiepileptic drug level monitoring. *JAMA* 1995; 274: 1622-6.
28. Jannuzzi G, Cian P, Fattore C, *et al.* A multicenter randomized controlled trial on the clinical impact of therapeutic drug monitoring in patients with newly diagnosed epilepsy. The Italian TDM Study Group in Epilepsy. *Epilepsia* 2000; 41: 222-30.
29. Fröscher W, Eichelbaum M, Gugler R, Hildenbrand G, Penin H. A prospective randomized trial on the effect of monitoring plasma anticonvulsant levels in epilepsy. *J Neurol* 1981; 224: 193-201.
30. Harden CL, Pennell PB, Koppel BS, *et al.* American Academy of Neurology; American Epilepsy Society. Management issues for women with epilepsy - focus on pregnancy (an evidence-based review): III. Vitamin K, folic acid, blood levels, and breast-feeding: report of the Quality Standards Subcommittee and Therapeutics and Technology Assessment Subcommittee of the American Academy of Neurology and the American Epilepsy Society. *Epilepsia* 2009; 50: 1247-55.
31. Marasco RA, Ramsay RE. Epilepsy in the elderly: medications and pharmacokinetics. *Consult Pharm* 2009; 24 (Suppl A): 10-6.
32. Feldman RG, Pippenger CE. The relation of anticonvulsant drug levels to complete seizure control. *J Clin Pharmacol* 1976; 16: 51-9.
33. Shorvon SD, Chadwick D, Galbraith AW, Reynolds EH. One drug for epilepsy. *Br Med J* 1978; 1: 474-6.
34. Schmidt D, Haenel F. Therapeutic levels of phenytoin, phenobarbital, and carbamazepine: individual variation in relation to seizure frequency and type. *Neurology* 1984; 34: 1252-5.
35. Johannessen SI, Tomson T. Pharmacokinetic variability of newer antiepileptic drugs: when is monitoring needed? *Clin Pharmacokinet* 2006; 45: 1061-75.
36. Woo E, Chan YM, Yu YL, Chan YW, Huang CY. If a well-stabilized epileptic patient has a subtherapeutic antiepileptic drug level, should the dose be increased? A randomized prospective study. *Epilepsia* 1988; 29: 129-39.
37. Gannaway DJ, Mawer GE. Serum phenytoin concentration and clinical response in patients with epilepsy. *Br J Clin Pharmacol* 1981; 12: 833-9.
38. St Louis EK. Monitoring antiepileptic drugs: a level-headed approach. *Curr Neuropharmacol* 2009; 7: 115-9.
39. Kwan P, Brodie MJ. Early identification of refractory epilepsy. *N Engl J Med* 2000; 342: 314-9.
40. Lossius MI, Hessen E, Mowinkell P, *et al.* Consequences of antiepileptic drug withdrawal: a double-blind, randomized study (Akershus Study). *Epilepsia* 2008; 49: 455-63.
41. Medical Research Council (MRC) Antiepileptic Drug Withdrawal Group. Randomised study of antiepileptic drug withdrawal in patients in remission. *Lancet* 1991; 337: 1175-80.
42. Overweg J, Binnie CD, Oosting J, Rowan AJ. Clinical and EEG prediction of seizure recurrence following antiepileptic drug withdrawal. *Epilepsy Res* 1987; 1: 272-83.
43. Callaghan N, Garrett A, Goggin T. Withdrawal of anticonvulsant drugs in patients free of seizures for two years. A prospective study. *N Engl J Med* 1988; 318: 942-6.
44. Matricardi A, Bertamino F, Risso D. Discontinuation of anti-epileptic therapy: a retrospective study of 86 children and adolescents. *Ital J Neurol Sci* 1995; 16: 613-22.
45. Specchio LM, Tramacere L, La Neve A, Beghi E. Discontinuing antiepileptic drugs in patients who are seizure free on monotherapy. *J Neurol Neurosurg Psychiatry* 2002; 72: 22-5.
46. Sillanpää M, Schmidt D. Prognosis of seizure recurrence after stopping antiepileptic drugs in seizure-free patients: a long-term population-based study of childhood-onset epilepsy. *Epilepsy Behav* 2006; 8: 713-9.

47. Berg AT, Shinnar S. Relapse following discontinuation of antiepileptic drugs: a meta-analysis. *Neurology* 1994; 44: 601-8.

48. Schmidt D, Löscher W. Uncontrolled epilepsy following discontinuation of antiepileptic drugs in seizure-free patients: a review of current clinical experience. *Acta Neurol Scand* 2005; 111: 291-300.

49. Sirven J, Sperling MR, Wingerchuck DM. Early versus late antiepileptic drug withdrawal for people with epilepsy in remission. *Cochrane Database Syst Rev* 2001; 3: CD001902.

50. Jacoby A, Johnson A, Chadwick D. Psychosocial outcomes of antiepileptic drug discontinuation. The Medical Research Council Antiepileptic Drug Withdrawal Study Group. *Epilepsia* 1992; 33: 1123-31.

51. Specchio LM, Beghi E. Should antiepileptic drugs be withdrawn in seizure-free patients? *CNS Drugs* 2004; 18: 201-12.

52. Chadwick D, Taylor J, Johnson T. Outcomes after seizure recurrence in people with well-controlled epilepsy and the factors that influence it. *Epilepsia* 1996; 37: 1043-50.

53. Ortinski P, Meador KJ. Cognitive side effects of antiepileptic drugs. *Epilepsy Behav* 2004; 5: S60-5.

54. Mula M, Monaco F. Antiepileptic drugs and psychopathology: an update. *Epileptic Disord* 2009; 11: 1-9.

55. Patsalos PN, Perucca E. Clinically important drug interactions in epilepsy: interactions between antiepileptic drugs and other drugs. *Lancet Neurol* 2003; 2: 473-81.

56. Nicoletti A, Sofia V, Vitale G, *et al.* Natural history and mortality of chronic epilepsy in an untreated population of rural Bolivia: a follow-up after 10 years. *Epilepsia* 2009; 50: 2199-206.

Chapter 2

Monitoring seizure frequency and severity in outpatients

Mark Quigg MD MSc, Professor of Neurology
Medical Director Clinical Neurophysiology: EEG, Neurological Sleep,
Evoked Potentials, and Intensive Monitoring
University of Virginia, Charlottesville, Virginia, USA

Introduction

Seizure occurrence is the primary outcome measure in the majority of epilepsy treatment trials. Whether the design measures seizure frequency reduction, seizure remission, or time to nth seizure, most treatment protocols depend on the gold standard of the outpatient seizure diary to monitor treatment effects. The self-maintained seizure diary, often formally or informally supplemented by family members or other observers, stands at the center of epilepsy research.

The advantages of diaries are obvious: they are cheap, they correspond closely to clinical practice and to patient experience, and they have the unquantified but appreciated benefit of a task with which the patient and family can illustrate their care and vigilance with a tangible product.

In this chapter, the advantages and limitations of the seizure diary and the conditions that may promote or limit accuracy will be reviewed. Attempts to address limitations of the seizure diary will also be briefly reviewed. The penultimate study in evidence-based medicine is the randomized, double-blinded controlled trial. The focus of this review, in contrast, is on the reliability of the outpatient seizure diary on which most randomized, controlled trials in epilepsy depend. There are no studies that directly evaluate the reliability of seizure diaries regarding their direct impact on patient outcomes; however, many studies have determined the reliability of patient recall and the correlations between recall and actual seizure occurrence.

History of the seizure diary

Since it is embedded in the history of epileptology, finding the first use of seizure diaries is difficult. The earliest studies that track seizure occurrence determined seizure frequency either by physician interview or by direct observation of seizures by medical staff. Early observational studies, such as the studies of the distributions of seizures by time of day based in the 'epileptic asylums' of the period, could be quite detailed in listing seizure type and the hour of their occurrence [1-3]. Studies of the chronobiology of seizures relied upon long-term seizure diaries at or exceeding a decade in duration [4]. A common feature is that seizure diaries were maintained by medical personnel; the degree of self-reporting of seizures is not documented in most of these institutionally-based or 'informed observer' studies.

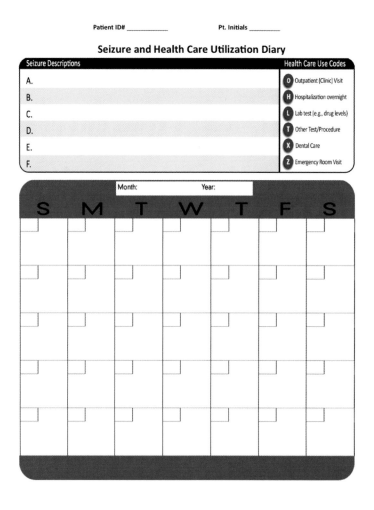

Figure 1. An example of an outpatient seizure diary used in a recent evaluation of epilepsy surgery. Patients are asked to maintain a record of seizure type as listed in a series of predetermined codes and to track medical interventions. A key to seizure types and medical intervention codes is provided for the patient's convenience.

Merritt and Putnam's 1938 landmark study on the effectiveness of phenytoin can be argued as the first 'modern' pharmacotherapy trial in epilepsy [5]. Although this study was outpatient-based (as opposed to asylum-based), Merritt and Putnam do not mention the use of seizure diaries. Regardless of the lack of explicit documentation, the features of seizure diaries have not drastically changed over the years. A typical seizure diary provided to patients in a treatment trial consists of a blank calendar into which the months/days are filled (Figure 1). Most studies require a coding of seizure type by some pre-defined criteria. An important job of the investigator is to translate the medically-acceptable seizure classification – 'complex partial seizures', 'secondarily generalized seizures' – to meaningful symptoms in the patient's own words – 'small seizures with confusion', 'big convulsions'. Modern trials may combine seizure diaries with other outpatient experiences such as medical care interventions or menstrual cycles [6, 7] among other study-specific data.

Patient recall reliability is high

Until recently, studies of seizure diaries centered on patient compliance and recall reliability. The goal of these studies was to demonstrate the ability of the patient to act as a truthful reporter who would maintain an accurate calendar record.

The first studies of the reliability of self-reported seizure diaries centered on the agreement of patient recollection with the written record. One of the first studies to examine diary reliability was reported by Neugebauer [8] who evaluated the ability of the patient to duplicate diary entries one day removed from entry **(III/B)**. For example, if a patient reported three seizures on his diary on Tuesday, he was asked to repeat his Tuesday diary entry on Wednesday. The patient was scored as accurate if he again counted three seizures. In this design, patients duplicated the previous day's diary entry with 95% accuracy.

Longer time spans were evaluated in another study of 32 patients who were asked to estimate the frequency of seizures for the preceding 2 months and asked to keep a seizure diary forward for the next month [9]. Patients were accurate in estimation of seizure frequencies for the preceding 2 months in comparison to the prospective seizure diary. Measurements of stress and changes in daily routines had no effect on the accuracy of retrospective estimates and in maintaining prospective seizure diaries. In this same study, about half of the subjects had observers – usually spouses or other family members – that provided independent retrospective estimates and maintained independent prospective seizure diaries. In contrast to patients, observers' diary counts did not agree with past estimates. The observers' diary counts were substantially lower than patients'. The authors concluded that patients, rather than observers, demonstrated high consistency between estimates of seizure frequency and seizure counts provided by diaries **(III/B)**.

These studies support the premise that seizure diaries are accurate reflections of a patient's perceptions of seizure occurrence. A major limitation of these studies, however, is that patient perception may not accurately reflect actual seizure recurrence.

Self-maintained seizure counts vary from EEG-confirmed seizures

Continuous video EEG (CV-EEG) created the opportunity for examining the accuracy of patient recall to the gold standard of EEG-confirmed seizures. Early studies in the validation of seizure-detection algorithms noted that seizures which the computer detected but were not reported by the patient occurred "without (the patient's) warning or memory for the seizure" [10].

Blum *et al* was the first to examine patient accuracy of self-reporting against the occurrence of seizures confirmed by CV-EEG [11] (IIa/B). In a prospective study of 32 consecutive patients, the investigators asked patients if they recently had a seizure when the patient had recovered sufficiently for a postictal interview (~30-60 minutes). As a control, they repeated the question at random times. After excluding some patients with no seizures or those with psychogenic pseudoseizure, only three patients of 27 (11%) accurately identified the occurrence of all seizures. On the other hand, seven of 27 (26%) were never aware of seizure occurrence. On average, 61% of seizures were unrecognized by the 27 patient sample. Not only were patients unreliable in recollection of a seizure, they were poor estimators of their own reporting accuracy. Although 44% of patients rated themselves as "always accurate", only 11% in fact were. Seizure frequency had an inverse correlation with seizure awareness; patients with the most seizures during monitoring had the worst accuracy. In contrast to the poor 'false negative' proportion of seizure recollection, there was not a single 'false positive', the inaccurate reporting of a seizure that didn't occur on CV-EEG.

Poor reliability in seizure awareness was corroborated by a large, retrospective study of ambulatory, outpatient EEG in which investigators matched computerized seizure detections with patient-activated push-button events signaling the occurrence of a perceived clinical seizure [12] (IIa/B). Out of >500 recordings, 47 had evidence of electrographically-confirmed partial seizures. Only 63% of these EEG-detected seizures were accompanied by patient confirmation. Calculating a 'false positive' rate in this study was not feasible since many patients underwent monitoring for diagnosis and may have had chronic, non-epileptic events (the authors note that 86% of patient reports contained non-epileptic events such as headache, dizziness, confusion, etc). The authors concluded that seizures were under-reported in patients undergoing 24-hour ambulatory EEG monitoring.

Subsequent studies of inpatient CV-EEG and short-term patient recollection agree with earlier studies that find that patient recollection is largely inaccurate. In a study of 31 patients admitted for inpatient CV-EEG for evaluation of medically intractable partial epilepsy, subjects were asked to fill out a seizure report every evening for the previous 24 hours [13] (IIa/B). For each seizure, they were asked to record specific premonitions and symptoms of seizures. Of the 138 seizures, 68 (49.3%) were recognized by patients, and 65 (46.8%) went unnoticed. In five (3.6%) events, patients were aware of the aura, but not of the complex partial seizure that followed. Eight patients (27.7%) were aware of all of their seizures; six subjects (20%) were not aware of any.

A prospective, consecutive sample of 91 patients evaluated with inpatient CV-EEG was specifically designed to determine the accuracy of self-maintained seizure diaries [14] (Ib/A).

In this study, patients were given a seizure diary to fill out, thus duplicating the outpatient experience. An additional randomized, controlled trial on the effect of patient reminders was added to determine if inaccuracy could be improved by encouraging compliance. Patients were randomized to 'reminded' and 'unreminded' groups; reminded patients were asked every morning of admission to document all seizures during the monitoring period. Finally, patients were asked to rate themselves on accuracy of seizure recollection on a 100-point scale; patients were then categorized into self-designated 'perfect documenters' and groups of self-perceived lesser reliability.

Patients failed to report 55% of all CV-EEG confirmed seizures. Only 30% of the patients who designated themselves perfect documenters were in fact perfect. The reminded group had no better accuracy than the unreminded group. Reminding patients did not improve the number of perfect documenters in either group.

These studies found that, in general, patient accounts of outpatient seizure occurrence should be treated, at best, as a minimum seizure count and, at worst, unreliable. These studies emphasized that under-reporting of seizures was not a matter of willful non-compliance, but a facet of the epileptic condition itself. These and other studies investigated what aspects of epilepsy were most likely to lead to inaccurate reporting of seizure occurrence.

Lack of diary accuracy varies with epilepsy syndrome and seizure type

In a study with a different design from the diary versus CV-EEG monitoring, patients with medically intractable partial seizures and their families were asked three questions in order to classify them into three reliability groups [15] **(IIb/B)**:

* 1. has the patient been aware of amnesic episodes (complex partial seizures) which occurred recently?;
* 2. family members were asked if the patient was capable of recalling seizures if they did not remind the patient; and if
* 3. seizures occurred which that patient denied their occurrence?

If answers were "No" for Questions 1 and 2 and "Yes" for Question 3, they were classified into the 'completely unaware' group. If answers were 1=Yes/2=Yes/3=No, patients were classified into the 'completely aware' group. Other combinations were assigned to the 'incompletely aware' group. The distribution of awareness classification was then evaluated across interictal EEG and neuroimaging findings. Of 134 patients, 17% were classified as completely unaware, 6% to the incompletely aware group (later combined with the unaware group), and 77% to the completely aware group. Patients in the unawareness group were older and had a later age of onset than patients in the awareness group. Temporal lobe foci defined by interictal epileptiform discharges (IEDs) were more frequent in the unawareness group (94%) than the awareness group (55%). Bilateral independent IEDs were found more frequently in the unawareness group than in the awareness group (48% vs. 13%).

Studies with corroborating CV-EEG emphasize, however, that chronic factors bare little relationship to inaccurate reporting. Neither age [11, 14], gender [14], duration of epilepsy [11, 14], the number or type of anticonvulsant medications [14], or cognitive performance [11, 14] were found as significant factors in diary or verbal reporting accuracy. Instead, most studies that compare diaries/recall versus CV-EEG monitoring find that factors associated with seizure characteristics are more important (IIb/B).

Primary generalized seizures are usually undersampled in CV-EEG studies since practice is focused on pre-surgical evaluation. The study of Blum et al [11] included three subjects with primary generalized epilepsy who achieved 100% accuracy with CV-EEG monitoring. The ambulatory EEG study of Tatum et al [12] found that 56% of generalized seizures were accurately identified by patients, and as the length of the generalized discharge decreased, accuracy decreased as well. Thirty-one recordings had evidence of generalized seizures. Only 56% of generalized seizures lasting for >3 seconds were labeled by patient confirmation. Bursts of seizures versus interictal epileptiform activity lasting more than 3 seconds were identified 39% of the time, and bursts shorter than 3 seconds were identified 26% of the time.

More data from CV-EEG studies are available for partial epilepsy. The extent of involvement of partial seizures (i.e. secondary generalization) may be important, but accuracy varies widely in the two studies that report it, ranging from 0%[11] to 83% [14]. The effects of temporal versus non-temporal localization of foci has also been undersampled due to the typical distributions of patients available to the epilepsy monitoring unit. Six of 27 patients in Blum et al's study [11] had extratemporal lobe epilepsy with an accuracy of 75%, a figure much higher than that of the 3-46% accuracy of their temporal lobe patients. On the other hand, subsequent studies with similarly small numbers found no statistically significant differences in accuracy between extratemporal and temporal lobe patients [13, 14].

Patients with temporal lobe foci have more consistent findings across CV-EEG studies. All three studies cited above found statistically rigorous greater degrees of inaccurate reporting and seizure unawareness in those patients with left compared to right temporal seizures. Blum et al found that patients with left temporal foci were less likely to recognize their seizures (96.7%) than patients with right temporal foci (56%) [11]. Kerling et al reported that patients with a left-sided focus were aware of only 34% of their left temporal seizures compared to right-temporal lobe patients' 72.1% accuracy. Although Hoppe et al found that the rate of left-sided patients lower than that of right-sided patients, their study found lateralization had modest effects that were less important than the occurrence of complex (versus simple) partial seizures and the vigilance state (wakefulness or sleep) during which the seizure occurred.

On that note, the vigilance state may have the most profound effect on accurate seizure recollection than any of the above factors discussed thus far (IIb/B). In limited circumstances, seizure counts may be accurate regardless of state. For example, in a case report of the circadian distribution of seizures as reported in a long-term seizure diary, the patient and family member were able to document the occurrence of nocturnal, sleep-associated seizures consisting of severe, focal ictal pain that interrupted sleep [16]; the timing and state of diary seizure occurrence were corroborated by CV-EEG with the use of intracranial electrodes. On the other hand, under more mundane circumstances, CV-EEG studies find that sleep-associated seizures appear at the greatest risk of under-reporting. Of a total of 582 seizures recorded from 91 patients, accuracy was 68% for seizures during wakefulness compared to only 14% for seizures during sleep [14]. These proportions agreed with those found in an earlier study (Kerling et al [13] awake accuracy = 61%; sleep = 13%).

Hoppe et al found a curious interaction of state with anticonvulsant use [14]. Patients taking levetiracetam, as opposed to other anticonvulsants, had a greater proportion of EEG-confirmed seizures that occurred during the awake state (1.9 seizures/monitoring day compared to 1.4/day). Since these patients had more seizures during wakefulness, their accuracy was enhanced.

Studies vary on the influence of auras on accurate seizure recollection. An important limitation on the use of auras as a hook by which to hang a memory is that auras are relatively uncommon among the seizures sampled and were not uniformly reported [11, 13, 14]. Blum et al found that patients often forgot the presence of aura preceding seizures. Hoppe et al subsumed auras under the designation "simple partial seizures" which had accuracy rates during wakefulness (88%) much higher than complex partial seizures (47%), but did not report accuracy of complex partial seizures with versus without auras. On the other hand, Kerling et al reported that 33% of seizures started with an aura. Sometimes patients remembered the aura but not the subsequent complex partial seizure. The question of the usefulness of auras in recollection was confounded by the fact that they most often occurred in right-sided temporal lobe seizures; there was no way to determine if aura recollection varied because of even distribution by lateralization or because of asymmetric recollection.

Alternatives to seizure diaries are limited

Although patient reports of seizure occurrence poorly reflect actual seizure frequency, patient testimony should not be ignored. For example, Kerling et al found that when patients reported that they may not be able to estimate seizure frequency, they should be believed [13]. Although comparison with CV-EEG results revealed that most of the patients slightly overestimated their ability to recognize seizures, there was a positive correlation between patients' perception and video/EEG findings. Many patients realize that they do not recognize each seizure, and this self-recognition is reliable.

Some studies may appear to devalue self-reported seizure frequency but have findings attributable to other mechanisms. For example, one study retrospectively evaluated the time for first event occurrence compared to self-reported seizure frequency in 155 consecutive patients admitted for evaluation in an inpatient epilepsy unit [17] (III/B). No correlation was found between these two factors, a finding attributable to accelerated seizure occurrence from anticonvulsant withdrawal [18] as well as self-report accuracy. Regardless of mechanism, outpatient seizure frequency is not an adequate criterion for inpatient epilepsy unit admission.

Finally, few studies have delineated the change in accuracy of seizure diaries to which family members contribute. Such a proposed study might randomize patients admitted to an epilepsy unit to family-aided versus non-aided arms, with appropriate measures to minimize inadvertent patient cueing. Both arms would be evaluated with CV-EEG to compare diary accuracy. From the available data, one may suspect that diary accuracy regarding 'false negatives' would improve at the possible expense of a rise in 'false positives' as family members identified non-epileptic sleep-associated movements such as sleep myoclonus or nightmares as possible seizures.

If seizure diaries have such problems, why do we continue to use them? In short, we lack alternatives and, maybe, accurate seizure counts as opposed to perceived seizure counts may not be that important.

Technologies to supplement or replace pen-and-paper diaries have been explored, but there are no trials in epilepsy that compare compliance rates or accuracy of traditional paper seizure diaries to electronic aids such as computerized online diaries, personal data assistants (PDAs), or other electronic equivalents. Certainly, online sources for both freeware and commercial seizure diaries abound. Outside of epilepsy a growing number of well-designed studies have compared paper versus electronic equivalents **(Ia/A)**. A recent review of randomized, controlled trials of PDAs in the management of chronic diseases concluded that PDA diaries appear to perform better than paper diaries in terms of compliance, time spent in data management, data accuracy, and patient preference. A major limitation, however, is inherent to electronic devices; PDA diaries continue to be fraught with technical failures [19]. How epilepsy patients, many of whom have cognitive impairments, could deal with technical challenges of these devices remains to be seen. Furthermore, it is unclear how a PDA or online application could overcome the physiological barriers to seizure awareness documented in the current review that prevent accurate seizure recall.

Ambulatory seizure monitoring devices may offer the ideal combination of safety, portability, reliability, and cost in the future. A host of devices under recent development – movement detectors based on actigraphy, or implantable electrode systems with seizure detection such as the Responsive NeuroStimulator [20] – are not yet commercially available and have yet to be validated by widespread study.

A small number of anticonvulsant trials have used inpatient EEG-confirmed seizures as the primary outcome measure as opposed to seizures logged in traditional diaries [21]. For example, the efficacy of levetiracetam was evaluated by comparing the cumulative duration of electrographic seizures per 24 hours during a pre-treatment baseline phase compared to a post-treatment sample. An expert review indicated that certain epileptic conditions, such as absence seizures or photosensitive epilepsies, could be assessed by the use of EEG surrogate markers in lieu of seizure diaries [22]. Notably, such inpatient studies may be feasible only with medications that can be quickly titrated to therapeutic levels to ensure that monitoring sessions remain tolerably short.

Perceived seizure occurrence has meaningful clinical outcomes in function and quality of life

No studies exist that directly tie the accuracy of seizure diaries to an outcome measure other than seizures; in other words, we don't know if an accurate seizure diary matters in terms of quality of life or functional outcomes measured in terms of employment, patient goals, etc. On the other hand, patient outcomes tied to perceived seizure frequencies are embedded in epilepsy literature and in numerous randomized, controlled trials in epilepsy treatment **(Ia/A)**.

A good example of an early use of secondary outcome measures in addition to seizure frequencies provided by diaries is a randomized controlled trial of lamotrigine [23]. The reduction in seizure frequency with lamotrigine, relative to placebo, was 29.7%. Quality of life measures were significantly higher for the lamotrigine group in subscales of 'mastery' and 'happiness'.

The surgical management of epilepsy has a rich literature of measuring secondary outcome measures relative to perceived seizure reduction or remission **(Ia/A)**. A review of eight controlled studies of psychological outcomes of epilepsy surgery (post-surgical patients compared to non-surgical controls) [24] and a subsequent controlled study [24] reveals that patients with seizure remission as determined by interview or diaries generally enjoy greater rates of full-time employment and driving, and score higher on quality-of-life measures.

Conclusions

The evidence suggests that patients are consistent and reliable in reporting their perceived seizure frequencies, but that the reliability of perceived seizure frequency compared to actual seizure frequency determined in EEG monitoring studies is poor. Poor accuracy is not a matter of laziness, but a feature of the peri-ictal morbidity of seizures themselves. Seizures that occur during sleep are the most likely to be inaccurately reported. Self-reported seizure frequency should be viewed as a minimum seizure frequency at best. Despite documented shortcomings, cost and lack of feasible alternatives ensure that seizure diaries will remain an important tool in clinical trials of epilepsy. Perceived seizure frequency and remission correspond to improved functional and psychological outcomes. Accordingly, clinical trials must be designed so that inaccuracies are evenly distributed across treatment arms.

Key points	Evidence level
◆ Patients' perceived seizure frequency recall is accurately reflected in seizure diaries.	III/B
◆ Perceived seizure counts in seizure diaries underestimate seizure frequency.	IIa/B
◆ Partial seizures that occur during sleep are the most inaccurately counted.	IIa/B
◆ Reminding patients to maintain an accurate seizure diary is ineffective.	Ib/A
◆ Self-reported seizure frequency does not predict the time to first seizure during inpatient EEG monitoring.	III/B
◆ Electronic diaries in chronic disease (outside of epilepsy) are preferred over paper diaries by patients and decrease time in data analysis, but have residual technical reliability problems.	Ia/A
◆ Better psychological outcomes after epilepsy surgery correspond to perceived seizure remission.	Ia/A

References

1. Langdon-Down M, Brain WR. Time of day in relation to convulsions in epilepsy. *Lancet* 1929; 1: 1029-32.
2. Griffiths GM, Fox JT. Rhythm in epilepsy. *Lancet* 1938; 2: 409-16.
3. Patry F. The relationship of time of day, sleep, and other factors to the incidence of epileptic seizures. *American J Psychiatry* 1931; 10: 789-813.
4. Halberg F, Howard RB. 24-hour periodicity and experimental medicine: examples and interpretation. *Postgraduate Medicine* 1958; 24: 349-58.
5. Merritt HH, Putnam TJ. Sodium diphenyl hydantoinate in the treatment of convulsive disorders. *JAMA* 1938; 111: 1068-73.
6. Herzog AG, Harden CL, Liporace J, *et al*. Frequency of catamenial seizure exacerbation in women with localization-related epilepsy. *Ann Neurol* 2004; 56: 431-4.
7. Quigg M, Fowler KM, Herzog AG. Circalunar and ultralunar periodicities in women with partial seizures. *Epilepsia* 2008; 49: 1081-5.
8. Neugebauer R. Reliability of seizure diaries in adult epileptic patients. *Neuroepidemiology* 1989; 8: 228-33.
9. Glueckauf RL, Girvin JP, Braun JR, Bochen JL. Consistency of seizure frequency estimates across time, methods, and observers. *Health Psychol* 1990; 9: 427-34.
10. Gotman J. Automatic seizure detection: improvements and evaluation. *Electroencephalography & Clinical Neurophysiology* 1990; 76: 317-24.
11. Blum DE, Eskola J, Bortz JJ, Fisher RS. Patient awareness of seizures. *Neurology* 1996; 47: 260-4.
12. Tatum WO, Winters L, Gieron M, *et al*. Outpatient seizure identification: results of 502 patients using computer-assisted ambulatory EEG. *J Clin Neurophysiol* 2001; 18: 14-9.
13. Kerling F, Mueller S, Pauli E, Stefan H. When do patients forget their seizures? An electroclinical study. *Epilepsy Behav* 2006; 9: 281-5.
14. Hoppe C, Poepel A, Elger CE. Epilepsy: accuracy of patient seizure counts. *Arch Neurol* 2007; 64: 1595-9.
15. Heo K, Han SD, Lim SR, Kim MA, Lee BI. Patient awareness of complex partial seizures. *Epilepsia* 2006; 47: 1931-5.
16. Quigg M, Straume M. Dual epileptic foci in a single patient express distinct temporal patterns dependent on limbic versus nonlimbic brain location. *Ann Neurology* 2000; 48: 117-20.

17. Eisenman LN, Attarian H, Fessler AJ, Vahle VJ, Gilliam F. Self-reported seizure frequency and time to first event in the seizure monitoring unit. *Epilepsia* 2005; 46: 664-8.

18. So N, Gotman J. Changes in seizure activity following anticonvulsant drug withdrawal. *Neurology* 1990; 40: 407-13.

19. Dale O, Hagen KB. Despite technical problems personal digital assistants outperform pen and paper when collecting patient diary data. *J Clin Epidemiol* 2007; 60: 8-17.

20. Morrell M. Brain stimulation for epilepsy: can scheduled or responsive neurostimulation stop seizures? *Curr Opin Neurol* 2006; 19: 164-8.

21. Stefan H, Wang-Tilz Y, Pauli E, *et al*. Onset of action of levetiracetam: a RCT trial using therapeutic intensive seizure analysis (TISA). *Epilepsia* 2006; 47: 516-22.

22. Binnie C. Proof of principle trials: EEG surrogate endpoints. *Epilepsy Res* 2001; 45: 7-11.

23. Smith D, Baker G, Davies G, Dewey M, Chadwick DW. Outcomes of add-on treatment with lamotrigine in partial epilepsy. *Epilepsia* 1993; 34: 312-22.

24. Jones JE, Berven NL, Ramirez L, Woodard A, Hermann BP. Long-term psychosocial outcomes of anterior temporal lobectomy. *Epilepsia* 2002; 43: 896-903.

Chapter 3

When to consider epilepsy surgery, and what surgical procedure?

Soheyl Noachtar MD, Neurologist and Psychiatrist
Associate Professor of Neurology and Head of the Epilepsy Center
Department of Neurology, University of Munich, Munich, Germany

Ingo Borggräfe MD, Pediatrician
Attending Physician and Head of the Pediatric Epilepsy Unit, Department of
Pediatric Neurology and Developmental Medicine, University of Munich,
Munich, Germany

Jan Rémi MD, Epilepsy Fellow at the Epilepsy Center
Department of Neurology, University of Munich, Munich, Germany

Introduction

Surgery is one of the cornerstones of epilepsy treatment. It should be considered in selected patients when medical treatment has failed. Patients for whom surgery is a viable and useful option should be identified quickly, because surgery may have a high success rate and possible seizure freedom will have several medical and social benefits for the patient.

This chapter discusses the indications for surgery, the timing of epilepsy surgery, which surgical approaches are available and which approach should be chosen for which syndrome. The necessary diagnostic steps and their contribution to the decision-making process are evaluated.

What is intractable epilepsy?

Medical intractability is a prerequisite of epilepsy surgery. The recurrence of seizures despite antiepileptic medication is well documented, but because of unstandardized definitions as well as misdiagnoses, the incidence and prevalence of intractable epilepsy (IE) are somewhat uncertain [1-3]. Patients with epilepsy whose seizures do not successfully respond to antiepileptic drug (AED) therapy are considered to have intractable epilepsy. This condition is also referred to as medically refractory or pharmacoresistant epilepsy. Whereas about 70-80% of epilepsy patients will enter 5-year remission [4], approximately 20-30% develop chronic intractable (pharmacoresistant) epilepsy [5, 6] **(IIa/B)**. Because of the need to individualize therapy, no rigid set of guidelines can be applied to determine medical intractability. The minimum criteria to determine medical intractability include failure of at least two to three antiepileptic drugs of first choice in monotherapy to control seizures [7] (IIa/B). Therapeutic ranges of serum drug levels are not acceptable as a criterion for drug failure as some patients will become seizure-free at serum drug levels above the therapeutic range without experiencing toxic side effects [8-10] (Ib/A). With several new AEDs available in recent years and recommendations developed to guide treatment [11, 12], it might have been expected that more, rather than fewer, drug trials would be recommended before determining intractability. However, several prospective case series have shown that a high likelihood of medical intractability can be identified after two unsuccessful trials [13, 14] (IIa/B). The first antiepileptic drug treatment is more likely to achieve seizure control than later alternative drug trials or combinations of AEDs independent of the particular AED [6] (IIa/B).

Population-based studies have provided information regarding the prognosis of intractable epilepsy that are helpful in making treatment decisions [7]. There is some evidence that a good prognosis is related to the rapidity with which seizures are brought under control. Poor prognostic factors include a high number of pretreatment seizures, long duration of epilepsy, family history of epilepsy, previous febrile seizures, traumatic brain injury as the cause of the epilepsy, intermittent recreational drug use, and prior or current psychiatric comorbidity, particularly depression [15] (III/B). The response to medication in terms of seizure control also depends on the etiology of epilepsy [16, 17] (III/B). Focal epilepsy due to stroke in adults is more likely to be controlled with antiepileptic drugs (AEDs) than mesial temporal sclerosis, cortical dysplasia or the combination of both [17]. Consideration of surgical therapy in appropriate candidates should not be delayed by repeated trials with adjunctive drugs since new AEDs control the seizures only in a minority of these patients.

Timing of epilepsy surgery

The rationale of early epilepsy surgical intervention is based on the notion that seizure freedom achieved by epilepsy surgery will improve the long-term quality-of-life outcome [18]. Intractable epilepsy is associated with increased mortality [19, 20], disability and diminished quality of life [21]. Examples include poor academic achievement, unemployment, and social isolation. Most patients with intractable seizures cannot drive. In one community-based survey of people with epilepsy, those with self-reported incomplete seizure control were more likely to express concerns about the feelings of fear, their quality of life, work, adverse effects of therapy, and the stigma associated with their condition, even when their seizures were relatively infrequent [21]. These complications of intractable epilepsy result from the combined effects of recurrent seizures, AED toxicity, as well as psychosocial factors such as excessive dependency [21]. Therefore, if acceptable seizure control is not achieved within 2 years, patients should be referred to an epilepsy surgery center for further evaluation [22].

The concern that recurrent seizures may have detrimental effects on the brain similar to kindling and secondary epileptogenesis [23] has led to a favor of early surgical intervention [24]. Whether the concept of secondary epileptogenesis, which is derived from animal studies, has clinical implications for human epilepsy remains controversial [25]. However, early surgical intervention in children with focal epilepsies offers the possibility to prevent the psychosocial morbidity and neuropsychological decline which are linked to intractable epilepsy [26-29] (IIa/B). The duration of epilepsy before surgery has been shown to correlate with the outcome of surgery; if the duration of epilepsy was less than 10 years, resective epilepsy surgery led to seizure freedom in 90% of patients, whereas only about one third became seizure-free after more than 30 years of epilepsy [26] (IIa/B). This result favors early surgical intervention. However, the complications of temporal lobe epilepsy surgery have to be considered. Dominant anterior temporal resection, for instance, is associated with a postoperative risk of verbal memory deficit, but that deficit levels off after 2 years, and non-dominant-side temporal lobe resection leads to a postoperative improvement that also levels off after about 2 years [27] (IIa/B).

Who are surgical candidates?

The results of epilepsy surgery depend on the localization of the epileptogenic zone (region of cortex that can generate seizures) and its complete removal [28]. If complete resection is not feasible, partial resection of epileptogenic cerebral tissue may also be worthwhile in selected patients, although the results are less favorable [29, 30] (IIb/B). Another approach has been the interruption of pathways of seizure spread, which was the rationale for resection of the anterior temporal lobe in isolated cases with posterior temporal or extratemporal seizure onset, although results were relatively unfavorable when compared to complete resection of the epileptogenic zone [31]. Presurgical evaluation should:

- select those patients who could benefit from surgery; and
- exclude those whom surgery would not help and may even harm.

A highly specialized multidisciplinary approach is required for this purpose. The diagnostic evaluation of approximately 80-90% of patients considered for epilepsy surgery can be based on non-invasive evaluations [32, 33]. The selection criteria for epilepsy surgery include [34]:

- confirmed diagnosis of epilepsy;
- medical intractability;
- disabling seizures;
- resectable focus (except callosotomy candidates, vagus nerve stimulation and deep brain stimulation);
- motivated patient;
- no progressive underlying cause (except Rasmussen's encephalitis);
- high probability that better seizure control will improve quality of life.

How to identify surgical candidates

Concordance of non-invasive results implicating a resectable focus allows one to proceed to epilepsy surgery based on non-invasive studies only in temporal lobe epilepsy, which is the most common focal epilepsy referred to epilepsy surgery centers [32, 35] **(IIb/B)**(Figure 1); otherwise, an invasive evaluation is required. These investigations are indicated and justified

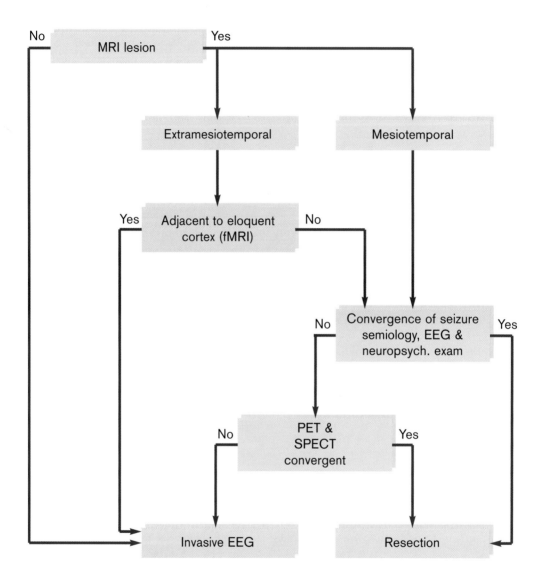

Figure 1. Flow chart of diagnostic evaluation in epilepsy surgery.

only if non-invasive studies are inconclusive or reveal discrepant results, but still support a testable hypothesis of a resectable focus. Under these circumstances, properly placed invasive electrodes frequently provide useful additional information about the localization and extent of the epileptogenic zone [28, 34, 36, 37]. If non-invasive evaluation reveals multifocality or diffuse epileptogenicity, resective surgery is very unlikely to be an option, but vagal nerve stimulation or corpus callosotomy can be considered.

The diagnostic evaluation includes the following (Figure 1):

- seizure description and patient history;
- EEG;
- EEG-video monitoring;
- MRI;
- PET/SPECT;
- neuropsychological evaluation.

Interictal EEG

Electroencephalography is the most specific method to define epileptogenic cortex. Interictal epileptiform discharges, particularly if consistent over time, can provide useful information [38, 39]. In temporal lobe epilepsy, consistently unitemporal interictal epileptiform discharges (IED) have a better prognosis for seizure freedom (85%) than bilateral IEDs [40] (IIb/B). Focal, particularly extratemporal, epilepsies in whom the EEG shows regional polyspikes are more likely associated with cortical dysplasia as the etiology of the epilepsy than patients with other IEDs [41] (IIb/B).

Ictal EEG-video monitoring

Ictal EEG-video recording is critical in localizing the epileptogenic zone. A careful analysis of the first clinical signs and symptoms of a seizure and of the evolution of the seizure symptomatology can provide important clues [42-44]. One must keep in mind, however, that often an epileptic seizure arises from a 'silent' region of the cortex and would remain asymptomatic unless it spreads to 'eloquent' cortex such as primary motor, primary sensory, or supplementary sensorimotor areas [45]. Invasive EEG techniques including stereotactically implanted multicontact depth electrodes or subdural strips and grids have been developed to further define the epileptogenic zone in selected patients (Figure 2).

Although surface EEG recordings are less sensitive than invasive studies, they provide the best overview and therefore the most efficient way to define the approximate localization of the epileptogenic zone. Invasive electrodes are subject to sampling errors if misplaced and should be used only after exhaustive non-invasive evaluations have:

- failed to localize the epileptogenic zone; and
- led to a testable hypothesis regarding this localization.

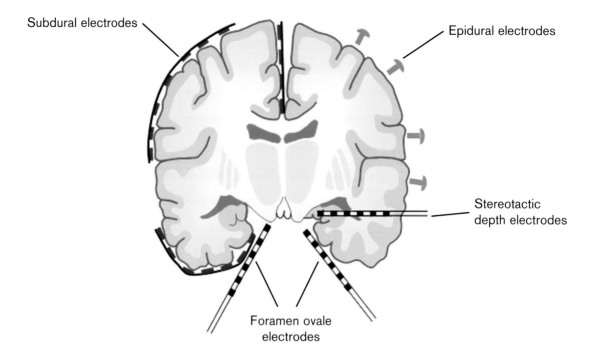

Subdural electrodes

Epidural electrodes

Stereotactic depth electrodes

Foramen ovale electrodes

Figure 2. Several types of invasive electrodes.

Invasive EEG studies are associated with additional risks [46] that are justifiable only if there is a good chance of obtaining useful and essential localizing information.

Electrical stimulation of the cortex can be performed either intra-operatively or extra-operatively and is useful to delineate the limits of cortical resection when the epileptogenic zone is adjacent to or overlapping with functional cortex [34, 47].

Structural imaging

Definition of the anatomic relationship of epileptogenic cortex to a lesion is a crucial issue in the evaluation of patients considered for epilepsy surgery (Figure 1). Structural imaging with high resolution MRI frequently provides essential information if performed adequately [48] (IIb/B). The concordance of interictal and ictal EEG localization with regard to the MRI lesion is good in temporal lesions but poorer in extratemporal lesions. If a structural lesion is found and its location is consistent with clinical and EEG data regarding the epileptogenic zone, removal of the lesion alone may be sufficient to control seizures [49] (IIb/B). In other cases, removal of additional cortex, identifiable with intra-operative or extra-operative invasive recording may be necessary. This is frequently the case in patients with epilepsy caused by cortical dysplasia, post-traumatic lesions, or perinatal stroke.

Functional imaging

Interictally, epileptogenic zones particularly in the temporal lobe are frequently associated with a reduced regional cerebral metabolism which can be detected by F-18-desoxy-glucose-PET [50]. Interictal SPECT may demonstrate a corresponding area of reduced cerebral blood flow, but is less sensitive than PET, and may provide misleading information [51]. Ictal SPECT studies particularly in temporal lobe epilepsy, however, are more reliable and show a region of increased cerebral perfusion [52]. In extratemporal epilepsies, ictal SPECT localizes better in patients with frontal than with parieto-occipital seizure onset [53]. Functional MRI is gaining relevance in the presurgical evaluation of epilepsy patients as it may help to localize language function in a non-invasive approach in adults and children [54, 55] **(IIb/B)**. More advanced techniques and paradigms are available to test for motor, sensory and cognitive functions, which may provide prognostic information with regard to postoperative functioning [56] **(III/B)**.

Neuropsychology

Neuropsychological testing is an integral part of the evaluation when considering epilepsy surgery. It is important to understand the pre-operative cognitive functioning level to adequately counsel about the risks of cognitive deficits and to plan post-surgical rehabilitation. Low IQ has been considered a poor prognostic factor for resective epilepsy surgery since it usually indicates diffuse brain damage which not infrequently is associated with a widespread epileptogenic zone [57]. However, many of the low-IQ patients benefit from surgery, especially patients with lesions. Low IQ should not exclude patients from resective epilepsy surgery, but is an important prognostic factor to consider in the counselling process. In selected children whose developmental delay appears to result at least in part from the effects of seizures, this delay may itself be a reason for surgical evaluation, as they may show a significant gain in developmental skills after resective epilepsy surgery [58, 59] **(IIb/B)**.

What kind of surgical procedures are available?

Several surgical procedures are available for treating patients with medically refractory epilepsy. These include focal resection of the epileptogenic cortex (anterior temporal lobectomy, focal cortical resection), as well as surgical interventions to remove or isolate the cortex of a grossly diseased hemisphere (functional hemispherectomy, multiple subpial transections, and anterior corpus callosotomy). In general, only complete resection of the epileptogenic brain region offers the possibility of cure. Other surgical procedures are palliative.

Temporal resections

Anterior temporal lobe resection can be performed on the basis of non-invasive studies only if clinical, EEG, and MRI data are convergent (Figure 1) [32, 33]. Non-invasive EEG monitoring includes sphenoidal electrodes, which are particularly sensitive to mesial temporal foci [60]. In many of the these patients, MRI demonstrates mesial hippocampal sclerosis [61], which is associated with a favorable postoperative outcome with regard to seizure control. The combination of anterior temporal lobectomy and medical treatment is clearly superior to medical treatment alone, which has been shown in the only available randomized controlled study on epilepsy surgery [62] **(Ib/A)** (see also Table 1).

Good results depend on the completeness of removal of mesial temporal structures [63] **(III/B)**. The persistence of postoperative IEDs is a poor prognostic factor for postoperative seizure outcome [64] **(III/B)**. More limited resection such as amygdalohippocampectomy is also a surgical option in selected patients [65]. Patients considered for dominant temporal lobectomy are at risk for verbal memory disturbances, particularly if their pre-operative mesial temporal structures are not atrophic and memory skills are above normal [66] **(III/B)**. It is yet not established whether more selective resections as amygdalohippocampectomy result in less cognitive deficits and are superior to anterior temporal lobe resections [67, 68].

Twenty to fifty percent of patients with medically intractable temporal lobe epilepsies will present with independent bitemporal interictal epileptiform EEG abnormalities and non-lateralized ictal surface recordings. It has been shown that these patients have a worse surgical outcome than patients with unitemporal interictal and ictal EEG abnormalities [40] **(III/B)**. In up to 77% of patients where bitemporal seizure patterns were recorded in non-invasive ictal EEG, invasive EEG recordings could still demonstrate the origin of all or most seizures in one temporal lobe and lead to successful epilepsy surgery [37] **(III/B)**. Depth electrodes in both temporal lobes are considered the most sensitive technique in these cases, but foramen-ovale electrodes provide an alternative semi-invasive recording technique with less risk [69] **(IV/C)**.

The outcome of mesial temporal resections has been investigated in several studies during the past years. The only randomized, semi-controlled trial of epilepsy surgery was conducted in 80 patients with temporal lobe epilepsy whose seizures were not controlled with medical treatment [70] **(Ib/A)**. Anterior temporal lobectomy and subsequent AED treatment in these patients was superior in achieving seizure control compared to medical therapy only [70]. Seizure freedom is achieved in up to 70% of patients after temporal resection and another 20% have a significant reduction of seizure frequency. In the remaining 10%, no improvement of seizure control is achieved [71]. No differences regarding seizure outcome are evident when comparing anterior temporal resection and selective amygdalohippo-campectomy. Depression and anxiety in patients with refractory epilepsy significantly improve after epilepsy surgery, especially in those who are seizure-free [72] **(IV/C)**. A decision analysis which used published data regarding seizure frequency and quality of life determined that temporal lobe resection in patients with intractable temporal lobe epilepsy provided substantial increases in life expectancy (5 years) compared to medical treatment [73] **(IIb/B)**.

The mortality of mesial temporal resections is low and accounts for less than 0.5%. The occurrence of complications leading to permanent neurological deficits such as hemianopsia, aphasia, motor or sensory deficit and cranial nerve palsy ranges between 0.4 and 4% [74].

Table 1. Outcome of temporal lobe epilepsy surgery.

Author	Year	Trial	n	Follow-up (yrs)	Sz-free (%)	Additional results	Evidence class
Controlled trials							
Wiebe et al [62]	2001	RCT	36	1	64	8% sz-free with medical treatment	Ib/A
Gilliam et al [127]	1999	CT	94	1	65	Health-related QoL better after surgery	IIb/B
Bien et al [128]	2001	CT	148	4.8	62	7.5% sz-free in medical treatment	IIb/B
Uncontrolled trials							
Radhakrishnan et al [129]	1998	UCT	175	3.6	77	Solely ipsilateral IED predict good outcome	III/B
Jeha et al [130]	1999	UCT	371	5.5	63	Recurrence of IED predict poor outcome	III/B
Jeong et al [131]	1999	UCT	93	1.5	84	Young age and lesion on MRI are good	III/B
Wieser et al [132]	2001	UCT	369	7.2	67	Proposal of new outcome score	III/B
Jutila et al [133]	2002	UCT	140	5.4	56	Rate of sz freedom at 1yr equals rate at 10 yrs	III/B
Alpherts et al [27]	2005	UCT	71	6	68	No effect of surgery on intelligence	III/B
Spencer et al [134]	2005	UCT	297	4.6	68	Delay to remission predicts relapse	III/B
Cohen-Gadol et al [135]	2006	UCT	372	6.2	74	Normal finding on histopathology predicts poor outcome	III/B
Al-Kaylani et al [136]	2007	UCT	150	6	78	42% off AED treatment, 68% of them remain sz-free	III/B
Asztely et al [137]	2007	UCT	54	12.2	65	69% have same long-term sz status as at 2-yr follow-up	III/B
Etiology-specific analysis: temporal tumors							
Zaatreh et al [138]	2003	UCT	68	9	65	Only tumor patients; gross resection of tumor tissue predicts good outcome	III/B
Radhakrishnan et al [139]	2006	UCT	23	4	83	Only ganglioglioma patients	III/B

RCT = randomized controlled trial; CT = controlled trial; UCT = uncontrolled trial; sz = seizure; number of patients given represents operated patients; evidence level is given for the highest level attained for any aspect of the study; yr = year

Extratemporal resections

The limits of resection for epilepsy surgery are more difficult to define in extratemporal epilepsies because the boundaries of the epileptogenic zones are more variable. Neocortical epilepsies are divided into lesional and non-lesional. In lesional extratemporal epilepsies, MRI can guide epilepsy surgery and frequently the epileptogenic zone lies in the vicinity of the structural lesion. Invasive studies may be needed to define the epileptogenic zone and its boundaries with regard to eloquent cortex. If surface EEG and imaging studies do not localize

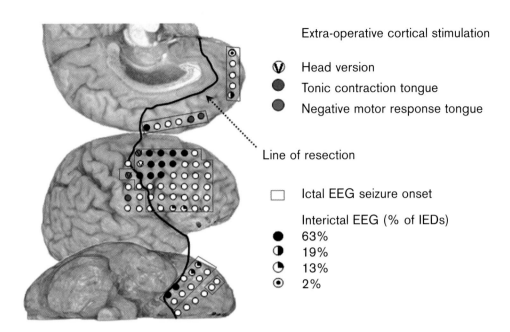

Extra-operative cortical stimulation

Head version

Tonic contraction tongue

Negative motor response tongue

Line of resection

Ictal EEG seizure onset

Interictal EEG (% of IEDs)

63%

19%

13%

2%

Figure 3. Results of invasive EEG-video monitoring in a patient with right frontal lobe epilepsy. Shown are the results of ictal and interictal EEG recording (IED = interictal epileptiform discharges), as well as the results of extra-operative cortical stimulation, which revealed only small areas of eloquent cortex. The frontal lobe resection caused transient side effects with loss of interest and psychomotor retardation for 3 months. All of the resected cortex showed signs of previous inflammation, suggesting an encephalitis as the etiology, which the patient had had no recollection of. Five years after surgery, the patient remains seizure-free and has no neuropsychological or behavioral deficits.

the epileptogenic zone with sufficient precision to guide invasive studies, semi-invasive EEG-recordings may be helpful, either in providing localizing information or in guiding placement of invasive electrodes (Figure 2) [75]. Improvement of imaging techniques such as MRI, PET and ictal SPECT, however, leads to less use of semi-invasive electrodes [75]. The relationship of the epileptogenic zone to functional cortex must be defined by intra-operative or extra-operative recording and stimulation techniques if the presumed epileptogenic zone lies near eloquent cortex such as the speech area or primary motor cortex [76] (Figures 1 and 3). The localization of the subdural electrodes in reference to anatomical structures is improved by fusing three-dimensional MRI data for brain anatomy and CT images for electrode location. This technique has been shown to be superior in terms of exact localization of the electrodes when compared to methods using the two-dimensional bicommissural reference system [77] (IIb/B). Based on invasive ictal recordings and results of electrical stimulation of the cortex, epilepsy surgery can be tailored individually by resecting the epileptogenic zone and sparing eloquent cortex (Figure 3).

The results of lesional epilepsy surgery are better because epilepsy surgery can be based on data from structural imaging as well as functional tests (EEG, SPECT, and PET), whereas in non-lesional epilepsy, surgery must rely on functional tests only [78]. Stereotactically-guided lesionectomies, which have the advantage of allowing resection of deep-seated lesions involving eloquent cortex with relatively low surgical morbidity, have been reported to achieve similar good results (56% Engel class I and 74% Engel class I and II) [49, 79] **(IIb/B)**. The presence of a lesion identified by neuroimaging predicts a good outcome in patients with neocortical epilepsy. These patients are seizure-free in 67% and have a reduction of seizure frequency in 22% of cases, whereas only 11% do not improve at all [80]. In patients with lesional frontal lobe epilepsy, freedom of disabling seizure and non-disabling daily seizures can be achieved in 72% of cases, whereas this is achieved in only 41% of patients with non-lesional frontal lobe epilepsy [81] **(III/B)** (see also Table 2).

Table 2. Outcome in extratemporal lobe epilepsy surgery.

Author	Year	Trial	n	Follow-up (yrs)	Sz-free (%)	Additional results	Evidence class
Meta-analysis							
Téllez-Zenteno et al [140]	2005	MA	772 XTLE	n.a.	31	Hemispherectomy, callosotomy and subpial transections excluded in this table	IIb/B
Ansari et al [141]	2007	MA	95 XTLE	n.a.	34	Children, mean age 4.5 yrs	IIb/B
Lerner et al [142]	2009	MA	854	n.a.	62	Only cortical dysplasia, TLE included	IIb/B
Uncontrolled trials							
Adler et al [143]	1991	UCT	35 XTLE	10	40	Mean age of onset 5.1 yrs;	III/B
Holmes et al [144]	2000	UCT	126 XTLE	3	43	Occurrence of exclusively ipsilateral IEDs predict better outcome	III/B
Janszky et al [145]	2000	UCT	61 FLE	1.8	49	Generalized EEG discharges predict poor outcome	III/B
Chung et al [146]	2005	UCT	74 XTLE	2.2	58	Only cortical dysplasia, poorest outcome in FLE (25% sz-free)	III/B
Cohen-Gadol et al [135]	2006	UCT	27 XTLE	6.2	42	Rate of sz-free patients at 1 yr equals rate at 10-yr follow-up	III/B
Mani et al [147]	2006	UCT	71 XTLE	2		Acute postoperative seizures predict poorer outcome	III/B
Boesebeck et al [148]	2007	UCT	81 XTLE	2	41	Low seizure frequency and tumor etiology predicts better outcome	III/B
Binder et al [149]	2008	UCT	52 OLE	6.7	69	42% had additional visual field defects after surgery (preop 36%)	III/B
Elsharkawy et al [150]	2008	UCT	218 XTLE	5	53	Cortical dysplasia predicts poor outcome	III/B

MA = meta-analysis; UCT = uncontrolled trial; sz = seizure; evidence level is given for the highest level attained; n.a. = not available; XTLE = extratemporal lobe epilepsy; FLE = frontal lobe epilepsy; OLE = occipital lobe epilepsy; yr = year

Hemispherectomy or when is one hemisphere better than two? [82]

Patients with intractable seizures and severe hemispheric damage may benefit from hemispherectomy or hemispherotomy [83]. A hemispherectomy is indicated only in patients who do not qualify for a more limited resection. Most patients who qualify for hemispherectomy suffer from medically intractable motor seizures with progressive motor impairment. With rare exceptions [84, 85] (IV/C) only children with severe hemiparesis and no remaining useful hand function qualify for this surgery. For hemispherectomy to be considered, clinical data, imaging and non-invasive EEG-video studies should show that seizures arise only or almost exclusively from the damaged hemisphere whereas the other hemisphere is relatively intact. Anatomic hemispherectomy was abandoned because of long-term complications, particularly superficial cerebral hemosiderosis which was almost invariably fatal. Functional hemispherectomy, which consists of total disconnection of one hemisphere but only a very limited resection of brain tissue (the frontal and occipital lobes actually remain in place) [86] or hemispherotomy, which is even less invasive but equally as effective, were introduced to reduce morbidity [83]. The risk of surgery must be weighed against the devastating and life-threatening effect of seizures and the chance for a marked developmental progress in these infants and young children postoperatively [74, 87]. If a hemispherectomy of the dominant side is considered, careful investigation of language representation is required. In young children, the intracarotid amobarbital test is difficult to perform to establish speech dominance. Several studies indicate, however, that language will almost invariably transfer to the contralateral hemisphere if the disease starts before 6 years of age [88] (III/B). The exact age limit is not yet known, but even after the age of 6 years language shift may still occur, although speech in these children is more likely to be impaired [89]. Early hemispherectomy may be considered in progressive hemispheric syndromes like Rasmussen's encephalitis, even before the neurological deficit is maximal to prevent the imminent intellectual deterioration [90]. Patients undergoing hemispherectomy will gain seizure freedom in 43-79% of cases [74, 91]. The best outcomes for this technique are reported for Rasmussen's encephalitis and Sturge-Weber syndrome with less favorable outcomes in diffuse cortical dysplasia. Mortality after hemispherectomy is mostly related to hemorrhage during surgery and occurs in 1-5% of patients [92]. Postoperative neurological complications include aphasia and deterioration of hemiparesis and sensory deficits [85].

Multiple subpial transections

The technique of multiple subpial transections (MSTs) was introduced as a surgical option for patients in whom the epileptogenic zone lies in functional essential cortex and cannot be resected [93]. The rationale is based on the concept that disruption of horizontal cortical interconnections with sparing of vertically oriented fibers will reduce seizure spread without causing functional deficits. This technique is generally considered a palliative technique although some authors have reported good results, when combining MSTs with resective surgery of some part of the epileptogenic zone [94, 95] (III/B).

Corpus callosotomy

Candidates for corpus callosotomy include patients with medically intractable symptomatic generalized epilepsies and multiple seizure types including tonic, atonic, generalized tonic-clonic seizures, absences, and less frequently, focal seizures. Most of these patients also have mental retardation and are diagnosed as Lennox-Gastaut syndrome. Non-invasive EEG-video recordings and imaging studies are sufficient in the evaluation of these patients. The rationale is based on the disruption of seizure spread from one hemisphere to the other.

Tonic and atonic seizures leading to injuries seem to respond better to callosotomy than other seizure types [96, 97] **(IIb/B)**. Refractory idiopathic generalized epilepsies with mild reduction in baseline IQ may benefit from callosotomy [98] **(IV/C)**. Because some patients after complete callosotomy suffer from a disconnection syndrome, a staged approach has been developed. A rostral 2/3 callosotomy is performed first. If this fails to improve seizure control, complete disconnection can be performed in a second step usually without producing a disabling disconnection syndrome [99, 100] **(IV/C)**. Focal EEG discharges with secondary bilateral synchrony and focal lesions in imaging studies have been considered as good prognostic signs for callosotomy (although resective surgery should first be considered in these patients), whereas severe mental retardation has been reported to be a poor prognostic factor [101] **(III/B)**. Postoperative neuropsychological complications usually improve sufficiently within several days to weeks; most patients actually demonstrate a neuropsychological improvement postoperatively, probably due to reduced seizure frequency and lower anticonvulsant levels, and is most marked in children [102] **(IIb/B)**. It has been suggested that patients whose language and hand dominance do not correspond (crossed dominance) may be greatly dependent on transfer of language through the corpus callosum, raising the concern that postoperative speech problems may occur. An intracarotid amobarbital test may be indicated in this situation [103] **(IIb/B)**. Corpus callosotomy was performed frequently in most major surgical epilepsy centers in the early 1990s. However, the use of ketogenic diet and vagal nerve stimulation in patients with Lennox-Gastaut syndrome has led most centers to abandon the technique of callosotomy or only perform it infrequently [104].

Vagal nerve stimulation

Vagus nerve stimulation (VNS) has been shown to significantly reduce seizures in controlled studies to an extent similar to newly marketed antiepileptic drugs [105-109] **(Ib/A)**. The reduction of seizure frequency may occur only after long-term treatment of more than one year [110]. However, only selected patients achieve a seizure control that significantly affects quality of life, and seizure freedom is extremely rare. Side effects are low, especially cardiac arrhythmias occur rarely, and then mostly during the intra-operative lead testing [111] **(III/B)**. Clinical observations of positive effects on mood, vigilance and drive led to the first studies with VNS in medically refractory depression [112].

Gamma knife radiosurgery

Gamma knife radiosurgery of mesial temporal lobe epilepsy has been shown to result in success rates similar to the rates reported for open surgery [113] **(III/B)**, but comparative studies are not yet available. The effect may take up to 1 year, as expected from radiation therapy. The target of gamma knife surgery is critical, because it seems effective in focal epilepsy caused by cavernomas in highly functional areas, particularly the central region, whereas cavernomas in mesial temporal regions do not respond well [114] (III/B). In patients with hypothalamic hamartomas, gamma knife radiosurgery was efficacious in improving gelastic seizures in about half of the patients (Engel classification I and II) in one recent study [115] (IIb/B).

Deep brain stimulation

There is renewed interest in deep brain stimulation (DBS) for the treatment of epilepsy. The anterior thalamic nucleus has been a target since the 1960s, but very little controlled data have been available [116], until a recent well-designed double-blind, randomized, controlled study demonstrated a 29% greater reduction with stimulation than control during the blinded phase of the trial and a 56% seizure reduction compared to baseline in the open label phase [117] (Ib/A). Electrical stimulation of the centromedian thalamic nucleus has been reported to reduce the frequency of generalized tonic-clonic seizures in severe epilepsy [118] (III/B), and to reduce overall seizure frequency in Lennox-Gastaut syndrome by up to 80% [119] (III/B). These results were not confirmed by a placebo-controlled study [120] (IIa/B), but the lack of effect was most likely due to the study protocol, where 3 months on/off stimulation blocks were used, but thalamic stimulation is considerably more effective in long-term stimulation [121]. Similarly, the use of electrical stimulation of the cerebellum, first performed in the 1970s, remains controversial. A controlled study failed to show reduction of seizure frequency [122] (IIa/B). The subthalamic nucleus is another potential target, but the evidence for efficacy of DBS is scarce [123] (III/B).

Epilepsy surgery turns medically refractory patients into medically controlled patients

It is not yet known how many and which patients can be withdrawn from antiepileptic drug treatment following epilepsy surgery. There are no prospective trials to demonstrate how many patients can be cured by epilepsy surgery. In a meta-analysis, about one third of surgically treated patients remained seizure-free off medication for more than 5 years following resective temporal lobe epilepsy surgery [124] (Ia/A). We need prospective studies to look for prognostic factors of surgical outcome with regard to seizure freedom. However, such studies are hampered by several social factors such as driving regulations which have a major impact on individual decisions to reduce AEDs following surgery.

Why does epilepsy surgery fail?

Failure of epilepsy surgery may be related to wrong localization of the epileptogenic zone, too widespread epileptogenic zones and too limited resection of the suspected epileptogenic zone. In patients with mesial temporal sclerosis, seizure patterns arise from neocortical regions after resective surgery rather than from residual hippocampal tissue [125]. These findings suggest the existence of a regional epileptogenicity in patients with mesial temporal sclerosis with the hippocampus representing the area of cortex with the lowest threshold for seizure generation. After hippocampal resection, the surrounding neocortical tissue also exhibiting epileptogenicity is then becoming the seizure onset zone. In addition, seizure onset on the contralateral temporal region can be detected in up to 25% of patients with mesial temporal sclerosis with postoperative seizure recurrence. Extensive re-evaluation of patients suffering from recurrent seizures after epilepsy surgery is mandatory and the possibility of a re-resection should be considered. In patients with recurrent seizures after a first resective epilepsy surgery, a second surgery may lead to seizure freedom in almost half of the patients and a reduction of seizure frequency by 90% can be achieved in one third of patients without increased mortality or morbidity [126].

Conclusions

Surgery is a viable option in selected epilepsy patients. The decision as to whether to refer patients to surgical treatment should be made early in the course of patients' epilepsy to maximize their benefit from surgery. Some patients may achieve seizure freedom; the chance for it will depend on the syndrome and on the available surgical techniques. Even when seizure freedom is not attainable, surgery may provide a palliative alleviation of the symptoms of epilepsy.

Key points	Evidence level
◆ Determine early whether patients are refractory to medical therapy. Typically, patients should be considered refractory to therapy when two AEDs in adequate doses have failed to control the seizures within 2 years.	Ib/A
◆ When patients are refractory, refer them early to specialized epilepsy centers.	
◆ In temporal lobe epilepsy, surgery is superior to medical treatment.	Ib/A
◆ In extratemporal lobe epilepsy, outcome differs greatly by location (poorer prognosis: frontal lobe epilepsy) and etiology (better prognosis: fully resectable benign tumor).	IIb/B
◆ Vagal nerve stimulation, callosotomy and multiple subpial transections are palliative procedures, but selected patients will benefit from them.	IIb/B
◆ One third of patients remain seizure-free without medication for more than 5 years after resective temporal lobe epilepsy surgery.	Ia/A
◆ Future developments will include improvement of gamma knife surgery and the use of deep brain stimulation.	

References

1. National Institutes of Health Consensus Conference. Surgery for epilepsy. *JAMA* 1990; 264: 729-33.
2. Hauser WA, Rich SS, Lee JR, Annegers JF, Anderson VE. Risk of recurrent seizures after two unprovoked seizures. *N Engl J Med* 1998; 338: 429-34.
3. Cockerell OC, Johnson AL, Sander JW, Shorvon SD. Prognosis of epilepsy: a review and further analysis of the first nine years of the British National General Practice Study of Epilepsy, a prospective population-based study. *Epilepsia* 1997; 38: 31-46.
4. Annegers JF, Hauser WA, Elveback LR. Remission of seizures and relapse in patients with epilepsy. *Epilepsia* 1979; 20: 729-37.
5. Sillanpaa M. Long-term outcome of epilepsy. *Epileptic Disord* 2000; 2: 79-88.
6. Kwan P, Brodie MJ. Early identification of refractory epilepsy. *N Engl J Med* 2000; 342: 314-9.
7. Berg AT, Kelly MM. Defining intractability: comparisons among published definitions. *Epilepsia* 2006; 47: 431-6.
8. Hermanns G, Noachtar S, Tuxhorn I, Holthausen H, Ebner A, Wolf P. Systematic testing of medical intractability for carbamazepine, phenytoin, and phenobarbital or primidone in monotherapy for patients considered for epilepsy surgery. *Epilepsia* 1996; 37: 675-9.
9. Lesser RP, Dinner DS, Luders H, Morris HH, 3d. Differential diagnosis and treatment of intractable seizures. *Cleve Clin Q* 1984; 51: 227-40.
10. Tomson T, Dahl ML, Kimland E. Therapeutic monitoring of antiepileptic drugs for epilepsy. *Cochrane Database Syst Rev* 2007: CD002216.
11. French JA, Kanner AM, Bautista J, et al. Efficacy and tolerability of the new antiepileptic drugs II: treatment of refractory epilepsy: report of the Therapeutics and Technology Assessment Subcommittee and Quality Standards Subcommittee of the American Academy of Neurology and the American Epilepsy Society. *Neurology* 2004; 62: 1261-73.
12. French JA, Kanner AM, Bautista J, et al. Efficacy and tolerability of the new antiepileptic drugs I: treatment of new onset epilepsy: report of the Therapeutics and Technology Assessment Subcommittee and Quality Standards Subcommittee of the American Academy of Neurology and the American Epilepsy Society. *Neurology* 2004; 62: 1252-60.
13. Brodie MJ, Kwan P. Staged approach to epilepsy management. *Neurology* 2002; 58: S2-8.
14. Kwan P, Arzimanoglou A, Berg AT, et al. Definition of drug resistant epilepsy: Consensus proposal by the ad hoc Task Force of the ILAE Commission on Therapeutic Strategies. *Epilepsia* 2010; 51: 1069-77.
15. Hitiris N, Mohanraj R, Norrie J, Sills GJ, Brodie MJ. Predictors of pharmacoresistant epilepsy. *Epilepsy Res* 2007; 75: 192-6.
16. Stephen LJ, Kwan P, Brodie MJ. Does the cause of localisation-related epilepsy influence the response to antiepileptic drug treatment? *Epilepsia* 2001; 42: 357-62.
17. Semah F, Picot MC, Adam C, et al. Is the underlying cause of epilepsy a major prognostic factor for recurrence? *Neurology* 1998; 51: 1256-62.
18. Gilliam F. The impact of epilepsy on subjective health status. *Curr Neurol Neurosci Rep* 2003; 3: 357-62.
19. Sperling MR, Feldman H, Kinman J, Liporace JD, O'Connor MJ. Seizure control and mortality in epilepsy. *Ann Neurol* 1999; 46: 45-50.
20. Mohanraj R, Norrie J, Stephen LJ, Kelly K, Hitiris N, Brodie MJ. Mortality in adults with newly diagnosed and chronic epilepsy: a retrospective comparative study. *Lancet Neurol* 2006; 5: 481-7.
21. Fisher RS, Vickrey BG, Gibson P, et al. The impact of epilepsy from the patient's perspective I. Descriptions and subjective perceptions. *Epilepsy Res* 2000; 41: 39-51.
22. National Institutes of Health Consensus Conference. Surgery for epilepsy. *JAMA* 1990; 264: 729-33.
23. Morrell F. Secondary epileptogenesis in man. *Arch Neurol* 1985; 42: 318-35.
24. Moshe SL, Shinnar S. Early intervention. In: *Surgical Treatment of the Epilepsies*, 2nd ed. Engel JJ, Ed. New York: Raven Press, 1993: 123-32.
25. Lüders HO. Clinical evidence for secondary epileptogenesis. In: *Brain Plasticity and Epilepsy.* Engel JJ, Schwartzkroin PA, Moshe SL, Lowenstein DH, Eds. San Diego: Academic Press, 2001: 469-80.
26. Janszky J, Janszky I, Schulz R, et al. Temporal lobe epilepsy with hippocampal sclerosis: predictors for long-term surgical outcome. *Brain* 2005; 128: 395-404.

27. Alpherts WC, Vermeulen J, van Rijen PC, da Silva FH, van Veelen CW. Verbal memory decline after temporal epilepsy surgery?: a 6-year multiple assessments follow-up study. *Neurology* 2006; 67: 626-31.
28. Rosenow F, Luders H. Presurgical evaluation of epilepsy. *Brain* 2001; 124: 1683-700.
29. Awad IA, Katz A, Hahn JF, Kong AK, Ahl J, Luders H. Extent of resection in temporal lobectomy for epilepsy. I. Interobserver analysis and correlation with seizure outcome. *Epilepsia* 1989; 30: 756-62.
30. Wyllie E, Luders H, Morris HH, 3d, *et al.* Clinical outcome after complete or partial cortical resection for intractable epilepsy. *Neurology* 1987; 37: 1634-41.
31. Fish D, Andermann F, Olivier A. Complex partial seizures and small posterior temporal or extratemporal structural lesions: surgical management. *Neurology* 1991; 41: 1781-4.
32. Sperling MR, O'Connor MJ, Saykin AJ, *et al.* A noninvasive protocol for anterior temporal lobectomy. *Neurology* 1992; 42: 416-22.
33. Winkler PA, Herzog C, Henkel A, *et al.* Noninvasive protocol for surgical treatment of focal epilepsies. *Nervenarzt* 1999; 70: 1088-93.
34. Noachtar S, Borggraefe I. Epilepsy surgery: a critical review. *Epilepsy Behav* 2009; 15: 66-72.
35. Thadani VM, Williamson PD, Berger R, *et al.* Successful epilepsy surgery without intracranial EEG recording: criteria for patient selection. *Epilepsia* 1995; 36: 7-15.
36. Noachtar S. Subdural electrodes in focal cortical dysplasia. *Epileptic Disord* 2003; 5 Suppl 2: S91-4.
37. So N, Gloor P, Quesney LF, Jones-Gotman M, Olivier A, Andermann F. Depth electrode investigations in patients with bitemporal epileptiform abnormalities. *Ann Neurol* 1989; 25: 423-31.
38. Engel J, Jr. A practical guide for routine EEG studies in epilepsy. *J Clin Neurophysiol* 1984; 1: 109-42.
39. Ojemann GA. Surgical therapy for medically intractable epilepsy. *J Neurosurg* 1987; 66: 489-99.
40. Schulz R, Luders HO, Hoppe M, Tuxhorn I, May T, Ebner A. Interictal EEG and ictal scalp EEG propagation are highly predictive of surgical outcome in mesial temporal lobe epilepsy. *Epilepsia* 2000; 41: 564-70.
41. Noachtar S, Bilgin O, Remi J, *et al.* Interictal regional polyspikes in noninvasive EEG suggest cortical dysplasia as etiology of focal epilepsies. *Epilepsia* 2008; 49: 1011-7.
42. Noachtar S. Seizure semiology. In: *Epilepsy: Comprehensive Review and Case Discussions.* Lüders HO, Ed. London: Martin Dunitz Publishers, 2000: 127-40.
43. Lüders HO, Noachtar S. *Atlas of Epileptic Seizures and Syndromes.* Philadelphia: Saunders, 2001.
44. Lüders H, Noachtar S. *Epileptic Seizures: Pathophysiology and Clinical Semiology.* New York: Churchill Livingstone, 2000.
45. Lüders HO, Awad IA. Conceptual considerations. In: *Epilepsy Surgery.* Lüders HO, Ed. New York: Raven Press, 1991: 51-62.
46. Van Buren JM. Outcome with respect to epileptic seizures. In: *Surgical Treatment of the Epilepsies.* Engel JJ, Ed. New York: Raven Press, 1987: 465-75.
47. Lüders H, Lesser RP, Dinner DS, Morris HH, Wyllie E, Godoy J. Localization of cortical function: new information from extraoperative monitoring of patients with epilepsy. *Epilepsia* 1988; 29 Suppl 2: S56-65.
48. Von Oertzen J, Urbach H, Jungbluth S, *et al.* Standard magnetic resonance imaging is inadequate for patients with refractory focal epilepsy. *J Neurol Neurosurg Psychiatry* 2002; 73: 643-7.
49. Cascino GD, Kelly PJ, Sharbrough FW, Hulihan JF, Hirschorn KA, Trenerry MR. Long-term follow-up of stereotactic lesionectomy in partial epilepsy: predictive factors and electroencephalographic results. *Epilepsia* 1992; 33: 639-44.
50. Engel J, Jr., Henry TR, Risinger MW, *et al.* Presurgical evaluation for partial epilepsy: relative contributions of chronic depth-electrode recordings versus FDG-PET and scalp-sphenoidal ictal EEG. *Neurology* 1990; 40: 1670-7.
51. Duncan R. SPECT in focal epilepsies. *Behav Neurol* 2000; 12: 69-75.
52. Duncan JS. Imaging and epilepsy. *Brain* 1997; 120: 339-77.
53. Noachtar S, Arnold S, Yousry TA, Bartenstein P, Werhahn KJ, Tatsch K. Ictal technetium-99m ethyl cysteinate dimer single-photon emission tomographic findings and propagation of epileptic seizure activity in patients with extratemporal epilepsies. *Eur J Nucl Med* 1998; 25: 166-72.
54. Gaillard WD, Pugliese M, Grandin CB, *et al.* Cortical localization of reading in normal children: an fMRI language study. *Neurology* 2001; 57: 47-54.
55. Gaillard WD, Balsamo LM, Ibrahim Z, Sachs BC, Xu B. fMRI identifies regional specialization of neural networks for reading in young children. *Neurology* 2003; 60: 94-100.

56. Janszky J, Jokeit H, Kontopoulou K, *et al.* Functional MRI predicts memory performance after right mesiotemporal epilepsy surgery. *Epilepsia* 2005; 46: 244-50.

57. Malmgren K, Olsson I, Engman E, Flink R, Rydenhag B. Seizure outcome after resective epilepsy surgery in patients with low IQ. *Brain* 2008; 131: 535-42.

58. Chugani HT, Shields WD, Shewmon DA, Olson DM, Phelps ME, Peacock WJ. Infantile spasms: I. PET identifies focal cortical dysgenesis in cryptogenic cases for surgical treatment. *Ann Neurol* 1990; 27: 406-13.

59. Loddenkemper T, Holland KD, Stanford LD, Kotagal P, Bingaman W, Wyllie E. Developmental outcome after epilepsy surgery in infancy. *Pediatrics* 2007; 119: 930-5.

60. Morris HH, 3d, Kanner A, Luders H, *et al.* Can sharp waves localized at the sphenoidal electrode accurately identify a mesio-temporal epileptogenic focus? *Epilepsia* 1989; 30: 532-9.

61. Jackson G, Berkovic S, Tress B, Kalnins R, Fabinyi G, Bladin P. Hippocampal sclerosis may be reliably detected by MRI. *Neurology* 1990; 40: 1869-75.

62. Wiebe S, Blume WT, Girvin JP, Eliasziw M. A randomized, controlled trial of surgery for temporal-lobe epilepsy. *N Engl J Med* 2001; 345: 311-8.

63. Nayel MH, Awad IA, Luders H. Extent of mesiobasal resection determines outcome after temporal lobectomy for intractable complex partial seizures. *Neurosurgery* 1991; 29: 55-60.

64. Hildebrandt M, Schulz R, Hoppe M, May T, Ebner A. Postoperative routine EEG correlates with long-term seizure outcome after epilepsy surgery. *Seizure* 2005; 14: 446-51.

65. Wieser HG, Yasargil MG. Selective amygdalohippocampectomy as a surgical treatment of mesiobasal limbic epilepsy. *Surg Neurol* 1982; 17: 445-57.

66. Chelune GJ, Naugle RI, Luders H, Awad IA. Prediction of cognitive change as a function of preoperative ability status among temporal lobectomy patients seen at 6-month follow-up. *Neurology* 1991; 41: 399-404.

67. Schramm J. Temporal lobe epilepsy surgery and the quest for optimal extent of resection: a review. *Epilepsia* 2008; 49: 1296-307.

68. Helmstaedter C, Richter S, Roske S, Oltmanns F, Schramm J, Lehmann TN. Differential effects of temporal pole resection with amygdalohippocampectomy versus selective amygdalohippocampectomy on material-specific memory in patients with mesial temporal lobe epilepsy. *Epilepsia* 2008; 49: 88-97.

69. Wieser HG, Elger CE, Stodieck SR. The 'foramen ovale electrode': a new recording method for the preoperative evaluation of patients suffering from mesio-basal temporal lobe epilepsy. *Electroencephalogr Clin Neurophysiol* 1985; 61: 314-22.

70. Wiebe S, Blume WT, Girvin JP, Eliasziw M. A randomized, controlled trial of surgery for temporal-lobe epilepsy. *N Engl J Med* 2001; 345: 311-8.

71. Engel JJ. *Epilepsy Surgery,* 2nd ed. New York: Raven Press, 1993.

72. Devinsky O, Barr WB, Vickrey BG, *et al.* Changes in depression and anxiety after resective surgery for epilepsy. *Neurology* 2005; 65: 1744-9.

73. Choi H, Sell RL, Lenert L, Muennig P, Goodman RR, Gilliam FG, *et al.* Epilepsy surgery for pharmacoresistant temporal lobe epilepsy: a decision analysis. *JAMA* 2008; 300: 2497-505.

74. Spencer S, Huh L. Outcomes of epilepsy surgery in adults and children. *Lancet Neurol* 2008; 7: 525-37.

75. Noachtar S. Epidural electrodes. In: *Epilepsy Surgery.* Lüders H, Comair Y, Eds. Lippincott Williams & Wilkins, 2001: 585-91.

76. Lüders H, Lesser RP, Dinner DS, *et al.* Commentary: chronic intracranial recording and stimulation with subdural electrodes. In: *Surgical Treatment of the Epilepsies.* Engel JJ, Ed. New York: Raven Press, 1987: 297-321.

77. Winkler PA, Vollmar C, Krishnan KG, Pfluger T, Bruckmann H, Noachtar S. Usefulness of 3-D reconstructed images of the human cerebral cortex for localization of subdural electrodes in epilepsy surgery. *Epilepsy Res* 2000; 41: 169-78.

78. Van Ness PC. Surgical outcome for neocortical (extrahippocampal) focal epilepsy. In: *Epilepsy Surgery.* Lüders HO, Ed. New York: Raven Press, 1991: 613-24.

79. Engel JJ, Van Ness PC, Rasmussen TB, Ojemann LM. Outcome with respect to epileptic seizure. In: *Surgical Treatment of the Epilepsies*, 2nd ed. Engel JJ, Ed. New York: Raven Press, 1993: 609-21.

80. Engel JJ. Presurgical evaluation protocols. In: *Surgical Treatment of the Epilepsies*, 2nd ed. Engel JJ, Ed. New York: Raven Press, 1993: 707-50.

81. Mosewich RK, So EL, O'Brien TJ, *et al.* Factors predictive of the outcome of frontal lobe epilepsy surgery. *Epilepsia* 2000; 41: 843-9.

82. Duchowny M. Hemispherectomy for epilepsy: when is one half better than two? *Neurology* 2004; 62: 1664-5.
83. Schramm J, Clusmann H. The surgery of epilepsy. *Neurosurgery* 2008; 62 Suppl 2: 463-81; discussion 481.
84. Steinhoff BJ, Staack AM, Bilic S, Kraus U, Schulze-Bonhage A, Zentner J. Functional hemispherectomy in adults with intractable epilepsy syndromes: a report of 4 cases. *Epileptic Disord* 2009; 11: 251-7.
85. McClelland S, 3rd, Maxwell RE. Hemispherectomy for intractable epilepsy in adults: the first reported series. *Ann Neurol* 2007; 61: 372-6.
86. Rasmussen T. Characteristics of a pure culture of frontal lobe epilepsy. *Epilepsia* 1983; 24: 482-93.
87. Basheer SN, Connolly MB, Lautzenhiser A, Sherman EM, Hendson G, Steinbok P. Hemispheric surgery in children with refractory epilepsy: seizure outcome, complications, and adaptive function. *Epilepsia* 2007; 48: 133-40.
88. Maehara T, Shimizu H, Kawai K, *et al*. Postoperative development of children after hemispherotomy. *Brain Dev* 2002; 24: 155-60.
89. Taylor LP. Neuropsychological assessment of patients with chronic encephalitis. In: *Chronic Encephalitis and Epilepsy: Rasmussen's Syndrome*. Andermann F, Ed. Boston: Butterworth, 1991: 111-21.
90. Villemure JG, Andermann F, Rasmussen TB. Hemispherectomy for the treatment of epilepsy due to chronic encephalitis. In: *Chronic Encephalitis and Epilepsy: Rasmussen's Syndrome*. Andermann F, Ed. Boston: Butterworth, 1991: 111-21.
91. Limbrick DD, Narayan P, Powers AK, *et al*. Hemispherotomy: efficacy and analysis of seizure recurrence. *J Neurosurg Pediatr* 2009; 4: 323-32.
92. Montes JL, Farmer JP, Andermann F, Poulin C. Hemispherectomy: medications, technical approaches, and results. In: *The Treatment of Epilepsy: Principles and Practice*. Wyllie E, Ed. Philadelphia: Lippincott Wiliams & Wilkins, 2006: 1111-24.
93. Morrell F, Whisler WW, Bleck TP. Multiple subpial transection: a new approach to the surgical treatment of focal epilepsy. *J Neurosurg* 1989; 70: 231-9.
94. Devinsky O, Romanelli P, Orbach D, Pacia S, Doyle W. Surgical treatment of multifocal epilepsy involving eloquent cortex. *Epilepsia* 2003; 44: 718-23.
95. Behdad A, Limbrick Jr DD, Bertrand ME, Smyth MD. Epilepsy surgery in children with seizures arising from the rolandic cortex. *Epilepsia* 2009; 50: 1450-61.
96. Gates JR, Rosenfeld WE, Maxwell RE, Lyons RE. Response of multiple seizure types to corpus callosum section. *Epilepsia* 1987; 28: 28-34.
97. Tanriverdi T, Olivier A, Poulin N, Andermann F, Dubeau F. Long-term seizure outcome after corpus callosotomy: a retrospective analysis of 95 patients. *J Neurosurg* 2009; 110: 332-42.
98. Cukiert A, Burattini JA, Mariani PP, *et al*. Outcome after extended callosal section in patients with primary idiopathic generalized epilepsy. *Epilepsia* 2009; 50: 1377-80.
99. Wilson DH, Reeves AG, Gazzaniga MS. 'Central' commissurotomy for intractable generalized epilepsy: series two. *Neurology* 1982; 32: 687-97.
100. Wilson DH, Reeves A, Gazzaniga M, Culver C. Cerebral commissurotomy for control of intractable seizures. *Neurology* 1977; 27: 708-15.
101. Spencer SS, Spencer DD, Williamson PD, Sass K, Novelly RA, Mattson RH. Corpus callosotomy for epilepsy. I. Seizure effects. *Neurology* 1988; 38: 19-24.
102. Lassonde M, Sauerwein C. Neuropsychological outcome of corpus callosotomy in children and adolescents. *J Neurosurg Sci* 1997; 41: 67-73.
103. Sass KJ, Novelly RA, Spencer DD, Spencer SS. Postcallosotomy language impairments in patients with crossed cerebral dominance. *J Neurosurg* 1990; 72: 85-90.
104. Smiths MC, Byrne R, Kanner AM. Corpus callosotomy and multiple subpial transections. In: *The Treatment of Epilepsy: Principles and Practice*. Wyllie E, Ed. Philadelphia: Lippincott Wiliams & Wilkins, 2006: 1159-68.
105. A randomized controlled trial of chronic vagus nerve stimulation for treatment of medically intractable seizures. The Vagus Nerve Stimulation Study Group. *Neurology* 1995; 45: 224-30.
106. Handforth A, DeGiorgio CM, Schachter SC, *et al*. Vagus nerve stimulation therapy for partial-onset seizures: a randomized active-control trial. *Neurology* 1998; 51: 48-55.
107. Salinsky MC, Uthman BM, Ristanovic RK, Wernicke JF, Tarver WB. Vagus nerve stimulation for the treatment of medically intractable seizures. Results of a 1-year open-extension trial. Vagus Nerve Stimulation Study Group. *Arch Neurol* 1996; 53: 1176-80.

108. DeGiorgio CM, Schachter SC, Handforth A, *et al*. Prospective long-term study of vagus nerve stimulation for the treatment of refractory seizures. *Epilepsia* 2000; 41: 1195-200.

109. Uthman BM, Reichl AM, Dean JC, *et al*. Effectiveness of vagus nerve stimulation in epilepsy patients: a 12-year observation. *Neurology* 2004; 63: 1124-6.

110. Chadwick D. Vagal-nerve stimulation for epilepsy. *Lancet* 2001; 357: 1726-7.

111. Ardesch JJ, Buschman HP, van der Burgh PH, Wagener-Schimmel LJ, van der Aa HE, Hageman G. Cardiac responses of vagus nerve stimulation: intraoperative bradycardia and subsequent chronic stimulation. *Clin Neurol Neurosurg* 2007; 109: 849-52.

112. George MS, Rush AJ, Marangell LB, *et al*. A one-year comparison of vagus nerve stimulation with treatment as usual for treatment-resistant depression. *Biol Psychiatry* 2005; 58: 364-73.

113. Barbaro NM, Quigg M, Broshek DK, *et al*. A multicenter, prospective pilot study of gamma knife radiosurgery for mesial temporal lobe epilepsy: seizure response, adverse events, and verbal memory. *Ann Neurol* 2009; 65: 167-75.

114. Bartolomei F, Regis J, Kida Y, *et al*. Gamma knife radiosurgery for epilepsy associated with cavernous hemangiomas: a retrospective study of 49 cases. *Stereotact Funct Neurosurg* 1999; 72 Suppl 1: 22-8.

115. Schulze-Bonhage A, Trippel M, Wagner K, *et al*. Outcome and predictors of interstitial radiosurgery in the treatment of gelastic epilepsy. *Neurology* 2008; 71: 277-82.

116. Fisher RS, Uthman BM, Ramsay RE, *et al*. Alternative surgical techniques for epilepsy. In: *Surgical Treatment of the Epilepsies*, 2nd ed. Engel JJ, Ed. New York: Raven Press, 1993: 549-64.

117. Fisher R, Salanova V, Witt T, *et al*. Electrical stimulation of the anterior nucleus of thalamus for treatment of refractory epilepsy. *Epilepsia* 2010; 51: 899-908.

118. Velasco F, Velasco M, Velasco AL, Jimenez F, Marquez I, Rise M. Electrical stimulation of the centromedian thalamic nucleus in control of seizures: long-term studies. *Epilepsia* 1995; 36: 63-71.

119. Velasco AL, Velasco F, Jimenez F, *et al*. Neuromodulation of the centromedian thalamic nuclei in the treatment of generalized seizures and the improvement of the quality of life in patients with Lennox-Gastaut syndrome. *Epilepsia* 2006; 47: 1203-12.

120. Fisher RS, Uematsu S, Krauss GL, *et al*. Placebo-controlled pilot study of centromedian thalamic stimulation in treatment of intractable seizures. *Epilepsia* 1992; 33: 841-51.

121. Velasco F, Velasco M, Jimenez F, *et al*. Predictors in the treatment of difficult-to-control seizures by electrical stimulation of the centromedian thalamic nucleus. *Neurosurgery* 2000; 47: 295-304; discussion 304-295.

122. Wright GD, McLellan DL, Brice JG. A double-blind trial of chronic cerebellar stimulation in twelve patients with severe epilepsy. *J Neurol Neurosurg Psychiatry* 1984; 47: 769-74.

123. Lee KJ, Jang KS, Shon YM. Chronic deep brain stimulation of subthalamic and anterior thalamic nuclei for controlling refractory partial epilepsy. *Acta Neurochir Suppl* 2006; 99: 87-91.

124. Schmidt D, Loscher W. How effective is surgery to cure seizures in drug-resistant temporal lobe epilepsy? *Epilepsy Res* 2003; 56: 85-91.

125. Hennessy MJ, Elwes RD, Binnie CD, Polkey CE. Failed surgery for epilepsy. A study of persistence and recurrence of seizures following temporal resection. *Brain* 2000; 123 Pt 12: 2445-66.

126. Awad IA, Nayel MH, Luders H. Second operation after the failure of previous resection for epilepsy. *Neurosurgery* 1991; 28: 510-8.

127. Gilliam F, Kuzniecky R, Meador K, *et al*. Patient-oriented outcome assessment after temporal lobectomy for refractory epilepsy. *Neurology* 1999; 53: 687-94.

128. Bien CG, Kurthen M, Baron K, *et al*. Long-term seizure outcome and antiepileptic drug treatment in surgically treated temporal lobe epilepsy patients: a controlled study. *Epilepsia* 2001; 42: 1416-21.

129. Radhakrishnan K, So EL, Silbert PL, *et al*. Predictors of outcome of anterior temporal lobectomy for intractable epilepsy: a multivariate study. *Neurology* 1998; 51: 465-71.

130. Jeha LE, Najm IM, Bingaman WE, *et al*. Predictors of outcome after temporal lobectomy for the treatment of intractable epilepsy. *Neurology* 2006; 66: 1938-40.

131. Jeong SW, Lee SK, Kim KK, Kim H, Kim JY, Chung CK. Prognostic factors in anterior temporal lobe resections for mesial temporal lobe epilepsy: multivariate analysis. *Epilepsia* 1999; 40: 1735-9.

132. Wieser HG, Blume WT, Fish D, *et al*. ILAE Commission Report. Proposal for a new classification of outcome with respect to epileptic seizures following epilepsy surgery. *Epilepsia* 2001; 42: 282-6.

133. Jutila L, Immonen A, Mervaala E, *et al*. Long-term outcome of temporal lobe epilepsy surgery: analyses of 140 consecutive patients. *J Neurol Neurosurg Psychiatry* 2002; 73: 486-94.

134. Spencer SS, Berg AT, Vickrey BG, *et al*. Predicting long-term seizure outcome after resective epilepsy surgery: the multicenter study. *Neurology* 2005; 65: 912-8.

135. Cohen-Gadol AA, Wilhelmi BG, Collignon F, *et al*. Long-term outcome of epilepsy surgery among 399 patients with nonlesional seizure foci including mesial temporal lobe sclerosis. *J Neurosurg* 2006; 104: 513-24.

136. Al-Kaylani M, Konrad P, Lazenby B, Blumenkopf B, Abou-Khalil B. Seizure freedom off antiepileptic drugs after temporal lobe epilepsy surgery. *Seizure* 2007; 16: 95-8.

137. Asztely F, Ekstedt G, Rydenhag B, Malmgren K. Long-term follow-up of the first 70 operated adults in the Goteborg Epilepsy Surgery Series with respect to seizures, psychosocial outcome and use of antiepileptic drugs. *J Neurol Neurosurg Psychiatry* 2007; 78: 605-9.

138. Zaatreh MM, Firlik KS, Spencer DD, Spencer SS. Temporal lobe tumoral epilepsy: characteristics and predictors of surgical outcome. *Neurology* 2003; 61: 636-41.

139. Radhakrishnan A, Abraham M, Radhakrishnan VV, Sarma SP, Radhakrishnan K. Medically refractory epilepsy associated with temporal lobe ganglioglioma: characteristics and postoperative outcome. *Clin Neurol Neurosurg* 2006; 108: 648-54.

140. Téllez-Zenteno JF, Dhar R, Wiebe S. Long-term seizure outcomes following epilepsy surgery: a systematic review and meta-analysis. *Brain* 2005; 128: 1188-98.

141. Ansari SF, Maher CO, Tubbs RS, Terry CL, Cohen-Gadol AA. Surgery for extratemporal nonlesional epilepsy in children: a meta-analysis. *Childs Nerv Syst* 2010l; 26: 945-51.

142. Lerner JT, Salamon N, Hauptman JS, *et al*. Assessment and surgical outcomes for mild type I and severe type II cortical dysplasia: a critical review and the UCLA experience. *Epilepsia* 2009; 50: 1310-35.

143. Adler J, Erba G, Winston KR, Welch K, Lombroso CT. Results of surgery for extratemporal partial epilepsy that began in childhood. *Arch Neurol* 1991; 48: 133-40.

144. Holmes MD, Kutsy RL, Ojemann GA, Wilensky AJ, Ojemann LM. Interictal, unifocal spikes in refractory extratemporal epilepsy predict ictal origin and postsurgical outcome. *Clin Neurophysiol* 2000; 111: 1802-8.

145. Janszky J, Jokeit H, Schulz R, Hoppe M, Ebner A. EEG predicts surgical outcome in lesional frontal lobe epilepsy. *Neurology* 2000; 54: 1470-6.

146. Chung CK, Lee SK, Kim KJ. Surgical outcome of epilepsy caused by cortical dysplasia. *Epilepsia* 2005; 46 Suppl 1: 25-9.

147. Mani J, Gupta A, Mascha E, *et al*. Postoperative seizures after extratemporal resections and hemispherectomy in pediatric epilepsy. *Neurology* 2006; 66: 1038-43.

148. Boesebeck F, Janszky J, Kellinghaus C, May T, Ebner A. Presurgical seizure frequency and tumoral etiology predict the outcome after extratemporal epilepsy surgery. *J Neurol* 2007; 254: 996-9.

149. Binder DK, Von Lehe M, Kral T, *et al*. Surgical treatment of occipital lobe epilepsy. *J Neurosurg* 2008; 109: 57-69.

150. Elsharkawy AE, Behne F, Oppel F, *et al*. Long-term outcome of extratemporal epilepsy surgery among 154 adult patients. *J Neurosurg* 2008; 108: 676-86.

Chapter 4

Optimizing decisions for treating women of childbearing potential before and during pregnancy

Joshua Mendelson MD, Fellow in Neurology
Kimford Meador MD, Professor of Neurology and Director of Epilepsy
Department of Neurology
Emory University
Atlanta, Georgia, USA

Introduction

There are over 500,000 women of childbearing age with epilepsy. With a birth rate of 3-5 per 1000 births, approximately 24,000 babies are born to women with epilepsy each year in the United States alone [1]. Generalized tonic-clonic seizures during pregnancy place both the mother and fetus at an increased risk of injury. Trauma involving the abdomen carries a possible risk of abruption, fetal intracranial hemorrhage, hypoxia or death [2]. Trauma was found to be the leading non-obstetrical cause of death in pregnant women with epilepsy [2]. A recent UK survey showed that there was a ten-fold greater risk of death in pregnant women with epilepsy, which appeared to be due primarily to seizures [2]. Seizure frequency increases during 17-33% of pregnancies [3]. The metabolism of antiepileptic drugs (AEDs) changes during pregnancy. This is largely due to metabolic changes associated with pregnancy including increased renal and hepatic clearance and changes in serum binding proteins, which result in alterations in AED blood levels [4]. The reduction in AED blood levels may result in increased seizure frequency during pregnancy [4]. Most women with epilepsy (WWE) require daily AED treatment and face a unique set of concerns when planning for pregnancy. This is largely due to the fact that in utero exposure to AEDs may result in both birth defects and cognitive complications. While the large majority of WWE on AEDs will have an uncomplicated pregnancy and delivery, preconception planning for those who wish to conceive is vital to minimize potential adverse outcomes for both mother and baby [5].

Teratogenesis and perinatal outcomes

The risk of fetal malformations for women with epilepsy taking an AED is approximately twice that of the general population [6]. Most women with epilepsy are unable to stop using AEDs since seizures themselves can be harmful to both mother and child. In utero AED exposure poses a risk of congenital malformations to the child, including orofacial clefts, heart abnormalities and skeletal, urological and neural tube defects [7]. Thus, the dilemma is to choose AEDs that control seizures and have the minimal potential for teratogenicity.

There have been reports of major congenital malformations as a result of AEDs used in the first trimester since the 1960s. In recent years, new information has become available from a number of pregnancy registries, which have been established to examine the risks that AEDs pose to the unborn. The new guidelines from the American Academy of Neurology and a recent meta-analysis determined that AEDs taken during the first trimester of pregnancy probably increase the risk of major congenital malformations in children born to women with epilepsy [8, 9].

Specific AEDs and their risk of congenital malformations have also been evaluated. Adverse effects to children born to women taking phenytoin were first described in 1973 by Loughnan *et al* and were given the name fetal hydantoin syndrome [10]. The syndrome consists of a constellation of malformations including growth retardation, microcephaly, developmental delay and multiple craniofacial anomalies. This terminology has since been replaced as these congenital malformations are seen with a wide array of AEDs. The Australian Registry of AEDs in pregnancy evaluated 292 women who were exposed to AEDs during pregnancy. There was a 10.5% incidence of birth defects in children with phenytoin exposure compared to a 4.3% incidence in children who were not exposed to AEDs (II/B) [11, 12]. A meta-analysis of 59 primary studies evaluating the risk of adverse effects of AED exposure during pregnancy by Meador *et al* revealed a 7.36% risk of major congenital malformations for phenytoin monotherapy compared to 3.26% in women not treated with AEDs, but this difference was not statistically significant (II/B) [9]. The UK registry reported a 3.7% overall rate of major congenital malformations for phenytoin compared to a 3.5% risk for no AED exposure in WWE (II/B) [13].

There is class II/B evidence that pregnant WWE who are treated with carbamazepine are probably not at substantial increased risk of major congenital malformations [8]. A study by Morrow *et al* found no increased risk in children born to WWE taking carbamazepine (II/B) [13]. Furthermore, the North American Pregnancy Registry found that treatment with carbamazepine resulted in a 2.6% increased risk of congenital malformations compared to 1.62% in the general population, which was not statistically different (II/B) [14]. This registry did report increased risks for cleft lip/palate and neural tube defects, but these risks remain to be confirmed by other registries. Of the first generation AEDs, carbamazepine has been shown over multiple studies to have no, or only a slight increased risk of major congenital malformations (II/B) [8, 15].

The risks associated with valproate therapy during pregnancy have been studied extensively. In a recent study it has been found that treatment with valproate resulted in a significant increased risk of major congenital malformations [8]; risks for specific malformations included neural tube defects, facial clefts and hypospadias, although other malformations may occur [13]. Multiple recent studies have found that valproate is associated with greater risk for congenital malformations **(II/B)** [8, 15]. Valproate's effect was found to be dose-dependent; doses greater than 1000mg per day appear to pose the greatest threat. Table 1 details the results of a recent meta-analysis, which indicates that treatment with valproate resulted in a 10.73% incidence of major congenital malformations **(II/B)** [9]. Furthermore, the risk of treatment with valproate monotherapy has been compared to treatment with other first and second generation AEDs. Samren *et al* found that valproate treatment carried a significantly higher risk of congenital malformation when compared to phenytoin monotherapy **(II/B)** [16]. The American Academy of Neurology practice parameters concluded that valproate monotherapy conveyed an increased risk of congenital malformations when compared to phenobarbital, carbamazepine, phenytoin and lamotrigine [8]. The AAN guidelines recommended avoidance of valproate use in the first trimester of pregnancy due to the potential risk of major congenital malformations [8].

Of the second generation AEDs, lamotrigine has the most data with regard to risk of major congenital malformations. A meta-analysis by Meador *et al* demonstrated that lamotrigine monotherapy is associated with a 2.91% incidence of major congenital malformation, which was not statistically significant **(II/B)** [9]. In one report on lamotrigine, an increased risk of cleft

Table 1. Pregnancy outcomes in women with epilepsy: meta-analysis. *Meador KJ, et al* [9].

Treatment	Malformations t (n)	Percentage	95% CI
Women without epilepsy	9 (108,084)	3.27	[1.37,5.17]
Carbamazepine	24 (4411)	4.62	[3.48, 5.76]
Lamotrigine	5 (1337)	2.91	[2.00, 3.82]
Phenobarbital	14 (945)	4.91	[3.22, 6.59]
Phenytoin	16 (1198)	7.36	[3.60, 11.11]
Valproate	19 (2097)	10.73	[8.16, 13.92]

95% CIs = 95% Confidence Intervals

lip/palate was observed [17], but another study found contradictory results for lamotrigine [18]. The most recent AAN guidelines indicate that treatment with lamotrigine has a probable lower rate of teratogenic outcomes when compared to valproate **(II/B)** [8]. At this time, there is insufficient data to fully evaluate most other AEDs (e.g. topiramate, zonisamide and levetiracetam). Recently, the FDA issued a warning for an increased risk of cleft defects (1.4%) for topiramate, but the detailed data supporting this warning have yet to be published [19]. A recent population-based cohort study of 837,795 liveborn infants in the Danish Medical Birth Registry from 1996 to 2008 examined 1532 infants exposed to lamotrigine, oxcarbazepine, topiramate, gabapentin, or levetiracetam during the first trimester [20]. They reported no increase in major congenital malformations for these new AEDs compared to the unexposed controls. However, only the lamotrigine group (n=1019) had adequate sample size. Thus, additional studies are needed for the other AEDs.

The most recent practice parameters suggest that there is a probable increased risk of major congenital malformation with AED polytherapy during the first trimester of pregnancy [8]. In a study by Kaaja *et al*, the risk of teratogenicity increased from 3.1%-7.8% in infants exposed to one AED, to 8.3%-13.5% in those exposed to two AEDs, and to greater than 13.5% in those exposed to three AEDs **(II/B)** [21]. Specific combinations of medications have not been fully evaluated, although it has been shown that polytherapy which includes valproate carries a higher risk of congenital malformations than does polytherapy without valproate **(II/B)** [8, 13].

Based on two class II/B studies, the AAN guidelines noted that there is probably an increased risk of small-for-gestational-age infants born to women with epilepsy [8]. In addition, a study published since the AAN guidelines has reported an increased risk for small-for-gestational-age babies [22]. However, the contributing factors, especially if differences exist across AEDs, remain uncertain. The AAN also concluded that there is probably no increased risk in perinatal death based on two class II/B studies, but a subsequent study reported an increased risk [23]. The AAN stated that there is possibly a lower APGAR score based on one class II/B study, and one subsequent study also found lower APGAR scores in children of WWE [24].

Cognitive deficits in children born to WWE

There are a variety of factors that may contribute to neurodevelopmental deficits in children of mothers with epilepsy. These include AED exposure, seizures during pregnancy, seizure type, heredity, maternal age/parity, and socioeconomic status. However, a recent study evaluated the cognitive outcomes of children born to pregnant women with epilepsy on monotherapy [25]. In utero valproate exposure was associated with significantly lower IQ scores. As illustrated in Table 2, children exposed to valproate, on average, had an IQ score 9 points lower than the score of those exposed to lamotrigine (95% confidence interval [CI], 3.1 to 14.6; p=0.009), 7 points lower than the score of those exposed to phenytoin (95% CI, 0.2 to 14.0; p=0.04), and 6 points lower than the score of those exposed to carbamazepine (95% CI, 0.6 to 12.0; p=0.04) **(II/B)** [25]. Similar to alcohol, the risk of cognitive effects is

Table 2. Cognitive effect of in utero AED exposure. *Meador KJ, et al* [25].

Treatment	N	Mean IQ	Mean (95% CIs) difference from valproate
Carbamazepine	73	98	6 (0.6 - 12.0)
Lamotrigine	84	101	9 (3.1 - 14.6)
Phenytoin	48	99	7 (0.2 - 14.0)
Valproate	53	92	-

95% CIs = 95% Confidence Intervals

thought to be mostly due to exposure during the third trimester. Thus, valproate exposure poses a risk to the child throughout the duration of pregnancy. This association between valproate use and IQ was found to be dose-dependent with doses greater than 1000mg per day posing the greatest risk **(II/B)** [25]. Similar to population studies, maternal IQ was strongly related to child IQ overall; this was true for each AED except valproate, suggesting that valproate disrupted this normally strong relationship.

The findings in this recent investigation are supported by prior studies. A retrospective study from the UK found a 7.9 point reduction in verbal IQ for children exposed to valproate **(II/B)** [2]. A prospective Finnish study reported 8-13 point verbal IQ reduction for valproate **(II/B)** [26]. This study was limited by its small valproate monotherapy sample (n=13). Valproate's effect on cognitive development was dose-dependent in all of these studies. The combined findings across these three studies strongly support an increased risk of cognitive impairment with fetal valproate exposure.

The effects of the other AEDs on cognitive outcome are less clear. There is class II/B evidence that carbamazepine exposure probably does not increase the risk of cognitive deficits [26]. Phenytoin, on the other hand, has been reported to impair cognitive function [27-29], but was not statistically worse than carbamazepine or lamotrigine according to the results of a prospective study that did control for maternal IQ **(II/B)**. A recent study which examined children under age 2 years old using the Griffiths Mental Development Scale found no cognitive deficits for children exposed in utero to levetiracetam compared to controls [30]. However, the study was limited by young age at assessment, retrospective collection of seizures, and alcohol and tobacco use during pregnancy, and a completer rate of only 58% for the levetiracetam group. At this point there are insufficient data for the potential cognitive effects of fetal exposure for all other AEDs.

Obstetrical complications/change in seizure frequency

Potential obstetrical complications in pregnant women with epilepsy have been evaluated for many years. Recent American Academy of Neurology practice guidelines have specifically addressed this issue [31]. Two prospective studies suggested that women with epilepsy are not at any increased risk of Cesarean section [32-33], but because of the lack of statistical precision in these two studies and contradictory evidence from multiple class III studies, the AAN concluded that a moderately increased risk of Cesarean delivery could not be ruled out [31]. Furthermore, a recent study has reported an increased risk of C-section [22]. Neither the AAN review nor these new studies have been able to address contributing factors. A study which evaluated the obstetrical and neonatal outcomes in 179 pregnancies of women with epilepsy found no increased risk of pre-eclampsia [32]. Similarly, pregnant patients with epilepsy do not appear to be at increased risk of developing premature contractions, premature labor, or pregnancy-related bleeding [32]. There are insufficient data to assess if any increased risk of spontaneous abortion exists.

There is insufficient evidence to determine if WWE are at risk for increased seizures during pregnancy [31]. However, seizures in women often vary with hormonal changes. Estrogen and progesterone are two hormones of particular importance. Estrogen has been shown to lower seizure thresholds whereas progesterone has the opposite effect [34]. Seizure frequency during pregnancy has been evaluated by multiple studies; however, no studies have compared seizure frequency in pregnant women to a non-pregnant control group of women with epilepsy, which is noted as a gold standard by the AAN guidelines [31]. The patient's seizure frequency prior to pregnancy has been used as a control group in multiple studies. In one class II/B study, seizure frequency before and after pregnancy was evaluated in 154 patients. Seizure frequency was unchanged in 54%, increased in 32% and decreased in 14% [35]. However, another study found that seizure frequency was unchanged in 72% of patients during pregnancy [36]. Two class II/B studies evaluated the predictive value of seizure control prior to pregnancy and found that 84-92% of patients who were seizure-free for 9 months prior to pregnancy remained so for the duration of their pregnancy [36, 37]. Thus, seizure control prior to pregnancy is predictive of seizure frequency during pregnancy.

Folate/Vitamin K

The mechanism by which the different AEDs cause malformations is an area that still requires research. However, it is known that some AEDs have properties that lower the serum level of folic acid. Folic acid is a B-vitamin that is necessary for the production and maintenance of new cells [38]. It is especially important during periods of rapid cell division and growth such as infancy and pregnancy. There is a relationship between folic acid deficiency and the presence of congenital malformations, including neural tube defects. The neural tube consists of an anterior and posterior neuropore, which close at 23 and 26 days gestation, respectively. Since pregnancy is frequently identified only after weeks of pregnancy, it is paramount for women, especially those on AEDs, to take daily folic acid supplementation prior to pregnancy. In women with past pregnancies which resulted in children with neural tube defects, a daily dose of 4mg of folic acid has been shown to decrease the risk of future neural tube defects by more than 70% [39]. However, the effect of preconception folate on congenital malformations has not been assessed directly in women with epilepsy taking AEDs. Preconception folate use has also been associated with higher IQ in children of WWE on AED monotherapy [23]. It is currently felt that all WWE should take supplemental folic acid prior to pregnancy to reduce the incidence of neural tube defects and neurocognitive deficits [40].

It has been postulated that treatment with enzyme-inducing AEDs may result in alterations in vitamin K metabolism in newborns and place them at higher risk of bleeding [41]. Prenatal administration of oral vitamin K to pregnant women with epilepsy taking AEDs is aimed at preventing hemorrhagic disease in newborns during their first day of life. There have been multiple case reports that suggest that the offspring of mothers using enzyme-inducing AEDs have vitamin K deficiency. There is class II/B evidence by Kaaja *et al* that did not find an association between enzyme-inducing AEDs and neonatal hemorrhage as long as the children receive intramuscular injection of vitamin K at the time of birth [42]. Thus, at this point there is inadequate data to support the need for prenatal vitamin K in WWE during pregnancy [40].

Breastfeeding is strongly recommended by the American Academy of Pediatrics [43]. The benefits of breastfeeding include promoting maternal-child bonding and has been associated with a reduced risk in the child of severe lower respiratory tract infections, atopic dermatitis, asthma, acute otitis media, non-specific gastroenteritis, obesity, type 1 and 2 diabetes, childhood leukemia, sudden infant death syndrome, and necrotizing enterocolitis [44]. Breastfeeding has also been associated in the mother with a reduced risk for type 2 diabetes, breast cancer, ovarian cancer, and maternal postpartum depression [44]. Observations in animals of adverse effects of some AEDs on the immature brain have raised concerns that breastfeeding may be detrimental when women are taking AEDs. Although AEDs cross into breast milk to variable extent, the levels in the child are usually at lower concentrations than in the maternal serum. Agents that are highly protein bound are less likely to cross into breast milk. These include phenytoin, phenobarbital, and valproic acid. According to recent AAN guidelines there is evidence that phenobarbital, valproate, carbamazepine and phenytoin do not cross into breast milk in clinically meaningful concentrations (class I – AAN classification) [40]. They also state there is class I evidence that levetiracetam crosses into breast milk and class II evidence that gabapentin, lamotrigine and topiramate cross over [40]. Data obtained from the NEAD Study provides evidence that breastfeeding when the child has already been exposed in utero to carbamazepine, lamotrigine, phenytoin or valproic acid during pregnancy creates no additional risk to the child's future cognitive status [45], but additional studies are needed. Data on breastfeeding while on other AEDs are limited or non-existent.

Conclusions

There is an increased risk of congenital malformations and cognitive deficits in WWE exposed to AEDs, especially those patients who are exposed to polytherapy and valproate. Most congenital malformations have already occurred by the time of pregnancy diagnosis. Thus, seizure control and planning prior to pregnancy are of paramount importance as it remains difficult to predict who will be adversely affected by AED exposure. However, greater than 90% of WWE exposed to AEDs will have an uncomplicated pregnancy. In the past, it was recommended that physicians simply choose the most effective AED for the individual woman; however, the recent increase in information concerning potential adverse effects of AEDs on pregnancy complicates therapeutic decisions. Although many gaps in our knowledge remain, physicians must consider factors related to the teratogenic risks including birth defects and cognitive deficits for specific AEDs from the evidence that is available.

Treatment with monotherapy as opposed to polytherapy is preferred. Folic acid supplementation should be initiated prior to pregnancy to reduce the risk of major congenital malformations. Given the definite risk of congenital malformations and cognitive deficits associated with valproate, it is recommended that it not be used as a first-line AED in women of childbearing potential. However, if valproate is necessary to control seizures in a woman with epilepsy of childbearing age, the lowest effective dose should be employed, as valproate's teratogenic risk is dose-dependent. A high intensity ultrasound is recommended at 18 weeks gestational age to evaluate for the presence of major congenital malformations. Medication levels should be checked at frequent intervals to help guide the need for dose escalations, as levels will likely decrease during pregnancy. After childbirth, medication doses will need to be decreased in most cases to avoid toxicity.

Information on teratogenesis for many AEDs remains inadequate, and additional studies are needed. Many children exposed to AEDs including valproate do not exhibit structural or behavioral teratogenesis. It is possible that teratogens interact with susceptible genotypes, to produce both anatomical and behavioral defects [46]. Additional research is critically needed to understand risks of other AEDs, underlying mechanisms, and causes for outcome variance.

Key points	Evidence level
◆ Antiepileptic drugs overall are associated with a probable increase in major congenital malformations.	II/B
◆ Valproate monotherapy is associated with an increased risk of major congenital malformation.	II/B
◆ Polytherapy is associated with a probable increased risk of major congenital malformations, but specific combinations of medications have not been adequately studied.	II/B
◆ Valproate polytherapy carries a probable increased risk of major congenital malformations.	II/B
◆ Children born to women with epilepsy who are untreated are not at a higher risk of cognitive deficits.	II/B
◆ Treatment with valproate probably increases the risk of cognitive deficits.	II/B
◆ Treatment with carbamazepine probably does not increase the risk of cognitive deficits.	II/B
◆ There is a possible increased risk of cognitive deficits with use of phenytoin, but valproate carries a higher risk.	II/B
◆ Polytherapy increases the risk of cognitive deficits.	II/B
◆ Children of women treated with antiepileptic drugs probably have a higher risk of being small for gestational age.	II/B
◆ There is no evidence for increased perinatal mortality in children of women with epilepsy.	II/B
◆ Women who were seizure-free for 9-12 months prior to pregnancy have an 84-92% chance of remaining seizure-free for the duration of their pregnancy.	II/B

References

1. Hirtz D, Thurman DJ, Gwinn-Hardy K, *et al*. How common are the common neurologic disorders? *Neurology* 2007; 68: 326-37.
2. Adab N, Kini U, Vinten J, *et al*. The longer-term outcome of children born to mothers with epilepsy. *J Neurol Neurosurg Psychiatry* 2004; 75: 1575-83.
3. Delgado-Escueta AV, Janz D. Consensus guidelines: preconception counseling, management, and care of the pregnant woman with epilepsy. *Neurology* 1992; 42: 149-60.
4. Betts T, Fox C. Proactive pre-conception counseling for women with epilepsy - is it effective? *Seizure* 1999; 8: 322-7.
5. Yerby MS, Leavitt A, Erickson DM, *et al*. Anti-epileptics and the development of congential anomalies. *Neurology* 1992; 42 (Suppl 5): 132-40.
6. Koch S, Loesche G, Jager-Roman E, *et al*. Major birth malformations and antiepileptic drugs. *Neurology* 1992; 42(suppl 5): 83-8.
7. Meador KJ. Effects of in utero antiepileptic drug exposure. *Epilepsy Curr* 2008; 8: 143-7.

8. Harden CL, Meador KJ, Pennell PB, *et al*. Practice parameter update: management issues for women with epilepsy. Focus on pregnancy (an evidence-based review): teratogenesis and perinatal outcomes. Report of the Quality Standards Subcommittee and Therapeutics and Technology Assessment Subcommittee of the American Academy of Neurology and American Epilepsy Society. *Neurology* 2009; 73: 133-41.

9. Meador KJ, Reynolds RW, Crean S, *et al*. Pregnancy outcomes in women with epilepsy: a systematic review and meta-analysis of published pregnancy registries and cohorts. *Epilepsy Research* 2008; 81: 1-13.

10. Loughnan PM, Gold H, Vance JC. Phenytoin teratogenicity in man. *Lancet* 1973; 1: 70-2.

11. Vajda FJ, Hitchcock A, Graham J, O'Brien T, Lander C, Eadie M. The Australian Register of Antiepileptic Drugs in Pregnancy: the first 1002 pregnancies. *Aust NZ J Obstet Gynaecol* 2007; 76: 468-74.

12. Vajda FJ, Hitchcock A, Graham J, *et al*. Foetal malformations and seizure control: 52 months data of the Australian Pregnancy Registry. *Eur J Neurol* 2006; 13(6): 645654.

13. Morrow J, Russell A, Guthrie E, *et al*. Malformations risks of antiepileptic drugs in pregnancy: a prospective study from the UK Epilepsy and Pregnancy Register. *J Neurology Neurosurgery Psychiatry* 2006; 77: 193-8.

14. Holmes LB, Wyszynski DF. North American antiepileptic drug pregnancy registry. *Epilepsia* 2004; 45: 1465.

15. Meador KJ, Pennell PB, Harden CL, *et al*. Pregnancy registries in epilepsy: a consensus statement on health outcomes. *Neurology* 2008; 71: 1109-17.

16. Samren EB, Van Duijn CM, Koch S, *et al*. Maternal use of antiepileptic drugs and the risk of major congenital malformations: a joint European prospective study of human teratogenesis associated with maternal epilepsy. *Epilepsia* 1997; 38: 981-90.

17. Holmes LB, Wyszynski DF, Baldwin EJ, *et al*. Increased risk for non-syndromic cleft palate among infants exposed to lamotrigine during pregnancy. *Birth Def Res (Part A): Clin Mol Teratol* 2006; 76: 318.

18. Dolk H, Jentink J, Loane M, Morris J, de Jong-van den Berg LT; EUROCAT Antiepileptic Drug Working Group. Does lamotrigine use in pregnancy increase orofacial cleft risk relative to other malformations? *Neurology* 2008; 71(10): 714-22.

19. FDA Drug Safety Communication: Risk of oral clefts in children born to mothers taking Topamax (topiramate). May 4, 2011. http://www.fda.gov/Drugs/DrugSafety/ucm245085.htm.

20. Mølgaard-Nielsen D, Hviid A. Newer-generation antiepileptic drugs and the risk of major birth defects. *JAMA* 2011; 305(19): 1996-2002.

21. Kaaja E, Kaaja R, Hiilesmaa V. Major malformations in offspring of women with epilepsy. *Neurology* 2003; 60: 575-9.

22. Kelly VM, Nelson LM, Chakravarty EF. Obstetric outcomes in women with multiple sclerosis and epilepsy. *Neurology* 2009; 73(22): 1831-6.

23. Mawer G, Briggs M, Baker GA, *et al*; Liverpool & Manchester Neurodevelopment Group. Pregnancy with epilepsy: obstetric and neonatal outcome of a controlled study. *Seizure* 2010; 19(2): 112-9.

24. Veiby G, Daltveit AK, Engelsen BA, Gilhus NE. Pregnancy, delivery, and outcome for the child in maternal epilepsy. *Epilepsia* 2009; 50: 2130-9.

25. Meador KJ, Baker GA, Browning N, *et al*. Cognitive function at 3 years of age after fetal exposure to antiepileptic drugs. *N Engl J Med* 2009; 360: 1597-605.

26. Gaily E, Kantola-Sorsa E, Hiilesmaa V, *et al*. Normal intelligence in children with prenatal exposure to carbamazepine. *Neurology* 2004; 62: 8-9.

27. Scolnick D, Nulman I, Rovet J, *et al*. Neurodevelopment of children exposed in utero to phenytoin and carbamazepine monotherapy. *JAMA* 1994; 271: 767-70.

28. Koch S, Titze K, Zimmerman RB, *et al*. Long-term neuropsychological consequences of maternal epilepsy and anticonvulsant treatment during pregnancy for school age children and adolescents. *Epilepsia* 1999; 40: 1237-43.

29. Losche G, Steinhausen HC, Koch S, Helge H. The psychological development of children of epileptic parents: II: the differential impact of intrauterine exposure to anticonvulsant drugs and further influential factors. *Acta Paediatr* 1994; 83: 961-6.

30. Shallcross R, Bromley RL, Irwin B, Bonnett LJ, Morrow J, Baker GA; Liverpool Manchester Neurodevelopment Group; UK Epilepsy and Pregnancy Register. Child development following in utero exposure: levetiracetam vs sodium valproate. *Neurology* 2011; 76(4): 383-9.

31. Harden CL, Hopp J, Ting TY, *et al*. Practice parameter update: management issues for women with epilepsy. Focus in pregnancy (an evidence-based review): obstetrical complications and change in seizure frequency.

Report of the Quality Standards Subcommittee and Therapeutics and Technology Assessment Subcommittee of the American Academy of Neurology and American Epilepsy Society. *Neurology* 2009; 73: 126-32.

32. Viinikainen K, Heinonen S, Eriksson K, Kalvianen R. Community-based, prospective, controlled study of obstetric and neonatal outcomes of 179 pregnancies in women with epilepsy. *Epilepsia* 2006; 47: 186-92.

33. Richmond JR, Krishnamoorthy P, Andermann E, Benjamin A. Epilepsy and pregnancy: an obstetric prospective. *American Journal of Obstetrics and Gynecology* 2004; 190: 371-9.

34. Jacono J, Robertson J. The effects of estrogen, progesterone and ionized calcium on seizures during the menstrual cycle of epileptic women. *Epilepsia* 2007; 28: 571-7.

35. Bardy AH. Incidence of seizures during pregnancy, labor and puerperium in epileptic women: a prospective study. *Acta Neurol Scand* 1987; 75: 356-60.

36. Gjerde IO, Strandjord RE, Ulstein M. The course of epilepsy during pregnancy: a study of 78 cases. *Acta Neurol Scand* 1988; 78: 198-205.

37. Tomson T, Lindbom U, Ekqvist B, Sundqvist A. Epilepsy and pregnancy: a prospective study of seizure control in relation to free and total plasma concentrations of carbamazepine and phenytoin. *Epilepsia* 1994; 35: 122-30.

38. Mills JL, Signore CC, Quinlivan EP, *et al*. Folic acid and the prevention of neural tube defects. *N Engl J Med* 2004; 350: 2209-11.

39. Prevention of neural tube defects: results of the Medical Research Council Vitamin Study. MRC Vitamin Study Research Group. *Lancet* 1991; 338: 131-7.

40. Harden CL, Pennell PB, Koppel BS, *et al*. American Academy of Neurology; American Epilepsy Society. Practice parameter update: management issues for women with epilepsy. Focus on pregnancy (an evidence-based review): vitamin K, folic acid, blood levels, and breastfeeding. Report of the Quality Standards Subcommittee and Therapeutics and Technology Assessment Subcommittee of the American Academy of Neurology and American Epilepsy Society. *Neurology* 2009; 73(2): 142-9.

41. Astedt B. Antenatal drugs affecting vitamin K status of the fetus and newborn. *Semin Thromb Hemost* 1995; 21: 364-70.

42. Kaaja E, Kaaja R, Matila R, Hiilesmaa V. Enzyme-inducing antiepileptic drugs in pregnancy and the risk of bleeding in the neonate. *Neurology* 2002; 58: 549-53.

43. Policy Statement: Breastfeeding and the use of human milk. *Pediatrics* 2005; 115: 496-506.

44. Ip S, Chung M, Raman G, Trikalinos TA, Lau J. A summary of the Agency for Healthcare and Research and Quality's evidence report on breastfeeding in developed countries. *Breastfeed Med* 2009; 4 Suppl 1: S17-30.

45. Meador KJ, Baker GA, Browning N, *et al*, for the NEAD Study Group. Effects of breastfeeding in children of women taking antiepileptic drugs. *Neurology* 2010; 75(22): 1954-60.

46. Duncan S, Mercho S, Lopes-Cendes I, *et al*. Repeated neural tube defects and valproate suggest a pharmacogenetic abnormality. *Epilepsia* 2001; 42: 750-3.

Chapter 5

Identification and management of depressive and anxiety disorders in epilepsy

Andres M. Kanner MD
Professor of Neurological Sciences and Psychiatry
Rush Medical College at Rush University
Director, Laboratory of EEG and Video-EEG-Telemetry
Associate Director, Section of Epilepsy and Rush Epilepsy Center
Rush University Medical Center, Chicago, Illinois, USA

Introduction

Psychiatric comorbidities are relatively frequent in people with epilepsy (PWE), having been identified in one out of every three patients in the course of their life [1]. Furthermore, the relation between some of the psychiatric disorders and epilepsy is complex [1-4]. For example, depressive disorders and epilepsy have been found to have a bidirectional relation as not only patients with epilepsy are at greater risk of developing mood disorders [1], but patients with mood disorders are at greater risk of developing epilepsy [2-4]. Depressive and anxiety disorders are the most frequent psychiatric comorbidities in PWE and more often than not, tend to occur together [1, 5]. These observations have significant implications with respect to the evaluation and management of these psychiatric comorbidities. Despite the relatively high frequency of psychiatric comorbidities, the available data on their clinical characteristics and treatment are based on limited high quality evidence. The purpose of this chapter is to review the level of evidence of epidemiologic, clinical and therapeutic aspects of comorbid depressive and anxiety disorders in PWE and to highlight the areas in need for research that can result in better quality evidence.

Epidemiologic data

Caveats

Prevalence rates of mood and anxiety disorders have ranged significantly in the literature from 10% to 60%, depending on the methodology used and the type of populations studied.

Some studies relied on screening instruments that identified symptoms of depression and anxiety in the previous 1-4 weeks, while others relied on structured interviews that aimed at generating a diagnosis based on well defined diagnostic criteria, according to the Diagnostic and Statistical Manual of Mental Disorders (DSM) [6]. While the former strategy identifies patients with 'possible' mood and anxiety disorders, the latter is suitable to establish a diagnosis of mood and anxiety disorders, yet only those that are identical to primary mood and anxiety disorders. On the other hand, the use of structured psychiatric interviews does not lend itself to identify the atypical presentations of mood disorders that have been commonly recognized in PWE (see below), resulting in their under-recognition.

Data

Population-based studies indicate that one in three to one in four PWE have experienced a mood disorder in the course of their life **(IIb/B)** [1]. For example, in a Canadian study, the lifetime prevalence of mood disorders was 24% in PWE compared to 13% in controls, while 17% had a lifetime history of a major depressive disorder compared to 10% of controls. Including dysthymia, the lifetime prevalence rate of depressive disorders increased to 34.2% (25.0-43.3) [1].

Population-based studies have identified a lifetime prevalence of anxiety disorders ranging from 11% to 30% **(IIb/B)**. In the Canadian study, the lifetime prevalence rate was 22.8% (14.8-30.9) in PWE vs. 11.2 (10.8-11.7) in non-epilepsy subjects, while that of panic disorder/agoraphobia was 6.6% (2.9-10.3) vs. 3.6% (3.3-3.9), respectively. In a British population-based study that used data from primary care medical records, the prevalence rate of anxiety disorders was 11% among 5834 PWE compared with 5.6% among 831,163 people without epilepsy [7]. Finally, comorbid occurrence of depressive and anxiety disorders is frequent. Thus, in the Canadian study, the lifetime comorbid anxiety and depressive disorders prevalence rate was 34.2% (25.0-43.3) in PWE vs. 19.6 (19.0-20.2) in non-epileptic people.

Data from tertiary centers

Studies carried out in patients seen at tertiary level epilepsy centers yield data that may not be generalizable to the entire population of PWE, but can provide important data of patients with more severe epilepsy. Data from such studies also reveal a high comorbid occurrence of depressive and anxiety disorders **(III/B)**. For example, using a structured psychiatric interview in a study of 188 consecutive outpatients with epilepsy from five tertiary epilepsy centers, 31 patients (16%) were found to have a current major depressive episode (MDE); 21 of these patients were also experiencing one or more anxiety disorders **(III/B)** [7]. In addition, 49 patients (29%) met criteria for one or more than one anxiety disorder. Among these 49 patients, 33 (67.5%) were also suffering from a depressive episode: 21 (43%) met criteria for an MDE and 12 (24.5%) for a sub-syndromic form of depression.

In people without epilepsy there are significant data based on class Ia level of evidence that also describes a relatively high comorbid occurrence of mood and anxiety disorders. For example, Dobson and Cheung, using data of a meta-analysis concluded that among patients with a primary depressive disorder, a mean of 67% (range: 42-100%) also experienced anxiety disorders concurrently or in their lifetime; conversely, in patients with anxiety disorders, a mean of 40% (range: 17-65%) also had a depressive disorder [8]. Furthermore, primary social phobia has been found as a comorbid anxiety disorder with both major depression and dysthymia in up to 70% of patients [9].

Clearly, inquiring about anxiety disorders is of the essence when investigating the existence of depressive disorders and vice versa. Failure to identify comorbid anxiety disorders (or symptoms) in patients being treated for a depressive disorder (and vice versa) can have a significant clinical impact on response to treatment. For example, in a study carried out in a general medical clinic setting, 112 (13%) of 880 patients were found to suffer from a primary depressive disorder; among these patients, 67% also were experiencing comorbid symptoms of anxiety of moderate severity **(III/B)**. After a follow-up period of 1 year during which symptoms of depression and anxiety were monitored at five time points, depressed patients who improved showed a significant decrease in severity of comorbid symptoms of anxiety, whereas depressed patients who worsened showed a significant increase in their anxiety index. The decrease in the anxiety index of patients in the no change group was not statistically significant [10]. On the other hand, no data are available in PWE, but there is no reason to expect that these patients may not be negatively affected by persistent symptoms of depression when attempting to treat an anxiety disorder and vice versa.

Suicidality

Suicidal ideation, attempts and completed suicide is a serious complication of mood and anxiety disorders **(IIb/B)**. In a population-based study carried out in Denmark, PWE had a two-fold higher risk of completed suicide compared to non-epilepsy controls, in the absence of any psychosocial problem. The risk increased by 32-fold in the presence of a mood disorder and by 12-fold in the presence of an anxiety disorder [11].

Clinical manifestations

In PWE, depressive and anxiety phenomena are categorized according to their temporal relation with seizure occurrence into peri-ictal (i.e. symptoms that precede, follow, or are the expression of the ictal activity) or interictal episodes (i.e. occur independently of seizure). Interictal depressive episodes are the most frequently recognized.

Caveats

As stated above, methodologically sound evidence exists with respect to population-based studies that investigated the existence of depressive and anxiety disorders in PWE that mimic primary disorders (see above). Yet, while atypical manifestations of mood disorders have been recognized since the early part of the 20th century, their presence has been accepted by a consensus of experts **(IV/C)** [12].

Depressive disorders

As stated above, in PWE, interictal depressive disorders can be identical to the primary mood disorders described in the DSM-IV-TR [1, 6], which are classified into four types: major depressive disorders, dysthymic disorders, minor depression, and depressive disorders not otherwise specified. The differences between a major depressive disorder and dysthymic disorder is based largely on severity, persistence, and chronicity, with symptoms in both disorders sharing common features, such as depressed mood, anhedonia, worthlessness, guilt, decreased concentration ability, recurrent thoughts of death, and neurovegetative symptoms (i.e. weight loss or gain, insomnia or hypersomnia, psychomotor agitation or retardation, fatigue). A diagnosis of a major depressive disorder is considered in patients with a recurrent MDE that lasts at least 2 weeks and consists either of a depressed mood or anhedonia, plus four of the other symptoms listed above **(IIb/B)**. Bipolar disorders will not be reviewed in this chapter.

Atypical depressive episodes

A significant number of PWE present depressive episodes that fail to meet DSM diagnostic criteria and are classified as atypical depression not otherwise specified **(IV/C)**. The atypical presentation of depressive episodes in PWE was initially recognized by Kraepelin [11] and later on confirmed by Bleuler [13] and Gastaut [14]. These authors described a pleomorphic pattern of symptoms that included affective symptoms consisting of prominent irritability intermixed with euphoric mood, fear, and symptoms of anxiety, as well as anergia, pain, and insomnia. Blumer coined the term 'interictal dysphoric disorder' to refer to this type of depressive episode **(IV/C)** [15]. More recently, Mula *et al* confirmed the presence of this entity, but observed that it was not specific to epilepsy as the clinical semiology was also evident in people with migraine **(III/B)** [16].

Some investigators have suggested that these atypical mood episodes may mimic dysthymic disorders, but fail to meet DSM-IV-TR diagnostic criteria because of the duration of symptoms **(IV/C)**. For example, in a study of 97 consecutive patients with refractory epilepsy and depressive episodes severe enough to merit pharmacotherapy, Kanner *et al* found that only 28 patients met DSM-IV criteria for MDE, while the remaining 69 patients (71%) failed to meet criteria for any of the DSM-IV categories and presented with a clinical picture consisting of anhedonia (with or without hopelessness), fatigue, anxiety, irritability, poor frustration tolerance, and mood lability with bouts of crying [17]. Some patients also reported changes in appetite and sleep patterns and problems with concentration. Most symptoms presented with a waxing and waning course, with repeated, interspersed symptom-free periods of 1 to several days' duration. The semiology most resembled a dysthymic disorder, but the intermittent recurrence of symptom-free periods precluded DSM criteria for this condition **(IV/C)**.

Peri-ictal episodes and symptoms of depression

Peri-ictal semiology includes signs and symptoms that are closely related to the seizure disorder. They have been recognized since the 19th century, but have remained poorly studied. There are no population-based data available and their existence and clinical manifestations have been accepted by a consensus of experts **(IV/C)** [18].

Pre-ictal depressive symptoms or episodes typically present as a dysphoric mood that precedes a seizure by several hours to days [19]; it becomes more accentuated during the 24 hours prior to the seizure and remits postictally though occasionally, they may persist for a few days after the seizure **(IV/C)**.

Postictal symptoms or episodes are typically identified 1 to 5 days after the seizure. This symptom-free period between seizure and onset of psychiatric symptoms may lead to their misdiagnosis as interictal phenomena. A systematic analysis of the clinical manifestation of postictal symptoms of depression was carried out so far in only one study of 100 consecutive patients with refractory epilepsy **(III/B)** [20], which demonstrated a relatively high frequency of postictal symptoms of depression. Indeed, 43% experienced a median of 5 postictal symptoms of depression occurring after more than 50% of their seizures for the previous 3 months and with a median duration of 24 hours (range 1 to 108 hours); 13% endorsed postictal suicidal ideation. Of note, among the 43 patients with postictal symptoms of depression, 27 (63%) had concurrent postictal symptoms of anxiety. Twenty-five patients had a prior history of mood disorder and 11 of anxiety disorder, while among the 13 patients with postictal suicidal ideation, 10 had a history of either major depression or bipolar disorder.

Ictal symptoms of depression, consisting of paroxysmal feelings of anhedonia, suicidal ideation, crying, feelings of helplessness and hopelessness are the second most frequent type of psychiatric symptoms after ictal fear **(IV/C)** [21]. Often both types of symptoms occur together. They typically present as simple partial seizures, which may or may not evolve into complex partial seizures. The short duration (less than 30 seconds) is often the pivotal clue that suggests the ictal nature of the depressive symptoms.

Anxiety disorders

As in the case of depressive disorders, anxiety disorders in PWE can be identical to the 11 anxiety disorders listed in the DSM-IV-TR in people without epilepsy. Phobias, generalized anxiety disorders (GAD) and panic disorders (PD) are the most frequently identified in PWE [1] **(IIb/B)**. The reader is referred to the DSM-IV-TR for a description of the different anxiety disorders. In contrast to the depressive disorders, no atypical manifestation of anxiety disorders has been identified in PWE.

Postictal anxiety symptoms or episodes

Postictal symptoms of anxiety are also relatively frequent among patients with refractory partial epilepsy **(III/B)**. In the study cited above [20], Kanner *et al* identified a median of two postictal symptoms of anxiety (range: 1 to 5) in 45 of the 100 patients with a median duration of 24 hours (range: 0.5 to 148 hours); 15 patients (33%) reported a cluster of four postictal symptoms of anxiety of at least 24 hours. Thirty-two patients reported symptoms of generalized anxiety and/or panic; an additional 10 patients also reported symptoms of compulsions and as stated above, 29 patients experienced postictal symptoms of agoraphobia. In 44 of these 45 patients, postictal symptoms of depression were also reported. A prior history of anxiety disorder was identified in 15 patients (33%).

Ictal anxiety symptoms or episodes

Ictal panic or fear is the most frequent psychiatric symptom that is the expression of a simple partial seizure and accounts for 60% of 'auras' of a psychiatric type **(IV/C)** [21, 22]. Ictal fear typically is the expression of simple partial seizures of mesial temporal origin, particularly involving the amygdala. Ictal activity originating in mesial frontal regions (cingulate gyrus) can yield symptoms of generalized anxiety, without the panic-type quality. Frequently, episodes of ictal fear are misdiagnosed as a panic disorder and the diagnosis is often reached only after the patient experiences a secondarily generalized tonic-clonic seizure. The following illustrates the clinical differences between panic attacks and ictal panic **(IV/C)** [23].

Ictal panic is typically brief (less than 30 seconds in duration), is stereotypical, occurs out of context to concurrent events, and may be followed by other ictal phenomena such as periods of confusion of variable duration and subtle or overt automatisms when and if the seizure evolves to a complex partial seizure. The intensity of the sensation of fear is mild to moderate and rarely reaches the intensity of a panic attack. On the other hand, panic attacks consist of episodes of five to 20 minutes' duration which at times may persist for several hours during which the feeling of fear or panic is very intense often described as a feeling of impending doom and is associated with a variety of autonomic symptoms, including tachycardia, diffuse diaphoresis, and shortness of breath. During a panic attack, patients may become completely absorbed by the panic-type experience to the point where they may not be able to report what is going on around them; nonetheless, there is no real confusion or loss of consciousness as in complex partial seizures. Finally, patients with panic attacks are more likely to develop agoraphobia, while this is rare among patients with ictal panic unless they suffer from interictal panic disorder as well. Given the relatively high comorbidity of interictal panic disorder in PWE, the concurrent occurrence of ictal fear and interictal panic disorder has to be investigated in all patients.

How to screen for depressive and anxiety disorders

Caveats

Screening instruments identify symptoms of depression and anxiety and suggest the possibility of a current depressive or anxiety disorder, but by themselves, do not establish a diagnosis. Scores yielding a suspicion of a depressive and/or anxiety disorder must prompt clinicians to conduct or refer for a formal psychiatric evaluation. Once the diagnosis of a mood disorder has been established by psychiatric evaluation, the self-rating screening instruments can be given at every visit to measure changes in symptom severity or document symptom remission.

In general, self-rating instruments are preferable, as they are easy to use in a busy clinic setting. The use of screening instruments in PWE with cognitive impairment may lead to unreliable data and, hence, the use of these instruments must be limited to patients of normal intelligence.

Depressive episodes

There are several self-rating screening instruments developed to identify symptoms of depression in the general population, such as the Beck Depression Inventory-II [24] and the Center of Epidemiologic Studies-Depression Scale [25], which have been found to be valid instruments to screen symptoms of depression in PWE **(III/B)** [26]. A six-item screening instrument, the Neurological Disorders Depression Inventory for Epilepsy (NDDI-E) was validated to screen for major depressive episodes specifically in PWE **(IIb/B)** [27]. It has the advantage of being constructed specifically to minimize confounding factors that plague other instruments, such as adverse events related to antiepileptic drugs or cognitive problems associated with epilepsy. Completion of the instrument takes less than 3 minutes. A score of >15 is suggestive of a major depressive episode and indicates that a more in-depth evaluation is necessary.

Anxiety disorders

There are several self-rating instruments available to identify anxiety symptoms. They include the Beck Anxiety Inventory (BAI) [28], the State-Trait Anxiety Scale (STAI) [29] and the Patient's Health Questionnaire, Generalized Anxiety Disorder-7 (GAD-7) [30]. None of these instruments have been validated in PWE, however. Yet, the GAD-7 has several advantages over the others including: its availability in multiple languages, ease of use (it takes 2 to 3 minutes to complete) and lack of physical items that can falsely elevate the score of the scale. A score of greater than 10 is suggestive of a generalized anxiety disorder.

There are two self-rating instruments that can screen for symptoms of depression and anxiety, but have yet to be validated in PWE. They include the Goldberg's Depression and Anxiety Scales [31] and the Hospital Anxiety and Depression Scale [32].

Treatment of depressive and anxiety disorders

There are almost no data on the treatment of mood and anxiety disorders based on controlled studies in PWE. Thus, the treatment strategies have been based on the management of primary depressive and anxiety disorders. Yet, given the large percentage of patients with atypical forms of depressive episodes among PWE, whether these data are applicable is yet to be established in controlled studies. At this point, most of the recommended treatment modalities have been reached by expert consensus **(IV/C)** and include pharmacotherapy, psychotherapy or a combination of both, depending on the individual needs of the patient.

Before starting any treatment, it is of the essence to rule out the following causes of psychiatric symptoms **(IV/C)**:

◆ administration of AEDs with negative psychotropic properties (e.g. barbiturates, topiramate, levetiracetam, zonisamide, vigabatrin and tiagabine);
◆ discontinuation of AEDs with anxiolytic (e.g. pregabalin, gabapentin) and/or mood stabilizing properties (e.g. valproic acid, carbamazepine, and lamotrigine) that were keeping an underlying anxiety/depressive disorder in remission. In addition, the aim of any type of treatment must be geared towards complete symptom remission, as persistence of symptoms, even in the presence of improvement, is associated with a significant risk of recurrence of MDE.

Neurologists and internists are expected to screen patients for depressive and anxiety disorders and often may prescribe psychotropic medications for their treatment. Yet it is important that non-psychiatrists recognize the circumstances in which to refer patients to a psychiatrist. These include **(IV/C)**:

◆ a depressive episode associated with suicidal ideation;
◆ major depressive episodes with psychotic features, which include 25% of cases, in which pharmacotherapy has to include antipsychotic and antidepressant drugs, and at times, electroshock therapy must be considered. Furthermore, the presence of psychotic symptomatology significantly increases suicidal risk;
◆ any major depressive or dysthymic episode that has failed to respond to two or more prior trials of selective serotonin reuptake inhibitors (SSRI) and/or serotonin-norepinephrine reuptake inhibitors (SNRI) at optimal doses;
◆ bipolar disorder, as the management is fraught with significantly lower therapeutic success and is associated with potentially serious complications that are beyond the therapeutic skills of conventionally-trained neurologists.

The use of antidepressant medication for a bipolar disorder can facilitate the development of manic and hypomanic episodes or of a rapid cycling bipolar disorder (i.e. four or more depressive, manic, or hypomanic episodes in a 12-month period). In fact, the American Psychiatric Association guidelines for the treatment of acute depression in bipolar disease advise against the initial use of antidepressant drugs [33]. Furthermore, a bipolar disorder can begin with recurrent major depressive episodes before the first manic or hypomanic episode occurs. Accordingly, before prescribing antidepressant medication for a major depressive, dysthymic, or minor depressive disorder, neurologists will need to inquire about a history of manic or hypomanic episodes as well as of a family history of bipolar disease and refer positively identified patients to a psychiatrist for management.

Pharmacotherapy

Choice of antidepressant drug

The first line of treatment of primary depressive and anxiety disorders includes the use of SSRIs or SNRIs (la/A) [34]. The same strategy should be followed in PWE (IV/C). Given the high comorbidity between the two conditions, the selected drug should have therapeutic efficacy in both types of conditions. The choice between SSRIs and SNRIs depends on the type of depressive episode: SNRIs are preferred for retarded depressive episodes (e.g. fatigue, slow thinking) (la/A in primary mood and anxiety disorders); otherwise, patients should be started on an SSRI. Other classes of antidepressants, including those of the tricyclic family and mono-amino-oxidase inhibitors (MAOI) have also been used in the management of depressive and anxiety disorders in PWE, but given their toxicity, have become a second-line treatment and will not be reviewed here. The reader is referred to other review articles [35, 36].

Among the six SSRI drugs, the choice must be based on:

- prior exposure and evidence of therapeutic profile (e.g. efficacy in mood and type of anxiety disorder);
- potential pharmacokinetic and pharmacodynamic interactions with concurrent AEDs; and
- the potential adverse event profile of the specific SSRI drug that could worsen underlying medical complications associated with the seizure disorder or other concurrent medical condition (i.e. obesity, sexual disturbances). These observations are based on level IV/C evidence.

Efficacy

To date, there has been only one controlled study that compared the safety and efficacy of the SSRI, sertraline, with that of cognitive behavior therapy (CBT) in a single-blind controlled study of 140 PWE with MDE (Ib/A) [37]. Both treatments were equally effective with symptom

Table 1. Efficacy of SSRIs and SNRIs in primary depressive and anxiety disorders.

Antidepressant drug	Depression	Panic disorder	Generalized anxiety	Starting dose	Maximal dose
Paroxetine*	+	+	+	10	60
Sertraline*	+	+	+	25	200
Fluoxetine*	+	+	-	10	80
Citalopram*	+	+	+	10	60
Escitalopram*	+	+	+	5	30
Fluvoxamine*	+	+	+	50	300
Venlafaxine^	+	+	+	37.5	300
Duloxetine^	+	+	+	20	120

* = SSRI; ^ = SNRI; + = used for the treatment of this condition. + = has FDA indication for this condition

remission found in 60% of each treatment arm at the end of the study. Of note, there was no worsening in seizure frequency among patients randomized to sertraline.

The efficacy of SSRIs and SNRIs in primary depressive and anxiety disorders is presented in Table 1.

If patients have already undergone a trial with an SSRI at optimal doses that failed to yield full remission of symptoms, a trial with an SNRI is the next step (IV/C). In fact, studies in primary depressive disorders have suggested that the use of SNRIs can yield symptom remission in patients in whom an SSRI had failed to do so (Ib/A). Referral to a psychiatrist should follow persistent symptoms despite two trials at optimal doses, one with an SSRI and one with an SNRI, as this is likely to represent a pharmacoresistant form of depressive/anxiety disorder.

Table 2. Common adverse events of SSRIs.	
Adverse events	Prevalence rate
Nausea*	35%
Insomnia*	25%
Diarrhea*	19%
Headache*	15%
Dry mouth*	13%
Sexual disturbances*	9%-20%
Osteopenia/osteoporosis	?
* also present in SNRIs	

Antiepileptic drugs

Given the fact that several AEDs have mood stabilizing (carbamazepine, valproic acid, lamotrigine), antidepressant (lamotrigine) or anxiolytic properties (gabapentin, pregabalin, tiagabine, benzodiazepines, valproic acid), it is reasonable to ask whether the use of one of these AEDs may be sufficient to treat the seizure disorder and the comorbid psychiatric condition. Unfortunately, there are sparse data limited to two open trials of lamotrigine in PWE which suggested an improvement in symptoms of depression **(IV/C)** [38, 39]. In double-blind placebo-controlled studies, pregabalin has been found to be efficacious in the treatment of primary GAD, while gabapentin was efficacious in primary social phobia **(Ia/A)** [40, 41]. Their efficacy in comorbid anxiety disorders in PWE is yet to be established, however.

Safety of antidepressant drugs in epilepsy

The common adverse events of SSRIs are listed in Table 2.

In addition to the adverse events listed in Table 2, SNRIs can be associated with excessive sweating. Hypertension and a syndrome of inappropriate antidiuretic hormone secretion, leading to hyponatremia, are potential adverse events identified in patients taking venlafaxine (but not duloxetine). Duloxetine should be used with great care in patients with a history of liver disease and should be avoided in those with glaucoma.

Are antidepressants proconvulsant drugs?

Concerns of antidepressant drugs causing seizures constitute one of the most frequent obstacles to treatment of mood and anxiety disorders. Yet, such concern is based on several misconceptions. First, any suspicion of proconvulsant properties of antidepressant drugs must factor in the existence of the bidirectional relation between epilepsy and depression, whereby not only are patients with epilepsy at higher risk of developing depression, but patients with depression have a four- to seven-fold higher risk of developing epilepsy (IIb/B) [2-4]. Thus, the occurrence of a seizure in a depressed patient may be the expression of the natural course of the mood disorder and not of an adverse event of the antidepressant drug. In fact, Alper et al reviewed data from the Food and Drug Administration Phase II and III clinical regulatory trials of several SSRIs and the SNRI, venlafaxine, and the α2-antagonist, mirtazapine, in patients with primary depression [42]. They found that the incidence of seizures was significantly lower among patients randomly assigned to antidepressants compared to those given placebo (standardized incidence ratio = .48; 95% CI, .36-.61). Of note, in both patients assigned to antidepressants and placebo, the seizure incidence was greater than the published incidence of unprovoked seizures in the general population (IIb/B). These data support the increased risk of depressed patients for the development of unprovoked seizures and epilepsy alluded to above, and suggests a protective effect of SSRIs and SNRIs.

There is a general consensus that antidepressant drugs can cause seizures at toxic doses and in fact, most reported seizures were in cases of overdose (IV/C). On the other hand, three antidepressants have been found to lower significantly the risk of seizures in patients without epilepsy. They include maprotyline (incidence: 15.6%, in a dose-dependent manner), clomipramine (incidence: 1-12.2% in a dose-dependent manner) and bupropion (0.5%-4.8% in a dose-dependent manner) (IV/C) [35, 36].

In PWE, the only controlled study was that of Gilliam et al, cited above, in which there was no difference in change in seizure frequency between patients randomized to CBT or sertraline [37]. Three open trials with SSRIs in patients with pharmacoresistant epilepsy suggested an improvement in seizure frequency [43-45], while in one study of 100 consecutive patients with pharmacoresistant epilepsy treated with sertraline, worsening of seizures occurred in only one patient [17].

Pharmacokinetic properties and interaction with AEDs

These data are derived from pre-clinical studies and small case series or isolated case reports (III/B). First-generation AEDs such as phenytoin, carbamazepine and phenobarbital are potent inducers of the cytochrome p450 (CYP) enzyme system. Oxcarbazepine and topiramate are much less potent inducers of CYP 3A4. Since the majority of antidepressant medications are substrates for one or more of the CYP isoenzymes, comedication with any of these AEDs would be expected to increase their systemic clearance, resulting in lower serum concentrations, specifically, those of sertraline, paroxetine, citalopram and escitalopram [46], and requiring increases in dosage in order to maintain a therapeutic antidepressant response [47]. In contrast to the enzyme-inducing drugs, the AED sodium valproate can inhibit certain CYP (2C9) and UDP-glucuronyltransferase enzymes, but no interaction with SSRIs or SNRIs have been reported.

By the same token, antidepressants of the SSRI family can inhibit several CYP isoenzymes (III/B) [46-48]. Fluoxetine has been shown to inhibit CYP 3A4, CYP 2C9, CYP 2C19, CYP 2D6, and CYP 1A2. Its metabolite, norfluoxetine, has also been shown to inhibit CYP 2D6, while fluvoxamine is an inhibitor of CYP 1A2, 3A4, CYP 2C9 and 2C19. Inhibition of CYP 3A4, CYP 2C9 and CYP 2C19 are of the most relevance when considering potential effects on the currently available AEDs, leading to increased phenytoin and carbamazepine serum concentrations [46, 47]. Conversely, SSRIs with the least potential for causing inhibitory interactions are citalopram and escitalopram. Although definitive studies are lacking, it has also been suggested that venlafaxine and duloxetine are unlikely to cause significant interactions with currently available AEDs [46].

Less clinical data are available regarding pharmacokinetic interactions between antidepressants and the newer generation AEDs. Given that the newer AEDs are in general less reliant upon the CYP isoenzyme system for their disposition, it is likely that there will be fewer opportunities for pharmacokinetic interactions.

Pharmacodynamic interactions between AEDs and antidepressants

One of the concerns that clinicians have to always keep in mind is the potential worsening of adverse events resulting from the combination of antidepressant drugs and AEDs that have common adverse events. Yet, the observations of this section are theoretical with limited data (IV/C). From a theoretical standpoint, the following potential synergistic adverse events have to be looked for carefully:

* potentiation of weight gain that can be caused by AEDs such as gabapentin, valproic acid, carbamazepine, pregabalin and antidepressant drugs such as sertraline and paroxetine;
* potentiation of sexual adverse events. Sexual adverse events, such as decreased libido, anorgasmia and sexual impotence can be relatively common with AEDs such as the barbiturates (phenobarbital and primidone), but can also be seen with other enzyme-inducing AEDs, related to the synthesis of the sex hormone-binding globulin, which binds the free fraction of sex hormones, and hence limits their access to the CNS. As mentioned above, the SSRIs and SNRIs are known to cause sexual adverse events. Whether the combination of this type of AED and antidepressants has a 'synergistic adverse effect' on sexual functions has yet to be established. The direct impact of the seizure disorder on sexual functions is an additional confounding variable which could, in fact, be the variable responsible for the decreased sexual drive independently of the exposure to the AEDs and/or antidepressant drugs;

◆ potentiation of osteopenia and osteoporosis between enzyme-inducing AEDs and SSRIs. Several population-based studies have suggested that exposure to SSRIs is associated with decreased bone mineral density (BMD) and bone fractures **(IIb/B)**. For example, one study found higher rates of bone loss at the hip for SSRI users, even after controlling for possible confounders, like depression [49]. In a Canadian population study, the adjusted odds ratio for hip fracture was 2.4 (95% CI, 2.0-2.7) for exposure to SSRIs compared to non-users [50]. A third population-based study carried out in the Netherlands found the risk of non-vertebral fracture to be 2.35 (95% CI, 1.32-4.18) for current users of SSRIs compared with non-users of antidepressants, after adjustment for age, sex, lower-limb disability, and depression [51]. The pathogenic mechanisms by which SSRIs may cause osteopenia have been suggested in preclinical studies of the serotonin transporter (which has been demonstrated in human osteoclasts, osteoblasts and osteocytes). Investigators have found that bone mineral accrual was impaired in growing mice treated with an SSRI [52]. Clearly, these data raise the question of whether the use of SSRIs increases the risk of osteopenia and osteoporosis recognized for a long time with enzyme-inducing AEDs.

Additional treatments for anxiety disorders

Benzodiazepines have been used in the treatment of GAD and PD, and anxiety secondary to life stressors or medical conditions. Yet, the risk of physical dependence and development of tolerance have limited their use to short-term trials **(IV/C)**. Typically they are used in GAD and PD at the start of pharmacotherapy with antidepressants until the latter agents' therapeutic effect takes over. Alprazolam is the benzodiazepine preferred for PD while clonazepam is used in GAD.

Buspirone is a serotonin-1A (5HT1A) agonist agent that has been found to be effective for the treatment of primary GAD **(III/B)** [53]. It is favored over the use of benzodiazepines because it does not cause drug dependence or withdrawal with long-term use and its lack of any significant pharmacokinetic interactions with other agents. Its onset of efficacy is delayed by several weeks, like that of antidepressant drugs.

Non-pharmacologic treatments

As shown above, CBT is effective in the treatment of MDE in PWE [37]. While there are no controlled data on the efficacy of CBT and behavior therapy in anxiety disorders in PWE, these forms of therapy are known to be very effective in the treatment of primary anxiety disorders, particularly panic disorders with agoraphobia, phobias and compulsions in obsessive-compulsive disorders **(III/B)** [54]. Often patients may require the combination of pharmacotherapy and non-pharmacologic interventions **(IV/C)**.

Conclusions

Despite the relatively high prevalence of depressive and anxiety disorders in PWE, there has been very little methodologically sound research focused on the treatment of these conditions. The studies reviewed in this chapter indicate the existence of high quality evidence supporting only certain aspects of depressive and anxiety disorders in epilepsy. These include:

◆ the high prevalence of these psychiatric disorders in population-based studies;
◆ the existence of depressive and anxiety disorders that mimic primary mood and anxiety disorders.

On the other hand, the long-held observation of atypical manifestations of depressive episodes in PWE is only supported by uncontrolled observational studies and while there is a consensus among the experts that such type of depressive episodes exist, many questions remain unanswered. These include:

◆ are these atypical manifestations specific to epilepsy or can they be identified in other neurologic disorders?;
◆ do they occur in PWE that suffer from more severe seizure disorders or can they be identified in patients with well controlled seizures?;
◆ are the atypical depressive episodes associated with certain types of epileptic syndromes (epilepsy of temporal lobe origin versus juvenile myoclonic epilepsy)? Is their response to treatment different than those of typical depressive disorders? Clearly, future studies with sound methodology are necessary to confirm these observations using population-based cohorts.

The existence of peri-ictal depressive and anxiety episodes has been recognized for a very long time but remains accepted by consensus only with very few methodologically sound studies available to document their clinical manifestations, real prevalence and course.

Finally, this review demonstrates the paucity of good evidence-based data on the treatment of depressive and anxiety disorders in PWE, as there has been only one randomized controlled study evaluating the efficacy of the SSRI, sertraline, and CBT for the treatment of MDE [37]. It is not surprising that the treatment of these psychiatric conditions remains empirical, and while a few open trials with various SSRIs have yielded encouraging data, this area is in desperate need of methodologically sound research. Such research should include:

◆ multicenter, randomized, double-blind placebo-controlled studies to evaluate the efficacy of SSRIs and SNRIs in the management of typical and atypical forms of depression and anxiety disorders;

◆ controlled studies aimed at evaluating the efficacy of CBT in the treatment of various types of depression and anxiety disorders in PWE and its impact on seizure reduction.

Finally, the empirical nature of the treatment of depressive and anxiety disorders in PWE should not be an excuse to refrain from treating these patients, following the same principles applied to the management of primary mood and anxiety disorders.

Key points	Evidence level
◆ Population-based studies indicate that one in three to one in four PWE have experienced a mood disorder in the course of their life.	IIb/B
◆ Population-based studies have identified a lifetime prevalence of anxiety disorders ranging from 11% to 30%.	IIb/B
◆ Comorbid occurrence of depressive and anxiety disorders is frequent.	IIb/B
◆ Suicidal ideation, attempts and completed suicide are serious complications of mood and anxiety disorders.	IIb/B
◆ Interictal depressive and anxiety disorders can be identical to the primary mood and anxiety disorders described in the DSM-IV-TR (IIb/B), but in a significant number of PWE, depressive episodes have atypical manifestations (IV/C).	IIb/B & IV/C
◆ Postictal depressive and anxiety episodes are relatively frequent in patients with poorly controlled seizure disorders.	III/B
◆ Ictal fear is the most common type of aura with psychiatric symptoms. Failure to recognize it often leads to misdiagnosis as panic attacks.	IV/C
◆ Antidepressant drugs of the SSRI and SNRI families are safe in the treatment of depressive and anxiety disorders in PWE.	IV/C
◆ Pharmacologic treatments with the SSRI, sertraline, and CBT have been found to be equally effective in the treatment of MDE in PWE.	Ib/A
◆ The choice of antidepressant drug depends on the type of depressive and anxiety disorder, their comorbid occurrence, concomitant medications and safety profile.	IV/C
◆ CBT and behavior therapy have been found to be effective in the treatment of primary anxiety disorders, and thus should be considered in PWE, particularly panic disorders with agoraphobia, phobias and compulsions in obsessive-compulsive disorders.	III/B

References

1. Téllez-Zenteno JF, Patten SB, Jetté N, Williams J, Wiebe S. Psychiatric comorbidity in epilepsy: a population-based analysis. *Epilepsia* 2007; 48: 2336-44.
2. Hesdorffer DC, Hauser WA, Ludvigsson P, Olafsson E, Kjartansson O. Depression and attempted suicide as risk factors for incident unprovoked seizures and epilepsy. *Ann Neurology* 2006; 59: 35-41.
3. Forsgren L, Nystrom L. An incident case-referent study of epileptic seizures in adults. *Epilepsy Res* 1990; 6: 66-81.
4. Hesdorffer DC, Hauser WA, Annegers JF, Cascino G. Major depression is a risk factor for seizures in older adults. *Ann Neurol* 2000; 47: 246-9.
5. Hesdorffer DC, Ludvigsson P, Olafsson E, Gudmundsson G, Kjartansson O, Hauser WA. ADHD as a risk factor for incident unprovoked seizures and epilepsy in children. *Arch Gen Psychiatry* 2004; 61(7): 731-6.
6. *Diagnostic and Statistical Manual of Mental Disorders*, 4th ed. Washington, DC: American Psychiatric Press, 2000.
7. Kanner AM, Barry JJ, Gilliam F, Hermann B, Meador KJ. Anxiety disorders, sub-syndromic depressive episodes and major depressive episodes: do they differ on their impact on the quality of life of patients with epilepsy? *Epilepsia* 2010; 51: 1152-8.
8. Dobson KS, Cheung E. Relationship between anxiety and depression: 479 conceptual and methodological issues. In: *Comorbidity of Mood and Anxiety Disorders*. Maser JD, Cloninger CR, Eds. Washington, DC: American Psychiatric Press, 1990.
9. Merikangas KR, Angst J. Comorbidity and social phobia: evidence from clinical, epidemiologic and genetic studies. *Eur Arch Psychiatry Clin Neurosci* 1995; 244: 297-303.
10. Zung WWK, Magruder-Habib K, Velez R, Alling W. The comorbidity of anxiety and depression in general medical patients: a longitudinal study. *J Clin Psychiatry* 1990; 51 (Suppl. 6): 77-80.
11. Christensen J, Vestergaard M, Mortensen P, Sidenius P, Agerbo E. Epilepsy and risk of suicide: a population-based case-control study. *Lancet Neurol* 2007; 6: 693-8.
12. Kraepelin E. *Psychiatrie*, vol 3. Leipzig: Johann Ambrosius Barth, 1923.
13. Bleuler E. *Lehrbuch der Psychiatrie*, 8th ed. Berlin: Springer, 1949.
14. Gastaut H, Morin G, Lesèvre N. Étude du comportement des épileptiques psychomoteurs dans l'intervalle de leurs crises: les troubles de l'activité globale et de la sociabilité. *Ann Med Psychol (Paris)* 1955; 113: 1-27.
15. Blumer D, Altshuler LL. Affective disorders. In: *Epilepsy: a Comprehensive Textbook*, v. II. Engel J, Pedley TA, Eds. Philadelphia: Lippincott-Raven, 1998: 2083-99.
16. Mula M, Jauch R, Cavanna A, *et al*. Clinical and psychopathological definition of the interictal dysphoric disorder of epilepsy. *Epilepsia* 2008; 49(4): 650-6.
17. Kanner, AM, Kozak AM, Frey M. The use of sertraline in patients with epilepsy: is it safe? *Epilepsy Behav* 2000; 1(2): 100-5.
18. Barry J, Ettinger AB, Harden CL, Gilliam F, Kanner AM. Depression Consensus Statement. *Epilepsy Behav* 2008; Suppl 1: S1-29.
19. Blanchet P, Frommer GP. Mood change preceding epileptic seizures. *J Nerv Ment Dis* 1986; 174: 471-6.
20. Kanner AM, Soto A, Gross-Kanner H. Prevalence and clinical characteristics of postictal psychiatric symptoms in partial epilepsy. *Neurology* 2004; 62: 708-13.
21. Weil A. Depressive reactions associated with temporal lobe uncinate seizures. *J Nerv Ment Dis* 1955; 121: 505-10.
22. Daly D. Ictal affect. *Am J Psych* 1958; 115: 97-108.
23. Kanner AM, Ettinger A. Anxiety disorders in epilepsy. In: *Epilepsy: A Comprehensive Textbook*. Engel J, Pedley T, Eds. Baltimore: Lippincott, Williams & Wilkins, 2008.
24. Beck AT, Steer RA. *Manual for the Beck Depression Inventory*. San Antonio: Psychological Corporation, 1993.
25. Baqar A. Husaini BA, Neff JA, Harrington JB, Hughes MD, Stone RH. Depression in rural communities: Validating the CES-D scale. *J Community Psychol* 1980; 8: 20-7.
26. Jones JE, Herman BP, Woodard JL, *et al*. Screening for major depression in epilepsy with common self-report depression inventories. *Epilepsia* 2005; 46(5): 731-5.
27. Gilliam FG, Barry JJ, Meador KJ, Hermann BP, Vahle V, Kanner AM. Rapid detection of major depression in epilepsy: a multicenter study. *Lancet Neurology* 2006; 5(5): 399-405.

28. Beck AT, Steer RA. *Manual for the Beck Anxiety Inventory*. San Antonio, TX: Psychological Corporation, 1990.

29. Hamilton M. The assessment of anxiety states by rating. *Br J Med Psychol* 1959; 32: 50-5.

30. Spitzer RL, Kroenke K, Williams JBW, Loewe B. A brief measure for assessing generalized anxiety disorder: the GAD-7. *Arch Intern Med* 2006; 166: 1092-7.

31. Goldberg D, Bridges K, Duncan-Jones P, Grayson D. Detecting anxiety and depression in general medical settings. *British Medical Journal* 1988; 297: 897-9.

32. HADS Zigmond AS, Snaith RP. The Hospital Anxiety and Depression Scale. *Acta Psychiatr Scand* 1983; 67: 361-70.

33. Hirschfield RMA, Bowden CL, Gitlin MJ, *et al.* Practice guideline for the treatment of patients with bipolar disorder. *Amer J Psychiatr* 2002; 159(4): 1-15.

34. Shelton RC, Lester N. Selective serotonin reuptake inhibitors and newer antidepressants. In: *Textbook of Mood Disorders*. Stein DJ, Kupfer DJ, Schatzberg AF, Eds. Washington, DC: The American Psychiatric Publishing, 2006: 263-80.

35. Kanner AM, Blumer D. Affective disorders in epilepsy. In: *Epilepsy: A Comprehensive Textbook*. Engel J, Pedley T, Eds. Baltimore: Lippincott, Williams & Wilkins, 2008.

36. Kanner AM. Depression in epilepsy: prevalence, clinical semiology, pathogenic mechanisms and treatment. *Biol Psychiatry* 2003; 54: 388-98.

37. Gilliam FG, Black KJ, Carter J, *et al.* Depression and Health Outcomes in Epilepsy: A Randomized Trial. Presented at the 61st annual meeting of the American Academy of Neurology: 25 April - 02 May 2009; Seattle, Washington, USA. http://www.abstracts2view.com/aan2009 seattle/view.php?nu=AAN09L_S26.002&terms.

38. Ettinger AB, Kustra RP, Hammer AE. Effect of lamotrigine on depressive symptoms in adult patients with epilepsy. *Epilepsy Behav* 2007; 10(1): 148-54.

39. Fakhoury TA, Barry JJ, Mitchell Miller J, Hammer AE, Vuong A. Lamotrigine in patients with epilepsy and comorbid depressive symptoms. *Epilepsy Behav* 2007; 10(1): 155-62.

40. Pande AC, Crockatt JG, Feltner DE, *et al.* Pregabalin in generalized anxiety disorder: a placebo-controlled trial. *Am J Psychiatry* 2003; 160: 533-40.

41. Bech P. Dose-response relationship of pregabalin in patients with generalized anxiety disorder. A pooled analysis of four placebo-controlled trials. *Pharmacopsychiatry* 2007; 40(4): 163-8.

42. Alper KR, Schwartz KA, Kolts RL, Khan A. Seizure incidence in psychopharmacological clinical trials: an analysis of Food and Drug Administration (FDA) summary basis of approval reports. *Biological Psychiatry* 2007; 62: 345-54.

43. Favale E, Audenino D, Cocito L, Albano C. The anticonvulsant effect of citalopram as an indirect evidence of serotonergic impairment in human epileptogenesis. *Seizure* 2003; 12: 316-8.

44. Favale E, Rubino V, Mainardi P, Lunardi G, Albano C. Anticonvulsant effect of fluoxetine in humans. *Neurology* 1995; 45: 1926-7.

45. Specchio LM, Ludice A, Specchio N, *et al.* Citalopram as treatment of depression in patients with epilepsy. *Clin Neuropharmacol* 2004; 27: 133-6.

46. Patsalos P, Perucca E. Clinically important drug interactions in epilepsy: interactions between antiepileptic drugs and other drugs. *Lancet Neurology* 2003; 2: 473-81.

47. Trimble MR, Mula M. Antiepileptic drug interactions in patients requiring psychiatric drug treatment. In: *Antiepileptic Drugs: Combination Therapy and Interactions*. Majkowski J, Bourgeois B, Patsalos P, Mattson R, Eds. Cambridge: Cambridge University Press, 2005, 350-68.

48. Nelson MH, Birnbaum AK, Remmel RP. Inhibition of phenytoin hydroxylation in human liver microsomes by several selective serotonin re-uptake inhibitors. *Epilepsy Res* 2001; 44: 71-82.

49. Haney EM, Warden SJ, Bliziotes MM. Effects of selective serotonin reuptake inhibitors on bone health in adults: time for recommendations about screening, prevention and management? *Bone* 2010; 46(1): 13-7.

50. Diem SJ, Blackwell TL, Stone KL, *et al.* Use of antidepressants and rates of hip bone loss in older women: the study of osteoporotic fractures. *Arch Intern Med* 2007; 167(12): 1240-5.

51. Liu B, Anderson G, Mittmann N, To T, Axcell T, Shear N. Use of selective serotonin-reuptake inhibitors or tricyclic antidepressants and risk of hip fractures in elderly people. *Lancet* 1998; 351(9112): 1303-7.

52. Warden SJ, Robling AG, Sanders MS, Bliziotes MM, Turner CH. Inhibition of the serotonin (5-hydroxytryptamine) transporter reduces bone accrual during growth. *Endocrinology* 2005; 146: 685-93.

53. Davidson JRT, DuPont RL, Hedges D, Haskins JT. Efficacy, safety and tolerability of venlafaxine extended release and buspirone in outpatients with generalized anxiety disorder. *J Clin Psychiatry* 1999; 60: 528-35.

54. Linden M, Zubraegel D, Baer T, Franke U, Schlattmann P. Efficacy of cognitive behaviour therapy in generalized anxiety disorders. Results of a controlled clinical trial (Berlin CBT-GAD Study). *Psychother Psychosom* 2005; 74(1): 36-42.

Chapter 6

Methods for evaluating and treating the postictal state

Autumn M. Klein MD PhD, Director, Program in Women's Neurology
Brigham and Women's Hospital
Instructor in Neurology, Harvard Medical School
Boston, Massachusetts, USA

Steven C. Schachter MD, Professor of Neurology
Harvard Medical School, Beth Israel Deaconess Medical Center
Chief Academic Officer and Director of NeuroTechnology
Center for Integration of Medicine and Innovative Technology (CIMIT)
Boston, Massachusetts, USA

Introduction

Physicians often focus on seizures as the disabling event in epilepsy, but the postictal state can lead to immediate and delayed functioning as well as a prolonged recovery period. The postictal state can have medical and physical effects in addition to a significant impact on cognitive functioning and possible psychiatric symptoms. Postictal symptoms and electrophysiological recordings can help to localize seizure foci, while newer imaging techniques illustrate changes after seizures. Unfortunately, other than treating the seizures themselves, there is little known about reducing the impact of the postictal state or treating it directly.

This chapter reviews published clinical studies on the most common topics researched in the postictal state, including headache, psychosis, cardiac, cognitive symptoms, as well as electrophysiological findings, imaging changes, and differentiation from non-electrographic seizures (NES). Most studies are case series or case reports (III/B) with very few controlled studies (II/B). These findings illustrate the need for further investigation into the medical, psychiatric, and cognitive aspects of the postictal state and emphasize that there is very little known or studied about potential treatments of the postictal state.

Articles were searched via PubMed using a variety of search criteria including the search terms postictal, epilepsy, seizures, and searches that intersected these terms with specific conditions and symptoms (e.g. pulmonary edema, respiratory, nose wiping, etc.). Articles were not limited to the English language. Given the search criteria, all abstracts were reviewed and selected for content related to clinical aspects of the postictal state. Review articles that summarized particular aspects of the postictal state (e.g. imaging, electrophysiology) were screened for further citations. Given the variety of ways used to define the length of time after a seizure (e.g <6 hours, <24 hours, 7 days), papers were not excluded based on their definitions (or lack thereof). Animal studies were excluded as were case reports that were not describing a unique entity or those including only a few patients. Electrophysiological studies other than clinical EEG recordings were also excluded. There were very few randomized controlled clinical trials obtained through these search mechanisms. Most articles are case reports or small case series. Given this, case series presented were selected for those that had the largest numbers of patients and somewhat controlled or matched groups. Often, these were more recent reports. Small case series were reported where there was a unique clinically relevant finding.

Headache

Headache and epilepsy are known to be comorbidities. Additionally, headaches are known to be related to seizures and can be either pre-ictal, peri-ictal, or postictal. In patients who are not aware of their seizures, headache can be the only symptom that a seizure has occurred and therefore can be used to track seizures. This is especially helpful if it occurs postictally. Several studies have evaluated this overlap, but most are retrospective and evaluate adult clinic populations or inpatient monitoring units.

In Trondheim, Norway, 109 adult patients with epilepsy were given a semi-structured interview which showed that 52% had interictal headache, 20% of which fulfilled criteria for migraine [1]. Postictal headache was seen in 44% and in those with partial epilepsy, there was an association with side of headache and EEG abnormalities. Most patients with moderate intensity postictal headache used analgesics with 90% reporting good effect. Interestingly, those with headaches were more likely to be on a higher number of antiepileptic medications (III/B). Other studies capturing surgical or focal temporal lobe epilepsy patients evaluating with questionnaires showed that most patients reported postictal headache but that most also had interictal migraine. In one study, there was no clinical correlation between severity of seizures, localization of seizures, and number of antiepileptic drugs (AEDs) [2] (III/B). None went into detail about treatment of postictal headaches other than to note that analgesics were used [3, 4] (III/B). The largest study to date on headache and epilepsy included 32 Korean epilepsy centers where intake questionnaires were given to 579 new patients at their initial appointments [5]. Using International Headache Society criteria, 12.4% of patients had interictal migraines, 28.3% reported headache around the time of their seizures, with 24.5% being postictal, and 36.3% of those with postictal seizure-related headache met migraine diagnostic criteria.

Since patients were being evaluated at the first clinic visit, many had not yet been started on a seizure medication and other treatments including headache medications were not discussed **(IIb/B)**.

One of the most rigorous studies done looking at headache and seizures was a prospective study done at a pediatric epilepsy clinic in Brazil which followed 50 children with epilepsy and used their siblings without epilepsy as a control group [6]. Using International Headache Society criteria, 46% of the children with epilepsy interictally had baseline headaches and of these, 43% of headaches were classified as migraines. Almost 40% had headaches with their seizures and of these, two thirds of headaches were postictal. Children with all types of epilepsy were included, but ~63% of those with headache had a generalized epilepsy. Treatment of headaches was not addressed **(IIa/B)**. Another pediatric study of 101 Canadian children with generalized and focal epilepsy used a structured questionnaire and chart review and showed that 41% of headaches were peri-ictal with most of them (29%) occurring postictally [7]. Migrainous features were seen in 58% of postictal headaches, and 24% of interictal headaches. This is one of the few studies that comments on treatment of a postictal symptom and shows that most children just used simple analgesics and did not resort to daily prophylactic medication for headaches **(III/B)**.

In summary, many people with epilepsy manifest headache with seizure and most commonly in the postictal period. While there are many studies that document this overlap, treatment of the postictal headache has not been directly studied. Aside from typical acute medications (e.g. aspirin, ibuprofen, naproxen), treatment of seizures has been the mainstay of treatment in reducing postictal headache.

Cardiac

Significant cardiac and respiratory changes have been noted peri-ictally, but much attention has been recently devoted to cardiac changes due to the mysterious etiology of sudden unexplained death in epilepsy (SUDEP). Twenty-five patients with medically refractory epilepsy manifesting with both complex partial and generalized tonic-clonic seizures underwent video-EEG monitoring for presurgical evaluation and showed increased ictal heart rate, prolonged postictal tachycardia, and decreased heart rate variability after the seizure [8]. There was also significant QTc shortening in 17 patients, mostly in those with secondarily generalized convulsions, and 14 with benign cardiac arrhythmias postictally **(III/B)**. In a similar study of 31 patients undergoing presurgical evaluation, heart rate variability was decreased within the first 15 minutes after a seizure but remained decreased up to 5-6 hours after the seizure [9] **(III/B)**. While convulsive seizures had a greater decrease in heart rate variability, the findings suggest autonomic instability postictally that may contribute to the pathophysiology of SUDEP.

In a case-control study, 19 patients who had died from SUDEP after having had video-EEG monitoring for presurgical evaluation were matched with controls for same date of admission for video EEG. Peri-ictal and postictal heart rate, heart rate variability, and cardiac repolarization were all found to be similar between the two groups. The SUDEP group was less likely to have a lesion on MRI and less likely to have medications lowered during EEG testing, but had more generalized tonic-clonic seizures (GTCs) per year [10] (IIa/B). These findings argue that for patients with epilepsy who have noted cardiac abnormalities, particularly bradycardia, insertion of a pacemaker should be considered.

Some patients with prolonged seizures have been shown to develop pulmonary edema, but this is not always significant enough to cause death, suggesting that there may be a primary respiratory etiology of SUDEP. Using mice that were susceptible to postictal respiratory arrest, administration of selective serotonin reuptake inhibitors (SSRIs) prevented postictal respiratory changes [11], suggesting that serotonin was involved in these postictal respiratory changes that lead to SUDEP. A retrospective review of epilepsy patients admitted for video EEG showed that ictal oxygen desaturation was significantly reduced in patients taking SSRIs as compared to those who were not [12]. However, no difference was seen in generalized tonic-clonic seizures (III/B). While there is still no clear etiology of SUDEP, these studies suggest that SSRIs may be a potential therapy.

Cardiac markers have also been studied as a means to differentiate electrographic seizures from other events such as syncope and non-electrographic seizures (NES) and to determine the extent of myocardial damage with a seizure. In a prospective study of 22 patients with electrographic seizures and non-electrographic seizures who were admitted for video EEG, creatine kinase (CK) was collected daily to correlate with seizure type [13]. Half the patients with generalized tonic-clonic seizures had postictal CK elevations while none of the patients with other seizure types or non-electrographic spells had postictal elevations. Prolonged elevations up to 19 times baseline were seen in 15% of patients with generalized tonic-clonic seizures (IIa or IIb/B).

A more recent study compared serum creatine phosphokinase (CPK) in 20 patients with generalized tonic-clonic seizures, 22 with vasovagal syncope, 20 with NES, and 20 controls [14]. Serum CPK concentrations measured 12-15 hours after the event and at one time in the control group showed that CPK concentrations were significantly greater in patients with generalized tonic-clonic seizures. There was no significant difference in CK concentration in patients with vasovagal events, NES, or controls (IIa/B).

A similar study in 31 children and adolescents with seizures examined myocardial injury after convulsions as compared to 50 controls [15]. There was no difference in troponin levels 12 hours versus 7 days after convulsive seizures but creatine kinase-muscle brain (CK-MB) and brain naturietic factor (BNP) were significantly elevated in the postictal state as compared to baseline (IIa/B).

Another pediatric study compared 65 children with active epilepsy as compared to 31 children with epilepsy but no seizures for 2 months prior [16]. In the children with active epilepsy, the authors showed that BNP levels were significantly higher 4 hours postictally than 24-48 hours postictally. In addition, BNP was significantly higher compared to the control children or children with syncope or partial motor seizures **(IIb/B)**.

Psychiatric

Since psychiatric diagnoses are comorbid with epilepsy, it is reasonable to consider that postical behavioral changes are a reflection of an underlying predisposition toward psychiatric disease. Given the usual obvious nature of postictal psychiatric changes, they have been very well studied, perhaps moreso than almost any other postictal change. The difficulty in comparing these studies and drawing meaningful conclusions from them is in determining when the end of the postical period becomes the beginning of the interictal period. Behaviors attributable to the interictal period can be arbitrary and may only be determined after several seizures and prolonged observation of the time between seizures. While the EEG could help to differentiate whether psychiatric symptoms occur interictally versus postically, these behaviors can occur after a seizure and show a normal EEG. Psychosis is the most studied and many papers have been written about this. In 2001, Kanemoto suggested a definition of any psychotic episode within 7 days from the last generalized tonic-clonic seziure or cluster of complex partial seizures [17], but generally used definitions have not been established.

Summarizing the common findings of several case series on postictal psychosis (PIP), Kanner and Barry noted that there was a delay from the time of the last seizure to onset of psychosis, psychosis was of short duration, there was a clustering of generalized tonic-clonic seizures prior to the onset of psychosis, psychosis started after >10 years of epilepsy, and psychosis showed a quick response to medications [18]. Since then, there have been several other studies with larger numbers and a few with control populations (i.e. those with epilepsy but without PIP). These studies have primarily examined the prevalence of PIP in epilepsy, the characteristics of the postical psychotic state, and the risk factors for developing it, but treatment is rarely discussed.

Using 72 hours to define the postical period, 114 patients with refractory epilepsy were given a 42-item questionnaire to screen for postictal psychotic, depressive, and cognitive symptoms [19]. Over 3 months, postictal psychotic and cognitive symptoms occurred >50% after seizures in 100 of 114 patients. Thirty-eight patients reported that their interictal psychiatric and cognitive functions declined. A history of depression or anxiety worsened these postictal symptoms **(III/B)**. A subsequent study showed that of 18 partial epilepsy patients with PIP, 6 went on to develop interictal psychosis, whereas only one of 36 partial epilepsy patients went on to develop PIP **(IIb/B)** [20].

A review of 622 cases of patients undergoing surgical evaluation for complex partial seizures showed that 29 patients developed PIP on monitoring [21]. A risk factor for developing PIP was a history of mood disorders in first- and second-degree relatives, not a personal history of mood disorders (III/B). The same group later designed a case-control study including 59 patients with PIP and 94 controls with epilepsy and no PIP [22]. PIP was significantly associated with bilateral interictal epileptiform activity, secondary generalization, and a history of encephalitis, as well as a family history of psychiatric disorders and epilepsy (IIa/B). Similar findings were seen in a population of 57 patients with refractory partial epilepsy and psychotic disorders as compared to a control group of 56 patients with refractory partial epilepsy without psychoses [23]. Those who had psychosis with their epilepsy, of which 26% were postictal and 51% were interictal, had a longer seizure history and were more likely to have bilateral hippocampal sclerosis (IIa/B).

A well-done study with extensive follow-up examined 58 patients with epilepsy who had 151 episodes of postictal psychosis over a period of 12.8 years [24]. The average length of each postictal psychotic episode was 10.5 days with 95% resolving within 1 month. Patients vulnerable to psychosis were likely to have longer episodes. This is one of the few studies that directly studied treatment of the postictal state, and they showed that antipsychotic drugs were the only variable that affected the length of PIP (III/B). A case report with two patients implanted with bitemporal depths for possible temporal lobectomy demonstrated that both patients had postictal psychosis after a seizure cluster and that there was no associated electrographic discharges or seizures, nor was there associated postictal suppression [25]. In these cases, antipsychotics and benzodiazepines were given acutely, the patients quickly resolved, and ultimately had their intended surgery (III/B). However, these cases suggest that there is some other mechanism for the psychosis other than that directly related to electrographic changes. If this is the case, then other treatment options should be considered.

Postictal psychosis is somewhat common after seizures and can last days to weeks. If PIP occurs frequently enough, it can increase the risk of interictal psychosis. Risk factors for the development of PIP likely include temporal lobe involvement, perhaps moreso if bilateral, longer duration of epilepsy, a cluster of convulsive seizures, and a personal or family history of some mood disorders. While not many studies focused on treatment, the use of antipsychotics seemed to reduce the period of postictal psychosis.

Postictal psychosis leading to postictal suicide and suicide with the use of AEDs in epilepsy has become an increasing concern. One of the very first case reports of suicide in epilepsy presented two patients, one of which was a female with postictal depression who committed suicide by medication overdose soon after she had three staring spells [26]. Case series of suicide occurring in epilepsy patients first noted that postictal psychosis led to suicide in 7% of cases [27]. One study looking at 43 epilepsy patients who had died noted that six (14%) had died by suicide, three of whom died by jumping in front of a train while in a postictal state [28]. In another large case series of 10,739 patients with epilepsy seen at a large epilepsy center over 12 years, there were five suicides, none of which were clearly postictal [29] (III/B).

The topic of suicide and epilepsy has been scrutinized moreso recently since the US Food and Drug Administration (FDA) published a meta-analysis showing that patients taking AEDs were almost twice as likely to have suicidal ideation or behavior as patients taking placebo [30]. While there were many criticisms of this research, this led to the FDA warning on all AEDs about increased risks of suicidal thoughts and behaviors. A literature search yielded studies done on this topic, but they do not clearly indicate specifically if the suicidal risk is postictal. They showed that there is a significantly higher rate of suicide in patients who have frequent seizures and, for poorly explained reasons, after temporal lobe surgery [31]. This would indirectly suggest that patients with frequent seizures spend more time in the postictal state, and that this could increase the risk of postictal suicide. Subsequent studies reporting on database evaluations of suicide and AEDs did not have the ability to indicate when the suicide occurred in relation to the seizures [32-34] **(III/B)**. Overall, the high rate of suicide and depression in epilepsy patients indicates that treatment with antidepressants and more aggressive monitoring of depression and suicide risk as well as consultation with a psychiatrist is indicated.

Cognitive

Postictal cognitive difficulties are commonly observed and deeply concern patients, but the length, severity, and long-term impact are hard to determine. One study compared cognitive functioning in 31 patients with focal seizures to 14 controls [35]. Computerized memory testing was done prior to seizures, immediately after seizures, and after 30 minutes and 1 hour. Reorientation could take up to 45 minutes depending on generalization and temporal lobe seizures led to longer-lasting, high impact memory impairments **(IIa/B)**.

A study with 17 patients with pharmacoresistant epilepsy undergoing monitoring performed interictal and postictal neuropsychological testing. A significant improvement in focus localization was seen as compared to interictal neuropsychology testing alone [36] **(III/B)**. A more recent study of 126 adults with temporal lobe seizures (47 right and 79 left) admitted for video-EEG monitoring were given cognitive testing when it appeared that they were not postictal the day of or the day prior to testing as well as not apparently affected by medication changes [37] **(III/B)**. They showed a possible small adverse effect of medications on testing, no effect as to the time of seizures, but a relationship between side of seizures and testing results. While this was a large study, the time testing performed was left to the medical staff to judge if they were or were not affected.

In a randomized controlled trial testing to see if patients admitted to a video-EEG monitoring unit could recall seizures, all patients were reminded at the onset of testing to document seizures, but the test subjects were reminded daily to document seizures [38]. Of 582 seizures captured, patients could not document 55% of all seizures, 73.2% of complex partial seizures, 26.2% of simple partial seizures and 41.7% of secondarily generalized seizures, 85.8% of seizures during sleep and 32% of all seizures during wakefulness. There was no difference in documentation with the daily versus routine reminder. An ictal focus in the left hemisphere (not just temporal) contributed to lack of documentation **(IIa/B)**.

There have been some studies to determine if Apo E4 is linked to postictal confusion, but the associations are still not entirely clear. Medically refractory temporal lobe epilepsy patients with at least one epsilon4 allele were three times more likely to have postictal confusion than patients without epsilon4 [39] (IIb/B). A similar subsequent study in 77 patients with temporal lobe epilepsy suggests that there is no association with Apo E4 and those epilepsy patients who have postictal confusion [40] (IIb/B).

Localization

Ictal presentations have long been scrutinized as localizing features, but when the onset of a seizure is missed, the postictal period can provide clues for seizure origin as well. Since the time of the original descriptions of epilepsy, postictal paresis, or 'Todd's paralysis' has been one of the most well-described postictal findings, but few have systematically analyzed these findings until recently. Still though, many of the studies presented are retrospective observational case series, so the more recent, larger studies are included here.

Of 513 patients undergoing evaluation on video EEG for surgery, 328 were reviewed and showed that 13.4% of patients had postictal paresis (PP) [41]. It was always unilateral and always contralateral to the seizure focus. Almost 10% of seizures had no overt clinical activity, and the PP was longer if there was associated tonic-clonic seizure activity (III/B). Other case series have found similar findings [42, 43] (III/B), with one finding that 93% of patients had postictal hemiparesis contralateral to the seizure focus. In this study, a seizure focus could not be identified in a few with unclear lateralization of postictal weaknesses [43] (III/B).

In some cases, postictal paresis and aphasia occur together and provide information on localization. Examining 35 patients with good post-surgical outcomes, observers blindly reviewed postictal events to determine localization of seizure onset [44]. Seizures originating in the dominant hemisphere and spreading to Wernicke's or Broca's areas always led to postictal aphasia whereas those in the non-dominant hemisphere did not, even with generalization. Postictal paresis had a similar strong correlation (III/B). A pediatric study of 70 children with benign rolandic epilepsy revealed that in addition to aphasia, 11.5% had postictal paresis that lasted up to 1 hour after a seizure [45] (III/B).

Speech has long been known to localize to the dominant hemisphere in almost all cases and postictal language has also been shown to lateralize to the dominant hemisphere [46] (III/B). Using the Boston Naming Test, 60 patients undergoing video EEG for lesional temporal lobe epilepsy had 212 seizures which showed that patients with dominant lobe TLE had a longer postictal language delay and had more postictal paraphasic errors than non-dominant TLE [47] (III/B).

Automatisms generally suggest seizures with temporal lobe origin but lateralization is not always clear. Of 193 seizures in 55 patients with medically refractory temporal lobe epilepsy and postoperative seizure-free outcomes, postictal automatisms were seen in 36% of seizures [48]. Only speech automatisms lateralized to the left side (III/B). Many other case series have described postictal automatisms but lateralization is still not always definitive. Postictal nose wipe has been described as a predominantly ipsilateral finding [49], as has postictal face wiping behavior [50]. A variety of other postictal behaviors have also been described, including hypersalivation and cough [51], leaving behavior [52], biting [53], cough [54], and loss of consciousness [55]. Of these, cough and loss of consciousness were the only ones that seemed to show a left-sided predominance. Overall, postictal behaviors can provide just as much information about localization of seizures as ictal behaviors, but more studies need to be done to obtain more information.

EEG

Postictal EEG changes usually show slowing, at times focal if in a partial epilepsy, and/or some associated relative electrosuppression. These findings can be useful for surgical planning but can also give an indication of how well medications may be working. In 29 patients undergoing surgical evaluation, postictal polymorphic delta activity was found in 64% of EEGs. Of those, delta activity correlated with the side of surgery in 96% of EEGs [56] (III/B). In 35 absence seizures analyzed, interchannel synchrony was found in the postictal state significantly moreso than the interictal period [57] (III/B). A similar study using 87 studies of transcranial magnetic stimulation in 58 patients showed that there was increased excitability in the 24 hours prior to a seizure and decreased excitability in the 24 hours after a seizure [58] (III/B). These findings stayed ipsilateral in focal seizures and did not secondarily generalize. Another study used event-related potentials in temporal lobe epilepsy patients admitted to a video-EEG unit and showed that event potentials were significantly decreased up to 6 hours postictally on the ipsilateral side of the seizure focus as compared to an interictal or pre-ictal event potential (III/B).

Information on medications and the postictal state is less well known. In a randomized control trial with 23 patients undergoing video EEG, the 11 patients on levetiracetam were shown to have a significantly longer interhemispheric delay in seizure spread and a significantly shorter postictal recovery of background activity as compared to the 12 patients on placebo [59] (Ib/A).

Overall, electrophysiological evidence about the postictal state is largely confined to moderate-sized case series that study the excitability of the cortex and the localization of seizures. Little information exists on the effect of antiepileptic medications on the postictal period other than knowing that successfully treating seizures will avoid the postictal state.

Imaging

Imaging the postictal state may help determine localization as well as to differentiate between non-convulsive status epilepticus (NCSE) versus the postictal state. Given the high mortality of non-convulsive status epilepticus, imaging with perfusion CT or MRI may be a quick diagnostic tool. A small pilot study first done in 2006 showed that perfusion CT showed increased regional perfusion in three patients in status epilepticus while six patients who had a single seizure showed decreased perfusion [60] (III/B). A later, larger study examined 19 unresponsive patients after seizure activity [61]. They were imaged with perfusion CT and images were correlated with clinical and EEG information. As expected, there was focally increased cerebral blood flow and increased blood volume in those in NCSE as compared to the postictal state. The area of blood flow correlated with clinical and EEG findings (III/B). This technique can also be used in differentiating NCSE or the postictal state from stroke. Four patients suspected of having stroke showed increased cerebral blood flow and increased cerebral blood volume, thereby avoiding thrombolytic therapy [62] (III/B).

A variety of postictal MRI findings have been reported but focally increased T2 changes and a decreased apparent diffusion coefficient (ADC) are the most common. In 10 patients with complex partial status epilepticus, the diffusion-weighted coefficient (DWI) and ADC changes were seen focally with later noted atrophy [63] (III/B). In 14 non-lesional patients with temporal lobe epilepsy, decreased postictal ADC was seen in neocortical foci [64] (III/B).

Increased T2 changes have also been reported transiently in the splenium in two patients with bitemporal epilepsy [65]. In many cases, increases in T2 change are not only seen focally in the epileptogenic zone, but also in the pia and pulvinar. This can be hard to differentiate from underlying comorbid conditions such as cancer or encephalitis [66] (III/B). In three patients with brain tumors and focally increased T2, FLAIR, and gadolinium changes suggestive of disease progression imaged shortly after seizures, controlling seizures led to resolution of imaging within 3 weeks [67] (III/B). Finally, in 18 patients with intractable focal epilepsy, diffusion tensor imaging (DTI) showed 50% of patients had a decrease postictally in DTI and in most of these, the area of decrease correlated with the area of seizure onset [68] (III/B). These findings suggest that postictal DTI imaging can help with localization of seizure onset and potential tracts where seizure spreads.

Non-epileptic seizures (NES)

Even for the best of epileptologists, non-epileptic seizures (NES) can be difficult to distinguish from epileptic seizures, therefore clinical characteristics are critical to differentiation. Since observers may miss the onset of an event, the postictal period is a time when the patient can be observed and the diagnosis of NES can be considered. Many studies have been done to compare pre-ictal and peri-ictal states of NES, but few have been done specifically on the postictal state. Retrospective analysis using a clinical computer database at one institution compared 16 epilepsy patients with 23 NES patients, most of whom were female [69]. Patients with NES had a much lower rate of postictal headache (6/16 [38%] with epilepsy as compared to 1/23 [4.3%] with NES), as well as fatigue (9/16 [58%] with electrographic seizures and 3/23 [13%] with NES). Twelve NES patients had no postictal symptoms, whereas all epilepsy patients had one postictal symptom. Treatment of seizures or NES was not addressed (III/B). A very interesting study at one institution studied

100 consecutive patients on long-term EEG monitoring and tried to differentiate NES patients on the basis of postictal symptoms [70]. In the 24 patients diagnosed with NES, 75% showed postictal whispering or partial motor behaviors, while none of those diagnosed with epilepsy showed this **(III/B)**. Other electrophysiological testing in NES has shown that event-related potentials in patients with temporal lobe epilepsy show a difference pre-ictal and postictal, whereas those in patients with NES do not [71] **(III/B)**.

Another single institution study looked at postictal breathing patterns of long-term monitoring patients and evaluated 23 convulsions in 15 patients with epilepsy and 24 convulsive events in 16 patients with NES [72]. Epilepsy patients had more prolonged inspiration and expiration, a lower respiratory rate, louder breathing, and longer periods of altered breathing after a seizure, whereas NES patients had an increased respiratory rate with short inspiration and expiration as well as brief pauses and irregular patterns **(III/B)**. No brain functional imaging studies have been done of NES and while there are therapies used for NES including traditional antidepressants and cognitive behavioral therapy, none address specifically the postictal period of a non-epileptic seizure.

There are many patients admitted for video-EEG monitoring with both epileptic seizures and NES, but the two types of events are often separated in time. In some of these cases, NES is diagnosed in the postictal period of an epileptic seizure, presumably when symptoms of a partial electrographic seizure progress and the patient then has a conversion event that is diagnosed as NES. There has been one case series on this, suggesting that impaired self-inhibition and frontal lobe activity may contribute to this series of events [73] **(III/B)**. Very little is known or written about this phenomenon and there are no known treatments for this.

In summary, a lack of symptoms in the postictal state can be useful in supporting the diagnosis of NES. The diagnosis is further supported by a similar lack of findings on EEG and/or MRI imaging.

Conclusions

The postictal state may be more debilitating than seizures themselves. With better treatments for the postictal state, we can improve quality of life of our epilepsy patients. The majority of studies evaluating the postictal period are case series and case reports with very few controlled studies. Even fewer address treatment for the postictal period, and no study is designed to directly test treatment of the postictal period alone. Given that the postictal state is very difficult to observe and study, usually due to a patient's confusion or amnesia and inability to report events, it is not surprising that most findings are from inpatient video-EEG monitoring where the patient is observed by trained clinical staff. These limitations make randomized controlled trials harder to plan and execute. Future studies should focus further research and treatment on the postictal state in an effort to limit disability in patients with epilepsy.

Key points	Evidence level
◆ Interictal headache is common in people with epilepsy, and most peri-ictal headaches are postictal. The only treatments mentioned for postictal headache are analgesics.	III/B
◆ There are no definitive cardiac changes that seem to correlate with SUDEP, but tachycardia and heart rate variability are noted in many seizures. In addition, while no serum markers have been definitively associated with cardiac damage, elevations of cardiac markers such as CK and troponin are usually seen after generalized tonic-clonic seizures.	III/B
◆ Postictal psychosis has been shown in people with longer duration of epilepsy, those with a personal or family history of mood disorders, and in those with temporal lobe involvement, often bilateral, of seizures. Treatments have not been well studied and are largely antipsychotics.	III/B
◆ There is a great deal of information that can be obtained from postictal behaviors and, currently, postictal paresis and aphasia are the two postictal behaviors that have best localized postictal slowing to the contralateral hemisphere and the dominant hemisphere, respectively.	IIb/B & III/B
◆ EEG findings in the postictal state correlate with seizure focus. Depending on whether seizures are focal or generalized, there is focal slowing and/or diffuse relative electrosuppression.	III/B
◆ Imaging changes can show focally increased blood flow on perfusion CT and an increase in T2 change on MRI that, at times, may mimic tumor or stroke.	III/B
◆ An unremarkable postictal state is typical for non-epileptic seizures.	III/B

References

1. Syvertsen M, Helde G, Stovner LJ, Brodtkorb E. Headaches add to the burden of epilepsy. *J Headache Pain* 2007; 8(4): 224-30.
2. Förderreuther S, Henkel A, Noachtar S, Straube A. Headache associated with epileptic seizures: epidemiology and clinical characteristics. *Headache* 2002; 42(7): 649-55.
3. Yankovsky AE, Andermann F, Bernasconi A. Characteristics of headache associated with intractable partial epilepsy. *Epilepsia* 2005; 46(8): 1241-5.
4. Ito M, Adachi N, Nakamura F, *et al*. Characteristics of postictal headache in patients with partial epilepsy. *Cephalalgia* 2004; 24(1): 23-8.
5. HELP Study Group. Multi-center study on migraine and seizure-related headache in patients with epilepsy. *Yonsei Med J* 2010; 51(2): 219-24.
6. Yamane LE, Montenegro MA, Guerreiro MM. Comorbidity headache and epilepsy in childhood. *Neuropediatrics* 2004; 35(2): 99-102.

7. Cai S, Hamiwka LD, Wirrell EC. Peri-ictal headache in children: prevalence and character. *Pediatr Neurol* 2008; 39(2): 91-6.

8. Surges R, Scott CA, Walker MC. Enhanced QT shortening and persistent tachycardia after generalized seizures. *Neurology* 2010; 74(5): 421-6.

9. Toth V, Hejjel L, Fogarasi A, *et al*. Periictal heart rate variability analysis suggests long-term postictal autonomic disturbance in epilepsy. *Eur J Neurol* 2010; 17(6): 780-7.

10. Surges R, Adjei P, Kallis C, *et al*. Pathologic cardiac repolarization in pharmacoresistant epilepsy and its potential role in sudden unexpected death in epilepsy: a case-control study. *Epilepsia* 2010; 51(2): 233-42.

11. Tupal S, Faingold CL. Evidence supporting a role of serotonin in modulation of sudden death induced by seizures in DBA/2 mice. *Epilepsia* 2006; 47: 21-6.

12. Bateman L, Li C, Lin T, Seyal M. Serotonin reuptake inhibitors are associated with reduced severity of ictal hypoxemia in medically refractory partial epilepsy. *Epilepsia* 2010; 51(10): 2211-4.

13. Wyllie E, Lueders H, Pippenger C, VanLente F. Postictal serum creatine kinase in the diagnosis of seizure disorders. *Arch Neurol* 1985; 42(2): 123-6.

14. Petramfar P, Yaghoobi E, Nemati R, Asadi-Pooya AA. Serum creatine phosphokinase is helpful in distinguishing generalized tonic-clonic seizures from psychogenic nonepileptic seizures and vasovagal syncope. *Epilepsy Behav* 2009; 15(3): 330-2.

15. Alehan F, Erol I, Cemil T, Bayraktar N, Ogüs E, Tokel K. Elevated CK-MB mass and plasma brain-type natriuretic peptide concentrations following convulsive seizures in children and adolescents: possible evidence of subtle cardiac dysfunction. *Epilepsia* 2009; 50(4): 755-60.

16. Rauchenzauner M, Haberlandt E, Foerster S, *et al*. Brain-type natriuretic peptide secretion following febrile and afebrile seizures – a new marker in childhood epilepsy? *Epilepsia* 2007; 48(1): 101-6.

17. Kanemoto K, Kim Y, Miyamoto T, Kawasaki J. Presurgical postictal and acute interictal psychoses are differentially associated with postoperative mood and psychotic disorders. *J Neuropsychiatry Clin Neurosci* 2001; 13(2): 243-7.

18. Kanner AM, Barry JJ. Is the psychopathology of epilepsy different from that of nonepileptic patients? *Epilepsy Behav* 2001; 2(3): 170-86.

19. Kanner AM, Soto A, Gross-Kanner H. Prevalence and clinical characteristics of postictal psychiatric symptoms in partial epilepsy. *Neurology* 2004; 62(5): 708-13.

20. Kanner AM, Ostrovskaya A. Long-term significance of postictal psychotic episodes II. Are they predictive of interictal psychotic episodes? *Epilepsy Behav* 2008; 12(1): 154-6.

21. Alper K, Devinsky O, Westbrook L, *et al*. Premorbid psychiatric risk factors for postictal psychosis. *J Neuropsychiatry Clin Neurosci* 2001; 13(4): 492-9.

22. Alper K, Kuzniecky R, Carlson C, *et al*. Postictal psychosis in partial epilepsy: a case-control study. *Ann Neurol* 2008; 63(5): 602-10.

23. D'Alessio L, Giagante B, Ibarra V, *et al*. Analysis of psychotic disorders in patients with refractory partial epilepsy, psychiatric diagnoses and clinical aspects. *Actas Esp Psiquiatr* 2008; 36(3): 138-43.

24. Adachi N, Ito M, Kanemoto K, *et al*. Duration of postictal psychotic episodes. *Epilepsia* 2007; 48(8): 1531-7.

25. Schulze-Bonhage A, Tebartz van Elst L. Postictal psychosis: evidence for extratemporal functional precursors. *Epilepsia* 2010; 18: 308-12.

26. Mendez MF, Doss RC. Ictal and psychiatric aspects of suicide in epileptic patients. *Int J Psychiatry Med* 1992; 22: 231-7.

27. Kanemoto K Kawasaki J, Mori E. Violence and epilepsy: a close relationship between violence and postictal psychosis. *Epilepsia* 1999; 40(1): 107-9.

28. Fukucki T, Kanemoto K, Kato M, *et al*. Death in epilepsy with special attention to suicide cases. *Epilepsy Research* 2002; 51: 233-6.

29. Blumer D, Montouris G, Davies K, *et al*. Suicide in epilepsy: psychopathology, pathogenesis, and prevention. *Epilepsy Behav* 2002; 3: 232-41.

30. Statistical review and evaluation: antiepileptic drugs and suicidality. (May 23, 2008. http://www.fda.gov/ohms/dockets/ac/08/briefings/2008-4372b1-01-FDA.pdf).

31. Bell GS, Gaitatzis A, Bell CL, *et al*. Suicide in people with epilepsy: how great is the risk? *Epilepsia* 2009; 50 (8): 1933-42.

32. Lim H, Song H, Hwang Y, *et al*. Predictors of suicidal ideation in people with epilepsy living in Korea. *J Clin Neurol* 2010; 6: 81-8.

33. Patorno E, Bohn R, Wahl PM, *et al.* Anticonvulsant medications and the risk of suicide, attempted suicide or violent death. *JAMA* 2010; 303(14): 1401-9.

34. Oelesen JB, Hansen PR, Erdal J, *et al.* Antiepileptic drugs and the risk of suicide: a nationwide study. Pharmacoepidemiology and Drug Safety. *JAMA* 2010; 19: 518-24.

35. Helmstaedter C, Elger CE, Lendt M. Postictal courses of cognitive deficits in focal epilepsies. *Epilepsia* 1994; 35(5): 1073-8.

36. Pegna AJ, Qayoom Z, Gericke CA, Landis T, Seeck M. Comprehensive postictal neuropsychology improves focus localization in epilepsy. *Eur Neurol* 1998; 40(4): 207-11.

37. Dodrill CB, Ojemann GA. Do recent seizures and recent changes in antiepileptic drugs impact performances on neuropsychological tests in subtle ways that might easily be missed? *Epilepsia* 2007; 48(10): 1833-41.

38. Hoppe C, Poepel A, Elger CE. Epilepsy: accuracy of patient seizure counts. *Arch Neurol* 2007; 64(11): 1595-9.

39. Chapin JS, Busch RM, Janigro D, *et al.* APOE epsilon4 is associated with postictal confusion in patients with medically refractory temporal lobe epilepsy. *Epilepsy Res* 2008; 81(2-3): 220-4.

40. Kauffman MA, Pereira-de-Silva N, Consalvo D, Kochen S. ApoE epsilon4 is not associated with postictal confusion in patients with mesial temporal lobe epilepsy with hippocampal sclerosis. *Epilepsy Res* 2009; 85(2-3): 311-3.

41. Gallmetzer P, Leutmezer F, Serles W, Assem-Hilger E, Spatt J, Baumgartner C. Postictal paresis in focal epilepsies - incidence, duration, and causes: a video-EEG monitoring study. *Neurology* 2004; 62(12): 2160-4.

42. Loddenkemper T, Wyllie E, Neme S, Kotagal P, Lüders HO. Lateralizing signs during seizures in infants. *J Neurol* 2004; 251(9): 1075-9.

43. Kellinghaus C, Kotagal P. Lateralizing value of Todd's palsy in patients with epilepsy. *Neurology* 2004; 62(2): 289-91.

44. Adam C, Adam C, Rouleau I, Saint-Hilaire JM. Postictal aphasia and paresis: a clinical and intracerebral EEG study. *Can J Neurol Sci* 2000; 27(1): 49-54.

45. Dai AI, Weinstock A. Postictal paresis in children with benign rolandic epilepsy. *AJ Child Neurol* 2005; 20(10): 834-6.

46. Ficker DM, Shukla R, Privitera MD. Postictal language dysfunction in complex partial seizures: effect of contralateral ictal spread. *Neurology* 2001; 56(11): 1590-2.

47. Ramirez MJ, Schefft BK, Howe SR, Hwa-Shain Y, Privitera MD. Interictal and postictal language testing accurately lateralizes language dominant temporal lobe complex partial seizures. *Epilepsia* 2008; 49(1): 22-32.

48. Rásonyi G, Fogarasi A, Kelemen A, Janszky J, Halász P. Lateralizing value of postictal automatisms in temporal lobe epilepsy. *Epilepsy Res* 2006; 70(2-3): 239-43.

49. Hirsch LJ, Lain AH, Walczak TS. Postictal nosewiping lateralizes and localizes to the ipsilateral temporal lobe. *Epilepsia* 1998; 39(9): 991-7.

50. Meletti S, Cantalupo G, Stanzani-Maserati M, Rubboli G, Alberto Tassinari C. The expression of interictal, preictal, and postictal facial-wiping behavior in temporal lobe epilepsy: a neuro-ethological analysis and interpretation. *Epilepsy Behav* 2003; 4(6): 635-43.

51. Hoffmann JM, Elger CE, Kleefuss-Lie AA. The localizing value of hypersalivation and postictal coughing in temporal lobe epilepsy. *Epilepsy Res* 2009; 87(2-3): 144-7.

52. Jin L, Inoue Y. Spontaneous periictal leaving behavior: a potential lateralizing sign in mesial temporal lobe epilepsy. *Epilepsia* 2009; 50(6): 1560-5.

53. Tassinari CA, Tassi L, Calandra-Buonaura G, *et al.* Biting behavior, aggression, and seizures. *Epilepsia* 2005; 46(5): 654-63.

54. Fauser S, Wuwer Y, Gierschner C, Schulze-Bonhage A. The localizing and lateralizing value of ictal/postictal coughing in patients with focal epilepsies. *Seizure* 2004; 13(6): 403-10.

55. Lux S, Kurthen M, Helmstaedter C, Hartje W, Reuber M, Elger CE. The localizing value of ictal consciousness and its constituent functions: a video-EEG study in patients with focal epilepsy. *Brain* 2002; 125(Pt 12): 2691-8.

56. Jan MM, Sadler M, Rahey SR. Lateralized postictal EEG delta predicts the side of seizure surgery in temporal lobe epilepsy. *Epilepsia* 2001; 42(3): 402-5.

57. Aarabi A, Wallois F, Grebe R. Does spatiotemporal synchronization of EEG change prior to absence seizures? *Brain Res* 2008; 1188: 207-21.

58. Badawy R, Macdonell R, Jackson G, Berkovic S. The peri-ictal state: cortical excitability changes within 24h of a seizure. *Brain* 2009; 132(Pt 4): 1013-21.
59. Tilz C, Stefan H, Hopfengaertner R, Kerling F, Genow A, Wang-Tilz Y. Influence of levetiracetam on ictal and postictal EEG in patients with partial seizures. *Eur J Neurol* 2006; 13(12): 1352-8.
60. Wiest R, von Bredow F, Schindler K, *et al.* Detection of regional blood perfusion changes in epileptic seizures with dynamic brain perfusion CT - a pilot study. *Epilepsy Res* 2006; 72(2-3): 102-10.
61. Hauf M, Slotboom J, Nirkko A, von Bredow F, Ozdoba C, Wiest R. Cortical regional hyperperfusion in nonconvulsive status epilepticus measured by dynamic brain perfusion CT. *Am J Neuroradiol* 2009; 30(4): 693-8.
62. Masterson K, Vargas MI, Delavelle J. Postictal deficit mimicking stroke: role of perfusion CT. *J Neuroradiol* 2009; 36(1): 48-51.
63. Szabo K, Poepel A, Pohlmann-Eden B, *et al.* Diffusion-weighted and perfusion MRI demonstrates parenchymal changes in complex partial status epilepticus. *Brain* 2005; 128(Pt 6): 1369-76.
64. Oh JB, Lee SK, Kim KK, Song IC, Chang KH. Role of immediate postictal diffusion-weighted MRI in localizing epileptogenic foci of mesial temporal lobe epilepsy and non-lesional neocortical epilepsy. *Seizure* 2004; 13(7): 509-16.
65. Oster J, Doherty C, Grant PE, Simon M, Cole AJ. Diffusion-weighted imaging abnormalities in the splenium after seizures. *Epilepsia* 2003; 44(6): 852-4.
66. Hattingen E, Raab P, Lanfermann H, Zanella FE, Weidauer S. Postictal MR changes - a rare and important differential diagnosis. *Radiologe* 2008; 48(11): 1058-65.
67. Finn MA, Blumenthal DT, Salzman KL, Jensen RL. Transient postictal MRI changes in patients with brain tumors may mimic disease progression. *Surg Neurol* 2007; 67(3): 246-50; discussion 250.
68. Diehl B, Symms MR, Boulby PA, *et al.* Postictal diffusion tensor imaging. *Epilepsy Res* 2005; 65(3): 137-46.
69. Ettinger AB, Weisbrot DM, Nolan E, Devinsky O. Postictal symptoms help distinguish patients with epileptic seizures from those with non-epileptic seizures. *Seizure* 1999; 8: 149-51.
70. Chabolla DR, Shih JJ. Postictal behaviors associated with psychogenic nonepileptic seizures. *Epilepsy Behav* 2006; 9(2): 307-11.
71. Wambacq I, Abubakr A. Auditory event-related potentials (P300) in the identification of psychogenic nonepileptic seizures. *Epilepsy Behav* 2004; 5(4): 503-8.
72. Azar NJ, Tayah TF, Wang L, Song Y, Abou-Khalil BW. Postictal breathing pattern distinguishes epileptic from nonepileptic convulsive seizures. *Epilepsia* 2008; 49(1): 132-7.
73. Devinsky O, Gordon E. Epileptic seizures progressing into nonepileptic conversion seizures. *Neurology* 1998; 51: 1293-6.

Chapter 7

Strategies for closing the treatment gap of refractory epilepsy

Joseph I. Sirven MD, Professor of Neurology
Department of Neurology
Division of Epilepsy
Mayo Clinic Hospital
Phoenix, Arizona, USA

Introduction

There are numerous therapeutic options for the management of chronic seizures and epilepsy. Seventeen approved antiepileptic drugs in the United States, one stimulation device, vagus nerve stimulation (VNS), epilepsy surgery for certain localization-related epilepsies and the ketogenic diet are all available. Despite the plethora of surgical and medical treatments, there remains a need for better therapies that fundamentally stop and cure epilepsy. Psychosocial consequences of epilepsy along with comorbid conditions of cognitive dysfunction, mood disorders and other concerns limit the benefit of current therapy. The goal for this chapter is to try to outline the treatment gap of epilepsy. To accomplish this goal, the discussion will center on the current state of epilepsy care followed by identification of three gaps. This chapter will discuss the current best evidence supporting various therapeutic options with the goal of closing the treatment gap.

The state of epilepsy care in the United States

In 2005, the United States (US) Centers for Disease Control and Prevention (CDC) conducted surveillance work to assess the state of epilepsy and seizure care in the United States based on 19 reporting states [1] **(Ib/A)**. The US CDC worked with the Behavioral Risk

Factor Surveillance System and assessed a number of epilepsy and seizure-related variables to better characterize how well the US healthcare structure was handling epilepsy care. The Behavioral Risk Factor Surveillance System is an ongoing, state-based, random, digit-dialed telephone survey of non-institutionalized United States adults over the age of 18. The system collects information on health risk, behaviors, and preventive health services that relate to the leading causes of death and morbidity.

The surveillance system included a total of 2207 adults from 19 states, or 1.65% who reported a history of epilepsy [1]. 0.084% had active epilepsy defined as either a history of epilepsy and currently taking medications or reporting one or more seizures during the past 3 months [1]. 0.75% were classified as having inactive epilepsy or a history of epilepsy or seizure disorder but not currently taking medicine to control epilepsy and no seizures in the 3 months preceding the survey [1] **(Ib/A)**.

American adults with a history of chronic seizures were much more likely to report fair or poor health, being unemployed or unable to work. These individuals also lived in households with the lowest annual incomes, and had a history of concomitant disorders such as stroke or arthritis [1]. Adults with a history of epilepsy also reported significantly worse quality of life. Individuals with epilepsy were more likely to be obese, physically inactive and smoking [1]. In adults with epilepsy who have had recent seizures, 16.1% reported not taking their epilepsy medications and 65.1% reported having had more than one seizure in the past month [1] **(Ib/A)**.

Among adults with a history of seizures, almost 24% reported cost as a barrier to seeking care from a physician over the previous year [1]. A total of 35% of adults also reported not having seen a neurologist or an epilepsy specialist in the previous year [1] **(Ib/A)**. The study showed that seizures and epilepsy are frequent occurrences among the American population and there is a significant burden of disease that cannot be assessed from epidemiologic studies [1]. Even with multiple treatment options, a major gap exists between treatment and optimal quality of life.

How well do seizure medications work?

This question was addressed in a seminal study by Brodie and Kwan in 2000 [2] **(IIa/B)**. Using newer agents Brodie and Kwan investigated 523 untreated patients with epilepsy. Of those 523 patients, 470 were drug naïve, 47% responded to their first antiepileptic drug and 13% were seizure-free on the second antiepileptic drug [2] **(IIa/B)**. Of the individuals whose seizures failed to respond to the first two agents, seizures in only 1% responded to the third choice of drug [2] **(IIa/B)**.

The study uncovered that there are two groups of epilepsy patients. There are those whose seizures can be managed with any seizure medication and will likely respond to the first or second agent presented to them in monotherapy. However, there is another group of individuals which are much more difficult to identify at an early point and whose seizures fail to respond to any drug. These cases are defined as refractory epilepsy patients who may need to be assessed for surgical intervention at an earlier point in their course of epilepsy as opposed to committing them to multiple medication trials over extended periods of time.

To further underscore this point, the International League against Epilepsy recently created a new definition which better defines drug-resistant epilepsy [3] (IV/C). The new operational definition is that a patient's seizures must have failed to be completely controlled with two antiepileptic drugs used in informative trials [3] (IV/C). Success is defined as an appropriately selected antiepileptic drug used with complete cessation of seizures for more than 1 year or three times longer than the baseline inter-seizure interval, whichever is longer of the two with a minimum of a year to determine an effect [3] (IV/C). This particular definition helps to define when a patient is likely not to be responsive to a seizure medication and more aggressive treatment is necessary [3].

Defining gaps

If one were to best categorize the treatment gaps of refractory epilepsy, there would be three broad groups. The first is a diagnostic treatment gap, which pertains to identifying individuals with refractory epilepsy and denoting them at an earlier point in the course of the disease before the psychosocial problems have had life-altering consequences. Second is a medical treatment gap, defined as lack of use of new drug therapies. Lastly, a surgical treatment gap exists, which refers to leveraging potentially curative and disease-modifying tactics by the use of devices or surgery.

Diagnostic treatment gap

One of the essential strategies in closing the treatment gap is to distinguish the 'at risk' population that will merit extra resources in order to better help them. Put another way, what are the biomarkers that will denote patients who may be in need of extra attention with regards to their condition? Table 1 shows helpful clinical historical biomarkers. Clinical historical biomarkers are helpful in predicting seizure remission. Such biomarkers with class 1 evidentiary support include: normal neurological and intellectual abilities; age of seizure onset less than 12 years of age; and infrequent or easily controlled seizures. If all three are present, there is an 80% remission rate. If none are present then there is a 20% remission rate [4, 5] (I/A). Other consistent historical biomarkers for remission have included the presence of idiopathic epilepsy, a normal physical examination and an early response within 2 years of antiepileptic drug-induced remission [4, 5] (I/A). Thus, the absence of these markers may portend a more difficult prognosis for the patient.

Modalities such as imaging have helped to find epileptogenic lesions, particularly those associated with heterotopia, low-grade neoplasms, and hemorrhagic infarctions, which are highly related to refractory epilepsy. Combining historical biomarkers with imaging may be potentially useful. Another helpful biomarker is electroencephalography (EEG). Although the EEG is useful in predicting which patients are likely to have seizure recurrence based on the presence of epileptiform discharges, there is a lack of specificity for predicting which patients

Table 1. Clinical historical biomarkers suggesting seizure remission [4, 5].	
Historical variable	**Level of evidence**
Seizure onset less than 12 years of age	Ia/A
Infrequent seizures	Ia/A
Normal examination	Ia/A
Idiopathic epilepsy	Ia/A
Early response to AED	Ia/A

are likely to enter a seizure remission. In the future, it is possible that high frequency oscillations found on intracranial EEG recordings may be fruitful in helping to select which patients are likely to have ongoing seizures [6] **(IV/C)**.

One of the more exciting approaches to diagnostic aspects of closing the treatment gap is the concept of seizure detection and prediction (see also Chapter 8). Seizures are manifestations of increased network synchronies. Therefore, it is reasonable to assume that there are changes in activity potentially embedded within an EEG signal that will reflect these synaptic or network changes before an actual seizure occurs. Examination of interictal spikes has not convincingly shown that spike frequency increases prior to ictal initiations. However, there are subclinical seizures, bursts or 'chirps' that increase prior to clinical events [7]. The concept of these early changes, which could occur minutes or even hours before a clinical event, characterizes the pre-ictal state [7].

Thus a device could be created to link early seizure detection to therapeutic intervention. To provide meaningful benefit this would require an automated system with rapid response. Ideally the intervention would reduce seizure duration so that alteration of consciousness or secondary generalization did not occur. If a seizure prediction algorithm allowed identification of a pre-ictal state before a seizure, then a window for intervention could be noted, reducing the unpredictability of seizures.

Coupling a seizure detection device for early seizure detection to a drug delivery system could be a potent strategy. Using devices in rats, computerized detection of ictal onset triggered application of diazepam to experimental seizure foci [8, 9]. The application was administered quickly enough, less than 5 seconds after seizure onset, to produce a 64% reduction in seizure duration [8, 9]. If such a device could be coupled with a seizure prediction algorithm, greater reduction or even seizure prevention could result. Rapid cooling or hyperthermia has also been linked with early seizure detection devices [10].

There are thus a number of historical, electroencephalographic and potential imaging biomarkers which could help identify who are patients likely to have drug-resistant seizures early in their course, help to predict when seizures occur, and in essence transform the quality of life of patients with epilepsy.

AED treatment gap

As one examines the current plethora of options available for epilepsy, one notes that most AEDs have been approved based on a limited understanding as to the mechanism of action of these various compounds. The current era of antiepileptic drug discovery was ushered in by Merritt and Putnam in 1937 when they demonstrated the feasibility of using a maximal electroshock (MES) seizure, or a MES model, to identify the anticonvulsive potential of phenytoin [11]. A number of other animal models have been employed in the search for more efficacious and tolerable AEDs. In the early 1970s, the National Institute of Neurological Disorders and Stroke embarked on a mission to encourage basic research aimed at a greater understanding of the factors that contribute to the initiation, propagation and amelioration of seizures. As part of this effort the Anticonvulsive Drug Development Program (ADD) was created to foster the development of new drugs for the treatment of epilepsy.

Since 1975 the ADD has accessioned more than 25,000 investigational anticonvulsant drugs from the academic community and the pharmaceutical industry. This has led to the identification and development of several new antiepileptic agents. It has fostered significant understanding not only of the therapeutic nature of various agents but also the basic science associated with epilepsy. As the understanding of the pathophysiology of acquired epilepsy at the molecular genetic level leads to the development of a new therapeutic approach, it is likely that drug development models will need to be refined in order to find better approaches for the management of epilepsy. The current approach for drug development is to identify agents that are effective for treating seizures but not likely to be disease-modifying or anti-epileptogenic as say an antibiotic or chemotherapy for an infection or neoplasms are, respectively. A discussion on future animal models for better AED identification is beyond the scope of this chapter and the reader is referred to other sources for a more comprehensive review of the topic [12].

Complementary and alternative therapy for epilepsy

One strategy for potential benefit for refractory epilepsy is complementary and alternative medicine (CAM). CAM is defined by the National Institutes of Health (NIH) as "those health care and medical practices not currently an integral part of conventional medicine" [13]. It is estimated that anywhere between 42% of the US population, 48% of the Australian population and 70% of the Canadian population use complementary and alternative medicine for various health conditions [13-17]. There are 600 million visits to CAM practitioners per year in the United States at a relative cost of 30 billion dollars which is almost always paid as an out-of-pocket expense [13]. The NIH has created a national center for complementary and alternative medicine at an initial budget of $100M per year to investigate potential therapies [17]. As a result, CAM has obtained a measure of legitimacy.

Several studies have explored the extent of CAM treatments in the United States. Sirven and colleagues surveyed 3100 members of the Epilepsy Foundation in Arizona in one of the first studies to address this issue [18] **(IIb/B)**. The results showed that about 51% had tried CAM for non-seizure-related conditions. These non-seizure-related conditions included memory loss, headaches, chronic pain, diabetes, and prevention of cardiac, cerebrovascular and neurodegenerative diseases. Forty-four percent of the respondents had used CAM specifically for their seizure control.

Several therapies are being used as CAM for seizures in epilepsy. The most commonly cited CAMs included acupuncture, botanical therapies (see also Chapter 11), chiropractic care, magnet therapy, prayer, stress management and yoga. The most commonly cited CAM procedure was prayer with 44% of individuals stating that they use prayer as treatment for their seizures [18] **(IIb/B)**. When asked whether CAM therapy benefited seizures, almost all respondents stated that each of the mentioned CAMs had positively benefited their seizures.

Evidence-based medicine supporting CAM treatments

Table 2 illustrates the available evidence on CAM for epilepsy. No randomized controlled trials have evaluated the efficacy of various CAM treatments for epilepsy. This has been highlighted by several recent reviews on the topic showing the absence of evidence to support CAM efficacy despite the high prevalence of use of these treatments by epilepsy patients [19, 20]. Two Cochrane reviews highlighted this fact in assessing the current state of evidence for CAM treatments for epilepsy [19, 20] **(III/B)**. One Cochrane review examined five studies of yoga, none of which were randomized or controlled [19] **(III/B)**, and the other review evaluated 11 stress management studies [20] **(III/B)**. Stress management studies included aromatherapy, desensitization, relaxation, biofeedback, massage, yoga, and acupuncture. Based on observational data, there appears to be a beneficial effect on seizure frequency related to either yoga or stress management, but there was no level I/A evidence to support the use of either approach. A recent review of CAM treatment efficacy for epilepsy reported high response rates with therapies such as biofeedback, yoga, acupuncture and one

Table 2. Evidence supporting CAM for epilepsy.		
CAM	**Study**	**Level of evidence**
Yoga	Ramaratnam [19]	IV/C
Stress management	Ramaratnam [20]	IV/C

botanical (*Cyanchum porophylum*) [21] (IV/C). However, none of these response rates are based on randomized controlled trials. There is no evidence to support the use of other modalities such as chiropractic care or any of the current botanicals that are used by some patients for the management of epilepsy.

Surgical gap: new devices for epilepsy

There is considerable hope and promise in devices for epilepsy. This section will address two modalities in late-stage pivotal randomized controlled trials. Table 3 addresses the current available evidence for new devices for epilepsy.

Deep brain stimulation for epilepsy

Seizure suppression with electrical stimulation of deep brain structures is effective in animal models using various neural targets including the cerebellum, hippocampus, caudate nucleus, thalamus, subthalamic nucleus (STN), and mammillary nuclei. A randomized controlled trial investigated deep brain stimulation (DBS) of the anterior nucleus of the thalamus (ANT) [22, 23]. One hundred and ten patients were enrolled in the trial and randomized to treatment or control. Bilateral stimulation of the anterior nucleus of the thalamus resulted in a significant (29%) reduction of seizures in the treatment group compared to the placebo group. The effect lasted for at least 2 years [22, 23] (Ib/A).

Animal studies investigating the efficacy of the ANT DBS for epilepsy primarily reflect the work of Mirski and colleagues [24]. Bilateral electrolytic lesions of the tracks connecting the mammillary bodies to the ANT in guinea pigs resulted in essentially complete protection from

Table 3. Evidence supporting novel devices for epilepsy.		
Device	**Study**	**Level of evidence**
Deep brain stimulation of anterior thalamus	SANTE [23]	Ib/A
Closed-loop stimulation of cortex (RNS)	RNS pivotal [28, 29]	Ib/A
Transcranial magnetic stimulation	Vonck [30]	IV/C
Trigeminal nerve stimulation	DeGiorgio [31]	IV/C

pentylenetetrazole-induced seizure activity [24]. This finding was supported by observations of enhanced glucose metabolism in the ANT following administration of both pentylenetetrazole and ethosuximide in guinea pigs [24]. High frequency DBS of the ANT was shown to increase the clonic seizure threshold in a pentylenetetrazole-induced seizure model [25].

The SANTE trial evaluated patients with partial onset epilepsy with or without secondary generalization associated with frequent seizures, resulting in falls, injuries and impaired quality of life, refractory to at least two therapeutically dosed antiepileptic agents for a minimum of 12 to 18 months [22, 23] **(Ib/A)**. Patients were without evidence of progressive neurologic or systemic disease and many had not improved from surgical resection and/or vagal nerve stimulation. Pilot studies showed that there is significant individual variation in outcome but overall bilateral high frequency ANT DBS appears to be safe, well tolerated and effective in some subjects with inoperable refractory epilepsy. In a series of six various pilot studies with up to six patients, the reduction in seizure frequency ranged from 14% to 75% [26] **(III/B)**. The pivotal SANTE trial, as discussed above, however, identified that this modality was useful for refractory epilepsy [22, 23] **(Ib/A)**. Despite this positive trial, the US Federal Drug Administration requested further study. The European Union has approved the device for use in drug-resistant epilepsy.

Closed-loop stimulation in the control of focal epilepsy

The only currently approved device for epilepsy management is vagus nerve stimulation (VNS). VNS is a cyclical type of open loop stimulation that has been shown to reduce seizures with statistical significance **(Ia/A)**. In 1999, a study of brief stimulation of induced afterdischarges showed that induced afterdischarges could be aborted [27]. Based on that study, investigators conceived the possibility that an implanted closed-loop device could both detect and abort epileptiform activity as opposed to the VNS or DBS approach of aborting activity without seizure detection. Currently, there is a device being investigated which is a closed-loop neurostimulation device termed responsive neurostimulation (RNS) [28]. The RNS system is comprised of an implantable pulse generator, depth electrodes and a programmer. The salient features of the RNS system is electrocorticography storage and algorithmic analysis so that ictal EEG recordings from the intracranial electrodes can be detected [28].

The neurostimulator utilizes one of three seizure detection tools, operating on one or two detection channels. The system is designed to detect a seizure when it occurs. The neurostimulator system can then deliver an electrical charge by phasic pulses with amplitude programmable between 0.5 milliamps to 12 milliamps with a duration programmable from 40 to 1000 microseconds at a frequency programmable from 1 to 330Hz [28]. Any of the electric contacts or the pulse generator housing may be programmed as anode or cathode. After a pulse-trained therapy has been delivered, a re-detection algorithm determines if the epileptiform activity is still present and if so up to four additional therapies may be delivered per episode. The neurostimulator system has a built-in charge density limit that allows no more than 25 micro-coulombs\cm^2\phase charge density to be delivered [28].

Recently the RNS investigators reported results from their multi-centered, double-blinded, randomized, controlled pivotal investigation of the RNS system for treatment of intractable partial epilepsy in adults [29] **(Ib/A)**. Eligible subjects were 18 to 70 years of age, had an average of three disabling partial seizures a month, had seizures that failed to improve from two or more antiepileptic medications and had seizure foci localized to one or two regions. Subjects completed a 3-month baseline to determine eligibility based on seizure frequency and were then given the option to have the RNS system neurostimulator leads implanted.

The neurostimulator was programmed to detect data on seizure detection 1 month postoperatively. Subjects were randomized 1:1 to receive sham or active responsive stimulation. Physicians responsible for acquiring data for the primary and secondary safety and efficacy outcomes were blinded to the randomization status. Seizure frequency was considered over the 84 days beginning 2 months after implantation. At completion of this blinded efficacy evaluation period, all subjects were able to receive stimulation until 2 years post-implant, then could transition into a 5-year open-label, long-term treatment trial [29].

As of 2009, 191 subjects had been implanted with the RNS neurostimulator across 29 United States sites. The mean age was 36 years, range 18 to 67, and 48% were female. The mean age of seizure onset was 14 years. Subjects were taking an average of 2.8 AEDs, 34% had previously been treated with VNS and 33% with epilepsy surgery. Sixteen percent had been treated with both VNS and surgery. Sixty percent had prior intracranial monitoring for localization of the epileptic focus [29]. Forty-six percent had ictal onset from mesial temporal structures only and 82% of these subjects had bilateral mesial temporal ictal onsets [29].

The trial demonstrated a statistically significant reduction in seizure frequency in the treatment group as compared to the sham stimulation group. During the last 2 months of the 3-month blinded evaluation period of the study, the treatment group experienced a mean percentage reduction of 29% in their disabling seizures compared to a 14% reduction for those in the sham stimulation group [29] **(Ib/A)**. In the long-term open-label period of the trial at least 12 weeks of data were available for 171 study participants; 47% of these subjects experienced a 50% or greater reduction of their seizure frequency based on their most recent 12 weeks of data as compared to their baseline [29].

The trial also demonstrated a serious adverse event rate less than the comparative surgical procedures. There were no serious, unanticipated device-related adverse events reported in the trial. There were no differences between the treatment and sham stimulation groups when comparing the rates of adverse events, including depression, memory impairment and anxiety. In summary, this particular study showed that there is significant improvement in seizures and is now being considered by the FDA for potential approval for its use in refractory partial epilepsy treatment in the United States.

Other forms of stimulation

Transcranial magnetic stimulation is an extracranial form of neurostimulation therapy that transmits magnetic fields via a coil held over the scalp. This form of stimulation therapy influences both excitatory and inhibitory functions of the cerebral cortex and is currently being investigated as a possible treatment option for refractory epilepsy and depression [30] (III/B). Trigeminal nerve stimulation involves the transcutaneous or subcutaneous stimulation of the infra-orbital or supra-orbital branches of the trigeminal nerve. A small pilot study evaluated the safety and efficacy of trigeminal nerve stimulation among patients with epilepsy and showed that four of seven patients had at least a 50% reduction in seizure frequency after 3 months of trigeminal nerve stimulation without significant pain or discomfort [31] (III/B). Controlled and multicenter studies in larger patient groups are still necessary for all of these emerging therapies before their utility in the treatment of epilepsy can be established.

Summary

There are many therapeutic options which hold promise in the future for closing the treatment gap of epilepsy. The ultimate goal for the management of epilepsy is to completely stop seizures with minimal impact on quality of life from those treatments. It is through rapid and early identification of patients who struggle with epilepsy that aggressive management can be most effective to avert psychosocial problems that are so common to this population. The goal is to determine how we can best utilize and harness the power of technology and science so that we can best improve the lives of our patients who suffer from this disabling condition. Hopefully as we look to the future we will see marked improvements in our approach to closing the treatment gap for those patients with epilepsy. Lastly, although this chapter has focused on the best evidence-based approaches to management of epilepsy, system-based processes need to be considered as well. The financing and access to healthcare are still essential elements for any successful treatment program. It is of no use to develop treatments for epilepsy if they cannot be accessed by all patients who could potentially benefit, regardless of their socioeconomic status. It is only by making certain that the economic and financial barriers to healthcare are erased that the rest of the treatment gaps of epilepsy can be addressed and significant strides can be made at the public health level for the management of epilepsy.

Conclusions

The evidence suggests that reliable diagnostic markers for seizure remission include:

* seizure onset less than 12 years of age;
* infrequent seizures;

- normal examination;
- normal intellectual abilities.

There is an absence of randomized controlled data supporting the use of various CAMs for epilepsy.

There is evidence to support the use of vagus nerve stimulation and deep brain stimulation of the anterior thalamus for refractory epilepsy as adjunctive therapy. There is forthcoming evidence to address the use of the closed-loop stimulation system, RNS, for refractory epilepsy.

Key points	Evidence level
• There are clinical historical biomarkers that predict seizure remission. Absence of these factors may portend a poor prognosis.	Ia/A
• There is an absence of clinical evidence to support the use of CAM for epilepsy.	IV/C
• There is evidence to support the use of vagus nerve stimulation and deep brain stimulation of the anterior thalamus for refractory epilepsy as adjunctive therapy.	Ib/A
• There are forthcoming randomized controlled trials addressing the efficacy of a novel closed-loop system of cortical stimulation for epilepsy.	Ib/A
• There is no current evidence to support the use of transcranial magnetic stimulation or trigeminal nerve stimulation for epilepsy.	IV/C

References

1. Kobau R, Zahran H, Thurman D, *et al*. Epilepsy Surveillance Among Adults - Nineteen States. Behavioral Risk Factor Surveillance Risk System, 2005. Accessed at: www.cdc.gov\mmwr\preview\mmwrhtml\ss5706a1.htm?s_cid=5706al_e.
2. Kwan P, Brodie MJ. Early identification of refractory epilepsy. *N Engl J Med* 2000; 343(19): 1369-77.
3. Kwan P, Arzimanoglou A, Berg AT, *et al*. Definition of drug resistant epilepsy: consensus proposal by the ad hoc Task Force of the ILAE Commission on Therapeutic Strategies. *Epilepsia* 2010; 51(6): 1069-77.
4. Camfield P, Camfield C, Smith S, Dooley S, Smith E. Long-term outcome is unchanged by antiepileptic drug treatment after a first seizure: a 15-year follow-up from a randomized trial in childhood. *Epilepsia* 2002; 43(6): 662-3.
5. Camfield P, Camfield C. Childhood epilepsy: what is the evidence for what we think and what we do? *J Child Neurol* 2003; 18(4): 272-87.
6. Jacobs J, Zijlmani M, Zermane R, *et al*. Value of electrical stimulation and high frequency oscillations (80-500 hz) in identifying epileptogenic areas during intracranial EEG recordings. *Epilepsia* 2010; 51(4): 573-82.
7. Litt B, Estellar R, Echauz J, *et al*. Epileptic seizures may begin hours in advance of clinical onset: a report of 5 patients. *Neuron* 2001; 30: 51-64.

8. Fisher RS, Ho J. Potential new methods for antiepileptic drug delivery. *CNS Drugs* 2002; 16: 579-93.

9. Stein AG, Eder H, Blum D, Drachev A, Fisher R. An automated drug delivery system for focal epilepsy. *Epilepsy Res* 2000; 39: 103-14.

10. Yang XF, Duffy D, Morley R, Rothman S. Neocortical seizure termination by focal cooling: temperature dependence and automated seizure detection. *Epilepsia* 2002; 43: 240-5.

11. Putnam T, Merritt H. Experimental determination of the anticonvulsant properties of some phenyl derivatives. *Science* 1937; 85: 525-6.

12. White HS, Woodhead JH, Wilcox KS, Stables JP, Kupferberg H, Wolf H. Discovery and preclinical development of antiepileptic drugs. In: *Antiepileptic Drugs*. Levy R, Mattson R, Meldrum B, Perucca E, Eds. Philadelphia, USA: Lippincott, 2002: 36-48.

13. Eisenberg DM, Davis RB, Ettner S, *et al.* Trends in alternative medicine use in the United States, 1990-1997: results of a follow-up national survey. *JAMA* 1998; 280: 1569-75.

14. Astin J. Why patients use alternative medicine: results of a national study. *JAMA* 1998; 279: 1548-53.

15. Maclennan A, Wilson D, Taylor A. Prevalence and costs of alternative medicine in Australia. *Lancet* 1996; 347: 569-73.

16. Health Canada. Perspectives on complementary and alternative healthcare. A collection of papers prepared for Health Canada, 1996. Available at: www.hc-sc.gc.ca/hpppb/healthcare/cahc/. Accessed January 2, 2010.

17. National Center for Complementary and Alternative Medicine. Major domains of complementary and alternative medicine, 2006. Available at: http//nccam.nih.gov/health/whatiscam. Accessed January 1, 2010.

18. Sirven J, Drazkowski J, Zimmerman R, Bortz J, Shulman D, Macleish M. Complementary/alternative medicine for epilepsy in Arizona. *Neurology* 2003; 61: 576-7.

19. Ramaratnam S, Sridharan K. Yoga for epilepsy. The Cochrane Library. *Cochrane Database Syst Rev* 1999; 2: CD001524.

20. Ramaratnam S, Baker GA, Goldstein LH. Psychological treatments for epilepsy. The Cochrane Library. *Cochrane Database Syst Rev* 2008; 3: CD002029.

21. Elsas S. Epilepsy. In: *Complementary and Alternative Medicine in Neurology: An Evidence-Based Approach to Clinical Practice*. Oken BS, Ed. London, UK: Informa Healthcare, 2003: 265-77.

22. Lega BC, Halpern C, Jaggi J, Baltuch G. Deep brain stimulation in the treatment of refractory epilepsy: update on current data and future directions. *Neurobiol Dis* 2010; 38(3): 354-60.

23. Fisher R, Salanova V, Witt T, *et al*; SANTE Study Group. Electrical stimulation of the anterior nucleus of thalamus for treatment of refractory epilepsy. *Epilepsia* 2010; 51(5): 899-908.

24. Mirski MA, Ferrendelli J. Interruption of the mamillothalamic tract prevents seizures in guinea pigs. *Science* 1986; 226(4670): 72-4.

25. Mirski M, Rossell L, Terry J, Fisher R. Anticonvulsant effect of anterior thalamic high frequency electrical stimulation in the rat. *Epilepsy Res* 1997; 28(2): 89-100.

26. Casey H, Samodani U, Litt B, Jaggi J, Baltuch G. Deep brain stimulation for epilepsy. In: *Neuromodulation*. Krames ES, Peckham PH, Rezai A. Burlington: Academic Press, 2009: 339-649.

27. Lesser R, Kim S, Beyderman L, *et al.* Brief bursts of pulse stimulation terminate afterdischarges caused by cortical stimulation. *Neurology* 1999; 53(9): 2073-81.

28. Sun F, Morrell M, Wharen R. Responsive cortical stimulation for the treatment of epilepsy. *Neurotherapeutics* 2008; 5(1): 68-74.

29. Morrell M and the RNS System Pivotal Investigators. Results of a multicenter double-blinded randomized controlled pivotal investigation of the RNS System for treatment of intractable partial epilepsy in adults. [abstract]. Presented at the American Epilepsy Society Meeting, Boston, MA, 2009.

30. Vonck K, Boon P, Goossens L, *et al.* Neurostimulation for refractory epilepsy. *Acta Neurol Belg* 2003; 103: 213-7.

31. DeGiorgio C, Shewmon A, Murray D, Whitehurst T. Pilot study of trigeminal nerve stimulation for epilepsy: a proof-of-concept trial. *Epilepsia* 2006; 47: 1213-5.

Chapter 8

Clinically relevant specifications for seizure prediction and detection systems

Ivan Osorio MD
Professor of Neurology
University of Kansas Medical Center
Kansas, USA

Introduction

The clinical practice of epileptology probably more than any other field in neurology (with the notable exception of headaches) relies entirely on subjective, unverifiable and incomplete information (patient diaries) to assess efficacy of treatments and to dictate adjustments either in the type of anti-seizure drug(s) being prescribed or in the dosage(s). No medical approach could be farther from evidence-based than this one. In support of this assertion, one study [1] showed that patients failed to report 55.5% of all recorded seizures (complex partial: 73.2%; simple partial: 26.2%; secondarily generalized: 41.7%) with 85.8% of these seizures occurring during sleep and 32% during wakefulness **(IIb/B)**. Another study [2] reported that only 26% of the patients with epilepsy were always aware of their seizures, including complex partial and secondarily generalized and 30% were never aware of any seizures **(IIb/B)**; these authors concluded that self-reporting of seizures was unreliable and patients reporting the lowest baseline frequency of seizures had the highest fraction of unrecognized seizures. To compound the limitations in the practice of clinical epileptology, the accuracy of seizure descriptions by witnesses is also low and the descriptions also lack objectivity [3] **(IIb/B)**.

The inaccuracy and incompleteness of seizure diaries are mainly due to the fact that complex partial and generalized seizures impair awareness and recent memory leading to under-reporting. Additionally, as documented through prolonged continuous monitoring of subjects with pharmacoresistant seizures undergoing evaluation for epilepsy surgery with intracranial electrodes, a large number of seizures do not cause sensations/feelings nor visible changes in behavior, thus going unnoticed not only by the patient but also by expert observers.

It seems as if clinical epileptology has been built on shifting sands and that it requires proper mooring in the form of accurate metrics that should not be limited to seizure frequency but encompass seizure duration and intensity, as well as inter-seizure interval lengths. These metrics, which are likely to place epileptology on solid ground, must be derived using means for continuous quantification of cortical signals that reflect with high sensitivity and specificity the onset and termination of seizures. Until the past two to three decades, technological limitations precluded the development of portable or implantable devices to quantify seizures in real-time or off-line, but this is no longer the case. However, many other hurdles, not all under the control of epileptologists, lie in the path to development and commercialization of a seizure monitoring device with clinical applicability:

- the requirement that cortical electrical signals be recorded invasively, given their very low signal-to-noise ratio and the fact that only about one third of the cortical mantle, namely, its convexities, is amenable to scalp surveillance, which makes scalp recordings of limited value for seizure detection purposes;
- the high cost (monetary, in human resources and time) of intracranial devices and of the procedures required to safely and properly place them;
- the reluctance of a large group of patients to undergo 'brain surgery' which translates into a relatively small market which does not justify the large monetary investment in clinical studies required to eventually gain approval from regulatory agencies and acceptance by the medical community and patients.

The main objectives of this chapter are to:

- assess the state of the art in automated seizure detection and quantification and in the sub-field of prediction;
- provide criteria for a performance evaluation of a detection algorithm and for valid comparisons; and
- offer directions for expanding the scope of automated seizure detection to increase accessibility to patients by obviating the requirement for invasive brain monitoring.

Automated brain-based seizure detection, quantification and classification

A search in one database (Scirus) for 'automatic seizure detection' yielded 17,679 'hits', numbers that reflect the importance of this endeavor and the interest it sparks across different disciplines outside epileptology, such as engineering, computer sciences, physics and mathematics. Since to date the performance of thousands of seizure detection algorithms has been not carried out using uniform criteria and the same EEG/ECoG database, valid and meaningful comparisons are not pertinent.

In order for the contents of this chapter to be accessible to all readers, the fundamental operations required to detect seizures must be described. The objectives of a seizure detection algorithm are to:

- identify the time of onset and termination of an epileptic seizure and do this in real-time or contemporaneously with the arrival of the signal at the device's processor if automated warning and treatment are desired;
- quantify intensity, duration and extent of spread;
- grade and verify/validate detections;
- log to memory the date, time and relevant characteristics of each detected seizure, and of the actions taken (e.g. warning or delivery of a therapy such as electrical currents).

The steps required to detect seizures are:

- extract from the signal (EEG or ECoG) the ictal 'part' using any tools that are suitable for this purpose such as spectral 'filters'. Figure 1 illustrates the decomposition/filtering of an ECoG signal into its 'ictal' and 'non-ictal' components;

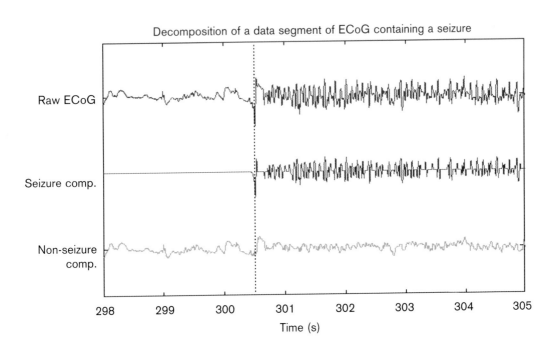

Decomposition of a data segment of ECoG containing a seizure

Figure 1. Decomposition/filtering of the raw signal into its seizure and non-seizure components. The top tracing (blue) is the unprocessed signal recorded from the epileptogenic zone using depth electrodes, showing a seizure with onset at 300.5s. The middle tracing (red) is the filtered seizure component, which in this case is 'zero', prior to onset. The bottom tracing (green) is mainly the non-seizure component.

◆ continuously quantify the ictal content as a function of time by comparing its present value (in a time window) to a past one known to correspond to the non-ictal or inter-ictal state; and

◆ issue a detection when the ictal content reaches or crosses a certain value or 'threshold' (Figure 2).

The intensity of the seizure is calculated by measuring, for example, the area under the curve or its maximal intensity, or computing the product of its duration by the time the ictal content spends above the 'threshold' (Figure 2, inset). The site of origin of a seizure and its

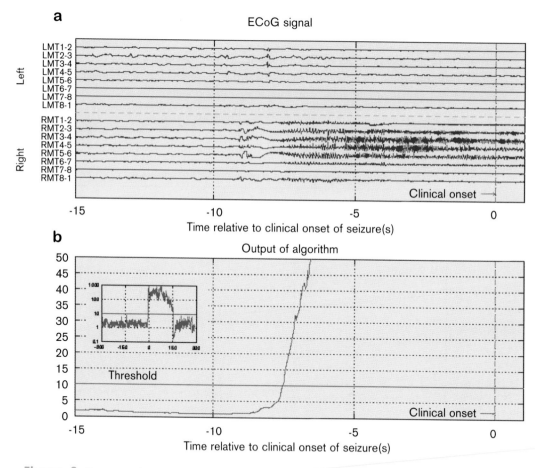

Figure 2. Top panel: Analog tracing of a seizure recorded using depth electrodes. The seizure originates from the right amygdalo-hippocampal region of a subject with pharmacoresistant epilepsy (x-axis: time in sec.; y-axis: electrode labels/locations). Bottom panel: The output of a seizure detection algorithm [5, 6] (red line) remains below the "threshold" (horizontal blue line) until 1 sec. after electrographic onset, at which time it crosses the threshold, signaling the onset of the seizure. The duration of this seizure is approximately 160 sec.; the area under the curve represents both the intensity and duration (x-axis: time in sec.; y-axis: intensity).

extent of spread are given by the location and number of electrode contacts where the ictal content reached or exceeded the pre-specified detection threshold. Details about automated seizure detection and the procedures for individualized algorithm adaptation and performance optimization are described in detail elsewhere [4-7] **(IIb/B)**.

Evidence-based medicine requires that the algorithms' performance be specified in terms of relevant metrics. For seizure detection algorithms (this also applies to prediction algorithms) performance is measured in terms of the following:

◆ sensitivity is defined as the number of seizures detected by the algorithm divided by the total number of seizures (detected and non-detected) over a period of time;
◆ specificity is defined as the number of correct detections (seizures in this case) divided by the total number of detections (correct and incorrect);
◆ speed of detection or the latency (in seconds) between electrographic onset and the issuance of a detection;
◆ computational complexity which may be measured as the number (million) of instructions per second (MIPS) required to make a decision regarding the ictal or non-ictal nature of the activity under consideration. The higher the algorithmic complexity, the higher the MIPS, bus and channel speed, bandwidth, memory speed, memory management techniques and system software required to maintain an adequate throughput. These features impact power consumption, whose magnitude determines the feasibility of implementation into an implantable device and the required battery half-life.

Definition of what range of values is satisfactory or acceptable for sensitivity, specificity and speed of detection features must take into account the clinical application (warning vs. treatment vs. event logging), the therapeutic ratio (narrow or broad) and the seriousness and tolerability of adverse events as well as the psycho-socio-economic profile of the intended user. If the detection algorithm is used exclusively for quantifying seizure frequency and severity, sensitivity and specificity must be the highest attainable (but no less than 90%) and if automated delivery of a treatment is the sole application, sensitivity should be at its highest (so as to treat the maximum number of events) possible, provided that treatment-related adverse events are neither serious nor intolerable; should this not be the case, then specificity of detection (treating only certain seizures) becomes the determining factor and sensitivity must be 'sacrificed'. Speed of detection is only important if the window (following electrographic onset) during which a therapy is efficacious is narrow. Data from a small but rigorously designed and conducted study [8] **(IIa/B)** suggest that in humans the therapeutic window for seizures of mesial temporal and dorsolateral frontal origin is about 5 seconds following electrographic onset. Automated warning for prevention of certain accidents in subjects with epilepsy imposes the stringent and heaviest demands on detection performance as sensitivity, specificity and speed of detection must be optimal. Operation of a motor vehicle, the activity most coveted by epilepsy patients in the US, may be enabled by an automated seizure detection device but possibly only if the sensitivity and specificity of a detection algorithm is consistently perfect (100%) and the warning is sufficiently long to allow the patient to get out of harm's way without endangering others or obstructing traffic. Notification (ex-post facto warning) that a fall to the ground occurred or that a seizure is exceeding its mean or median duration or severity are less exigent but valuable applications that may be more readily implemented than those required for the operation of motor vehicles or power equipment.

Proper evaluation of the performance of seizure detection algorithms must take into consideration that beyond a certain boundary or limit (which is unknown a-priori and possibly unique to each algorithm) improvements in one feature such as sensitivity will inevitably lead to performance degradation in the other(s). Case in point, increases in sensitivity of detection will lead to decreases in specificity and vice versa, and increasing the speed of detection will augment sensitivity but diminish specificity. The optimal choice of detection parameters requires incorporation into the analysis of at least two (sensitivity and specificity) and preferably all three dimensions (sensitivity, specificity and speed of detection) and the use of statistical tools such as receiver operator curves or cluster analysis or of quantitative visualization tools (e.g. surfaces or 3-D structures as in Figure 3).

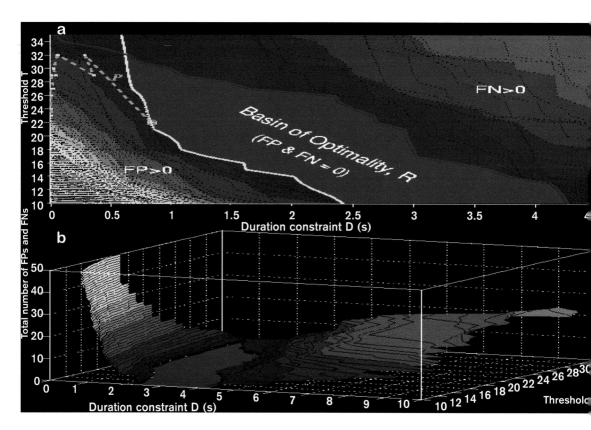

Figure 3. Top panel: Two-dimensional representation of the effects of changing the duration constraint D (x-axis), defined as the time the seizure energy must stay at or above the threshold T, before the algorithm issues a detection vs. the pre-specified value of the threshold T (y-axis) at which the detection is issued. False positive (FP) detections are below and to the left of the lower edge of the basin of optimality (blue region) and false negative (FN) detections are above and to the right of the upper edge of this region. There are no FPs or FNs in the basin of optimality. Bottom panel: 3-D representation of the basin of optimality and its relation to FPs (left wall) and FNs (right wall). Notice that decreases in the duration constraint D (x-axis) increase the number of FPs while increases in the duration of this constraint result in more FNs.

The lack of accurate and relevant seizure metrics has thwarted development of a conceptual framework and of a methodology to investigate the spatio-temporal behavior of seizures at different time scales (days to years) and the efficacy of anti-seizure therapies whether pharmacologic or non-pharmacologic (electrical stimulation, direct drug delivery to brain or application of thermal energy). Traditionally, frequency is the only metric of interest, even though it is obvious that seizures also have intensity (Si), duration (Sd), and extent of spread (Sc). These three variables or dimensions may be conflated into a single measure, *seizure severity*, that is validly represented by their standardized average [8] (Si + Sd + Sc)/3 **(IIa/B)**. Seizure severity takes into account the observation [9] **(IIa/B)** that intensity, duration and extent of spread are inter-correlated: the more intense, the longer the seizure and the longer the seizures, the higher the probability of spread. This and the fact that the distribution of these variables is not normal should influence the selection of tests for statistical analysis of therapeutic clinical trials.

Accurate knowledge of the type of seizures a patient has (simple partial, complex partial, secondarily or primarily generalized), which is not obtainable via seizure diaries [3] **(IIb/B)**, and of their frequency would allow for better assessment of efficacy that may be translated into safer, more efficacious and tolerable treatments. Automated classification of seizures may be accomplished using seizure severity. Preliminary results [6] **(IIb/B)** suggest that the severity as defined above is useful for the clinical classification of seizures into simple partial, complex partial or secondarily generalized as there appears to be a positive correlation between them: simple partial have the lowest, secondarily generalized the highest and complex partial an intermediate severity. A more fruitful and precise approach would be to assess reaction time (simple or complex) and certain other cognitive functions using tests automatically triggered by seizure detections. Complex reaction time tests which provide valuable information about a subject's level of responsiveness are robust against practice/learning effects and are implementable into handheld devices. Precise assessment of the time, degree and duration of cognitive dysfunction is done through measurements of the latencies (in milliseconds) between the presentation of stimuli and the responses (in the form, for example, of a button press) and the percentage of correct responses (type of button pressed) for seizure-triggered compared to interictal tests. Real-time administration of cognitive tests would enable the classification of seizures into two broad classes: associated or not associated with cognitive impairment or loss of awareness. This classification may be further refined by including in the analysis measures of severity based on EEG/ECoG, so that partial may be distinguished from generalized seizures and within partial, simple from complex.

Automated brain-based seizure detection, quantification and classification: assessment of therapeutic efficacy

Brain electrical stimulation (BES) for treatment of pharmacoresistant epilepsies is currently the subject of intense research interest. Two large clinical trials have been completed: one delivers electrical currents periodically to the thalamus [10] **(Ib/A)** and the other contingently to the epileptogenic zone [11] **(Ib/A)**. Despite the long history of use of electrical currents as a tool for probing into the properties of nervous tissue and controlling or modulating its activity, there is limited knowledge about the role that stimulation parameters such as frequency (in Hertz) or intensity (in milli-amperes) play in the triggering or abatement of seizures and whether differences in their relative magnitude (e.g. 'low' [<100Hz] versus 'high' [>100Hz] frequencies) favor seizure triggering or abatement. The most consistent result is that BES at a wide range of frequencies (3-100Hz) will, at certain intensities and under certain conditions, 'kindle' non-epileptogenic tissue in animals [12-14] **(IIa/B)** and trigger afterdischarges and seizures in potentially epileptogenic tissue in humans [15] **(IIa/B)**. However, the fact that at these frequencies (3-100Hz) BES may also suppress afterdischarges and seizures in humans [16-19] **(IIa/B)** and animals [20-23] **(IIb/B)**, makes it difficult to accurately predict its effect, at these frequencies, on epileptogenic neocortex, amygdala and hippocampus. This dual effect (pro-ictal and anti-ictal) suggests the therapeutic ratio of this modality at 3-100Hz could be narrow, making the search for safe, tolerable and efficacious stimulation parameters difficult and lengthy. The practice of BES for seizure control may, in the absence of objective and reproducible measures of seizure severity, be of limited clinical value.

A meta-analysis of the results of contingent delivery of high frequency (>100Hz) electrical currents to the epileptogenic zone (local closed loop) and to the anterior thalamic nuclei (remote closed loop) in humans [8] **(IIa/B)**, while in their totality beneficial, were multifarious intra- and inter-individually. Seizure severity (defined as the standardized average of intensity, duration and extent of spread) and time between seizures was significantly ($p < 0.05$) reduced in certain subjects, increased in others (but significantly only in one subject) and unchanged in some.

The existence of an effect of electrical stimulation that outlasts its duration ('carry-over') on severity and length of time between seizures [8] **(IIa/B)** that may be beneficial (see Figure 4) or deleterious could not have been uncovered without means for quantification of seizure severity. The duration and direction (beneficial or detrimental) of the carry-over effect is quantifiable and may be used to program the timing of delivery of electrical current to the target area(s); delivery of electrical currents may be avoided for the duration of the carry-over effect to minimize adverse reactions, maximize battery life (of an implantable device) while maintaining the protective effect.

The effect of BES which as stated above may be beneficial or detrimental (depending on site of delivery, stimulation parameters used, circadian and other factors) intra- and inter-individually, is not limited to seizure frequency but also to intensity, duration and extent of spread. Thus, therapy optimization (maximization of control and minimization of adverse effects) cannot be effectively nor efficiently accomplished without rigorous quantitative analyses that include clinical and subclinical seizures.

This evidence-based approach to seizure detection, quantification, classification and logging is directly translatable to any therapeutic modality (pharmacological, thermal, etc.) and is not restricted to subjects with pharmacoresistant epilepsies. The possibility of extending automated seizure detection and quantification to patients responsive to drug therapy that for obvious reasons are not candidates for device implantation and the strategies required to accomplish this important objective will be addressed below.

90th percentile of max ratio time-locked to detection (t=120s) (A26058) for both mild/severe seizures

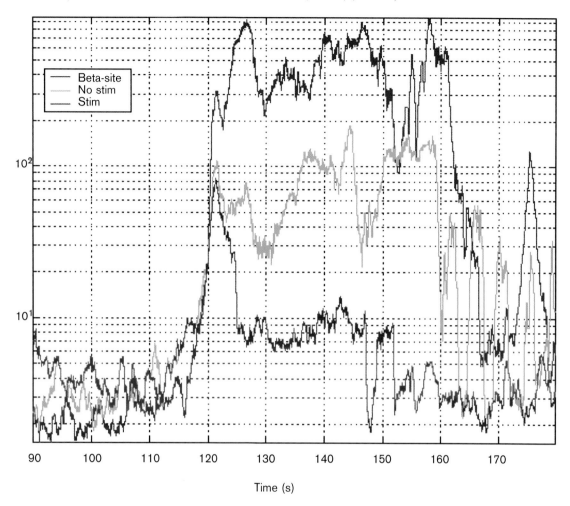

Figure 4. Seizure intensity (y-axis) and duration (x-axis) (same subject, same epileptogenic zone) of a baseline seizure (blue curve), a seizure treated with high frequency currents shortly after onset (red curve) and a seizure in the experimental phase that was not treated (green curve). (The experimental design called for stimulation of every other seizure.) The ability to quantify intensity and duration allowed identification of a 'carry-over' effect: the effect of high frequency stimulation outlasts its duration. This effect while beneficial is inferior to that of stimulation at seizure onset, which may suggest that contingent is superior to periodic stimulation as it not only abates seizures but has a protective effect that outlasts its duration.

It may be concluded that the practice of reliable and relevant evidence-based epileptology will force revisions of currently accepted concepts, strategies and approaches, and will help lay the foundations for the emergence of a clinical science.

Automated brain-based seizure prediction

The early optimism about the feasibility of predicting seizures in real time [24-29] (IIb/B) through the application of non-linear dynamic methods to the ECoG or EEG has been replaced by the sobering realization that these results could not be replicated [30-35] (Ib/A). Much more knowledge about the spatio-temporal behavior of seizures than is currently in existence is required to advance this important subfield.

Automated cardiac-based (EKG) seizure detection

Seizures originating from structures that are part of the central autonomic system [36] (IIa/B), such as the amygdalae and insulae, or from cortical regions that project to these autonomic structures which are distributed throughout the neuraxis, cause changes in heart rate that are not explainable by increases in motor activity, metabolic demands of the body or by changes in arterial gases. The most prominent and readily detectable alterations are cardiac chronotropic and manifest in the majority of seizures as tachycardia [37, 38] (III/B) and rarely as bradycardia [39] (III/B). Of clinical value is the observation that in certain epilepsies, seizure onset may be detected earlier with heart than with cortical electrical signal detection, as tachycardia precedes electrographic or behavioral manifestations [40] (IIb/B).

Heart rate may be measured automatically in real-time using a wide variety of existing algorithms and increases or decreases may be used to detect seizures in lieu of cortical activity (Figure 5). This approach would not only circumvent, in a large number of cases, the one that requires intracranial electrodes in order to overcome the important limitations that make the low yielding scalp recordings impracticable for long-term use, but by virtue of its lower demands on human and technical resources/procedures and consequentially cost, would have widespread applicability, so as to lessen, at a global scale, the medical and socioeconomic seizure burden on patients, their caregivers and the health systems.

Novel anti-seizure epilepsy therapies, dosing regimes and delivery modalities are being developed at a brisk pace, a welcome shift from the prototypical one (round-the-clock, periodic or non-contingent drug administration by mouth or parenterally). However, in order to fulfill their large potential, means to comprehensively and objectively assess their efficacy and proclivity to cause adverse events must be refined and adopted without further delay; it may be said that at this juncture, the medical impact of 21st century technology is being measured using ineffectual tools (patient seizure diaries). While myriad methods for detecting seizures in real time exist, their adoption into clinical practice must await the establishment of standards of performance (false positive and negative rates, speed of detection, computational cost), which require a large high-quality representative database urrently not available. Materialization of these steps will lay out the foundation for evidence-based epileptology and promote its growth into a mature clinical science.

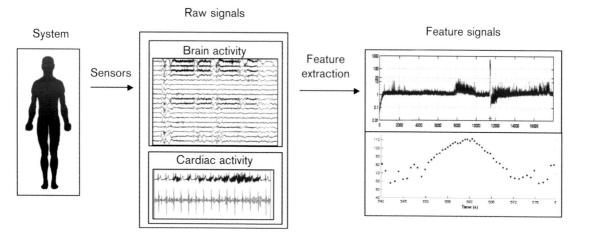

Figure 5. ECoG (middle panel, top graph) and EKG (middle panel bottom graph) recorded from a subject (left panel). Application of detection algorithms to the ECoG (right panel, top graph) and to the EKG (right panel, bottom graph) results in detection of the seizure as seen by the increase in the values of the extracted features.

Conclusions

To conclude, precise quantification of seizure frequency, severity and inter-seizure interval using cerebral or cardiac signals will allow evidence-based assessment of the state of the disease, its evolution and of the efficacy (or adverse effects) of therapeutic interventions. This approach will advance the field of epileptology and benefit patients in a cost-effective manner.

Acknowledgements

The graphics were generated by Mark Frei, PhD.

Key points	Evidence level
◆ Patients' seizure diaries are incomplete and inaccurate.	IIb/B
◆ Automated seizure detection using cortical signals is feasible.	IIb/B
◆ Automated seizure detection is clinically useful.	IIb/B
◆ Automated seizure quantification is feasible.	IIb/B
◆ Automated seizure quantification is clinically useful.	IIb/B
◆ Seizure severity is a clinically useful measure.	IIb/B
◆ Electrical stimulation triggers seizures.	Ia/A
◆ Electrical stimulation decreases seizure frequency.	Ib/A
◆ Automated seizure detection using heart rate is feasible.	III/B
◆ Automated seizure detection using heart rate is useful.	III/B

References

1. Hoppe C, Poepel A, Elger CE. Epilepsy: accuracy of patient seizure counts. *Arch Neurol* 2007; 64: 1595-9.
2. Blum DE, Eskola J, Bortz JJ, Fisher RS. Patient awareness of seizures. *Neurology* 1996; 47: 260-4.
3. Mannan JB, Wieshmann UC. How accurate are witness descriptions of epileptic seizures? *Seizure* 2003; 12: 444-7.
4. Qu H, Gotman J. Improvement in seizure detection performance by automatic adaptation to the EEG of each patient. *Electroencephalogr Clin Neurophysiol* 1993; 86: 79-87.
5. Osorio I, Frei MG, Wilkinson SB. Real-time automated detection and quantitative analysis of seizures and short-term prediction of clinical onset. *Epilepsia* 1998; 39: 615-27.
6. Osorio I, Frei MG, Giftakis J, *et al.* Performance reassessment of real-time seizure-detection algorithm on long ECoG series. *Epilepsia* 2002; 43: 1522-35.
7. Haas SM, Frei MG, Osorio I. Strategies for adapting automated seizure detection algorithms. *Med Eng Phys* 2007; 29: 895-909.
8. Osorio I, Frei MG, Sunderam S, *et al.* Automated seizure abatement in humans using electrical stimulation. *Ann Neurol* 2005; 57(2): 258-68.
9. Sunderam S, Osorio I, Frei MG. Epileptic seizures are temporally interdependent under certain conditions. *Epilepsy Res* 2007; 76: 77-84.
10. Fisher R, Salanova V, Witt T, *et al.* Electrical stimulation of the anterior nucleus of thalamus for treatment of refractory epilepsy. *Epilepsia* 2010; 51: 899-908.
11. Barkley GL, Smith B, Bergey G, *et al.* Safety and preliminary efficacy of a responsive neurostimulator. *Neurology* 2006; (Suppl 2): A387.
12. Goddard GV, McIntyre DC, Leech CK. A permanent change in brain function resulting from daily electrical stimulation. *Exp Neurol* 1969; 25: 295-330.
13. Corcoran ME, Cain DP. Kindling of seizures with low-frequency electrical stimulation. *Brain Res* 1980; 196: 262-5.
14. Lothman EW, Williamson JM. Influence of electrical stimulus parameter on afterdischarge threshold in the rat hippocampus. *Epilepsy Res* 1992; 13: 205-13.
15. Penfield W, Jasper H. Electrical stimulation and afterdischarge. In: *Epilepsy and the Functional Anatomy of the Human Brain*. Boston, MA: Little Brown, 1954: 200-8.
16. Lesser RP, Kim SH, Beyderman DL, *et al.* Brief bursts of pulse stimulation terminate afterdischarges caused by cortical stimulation. *Neurology* 1999; 53: 2073-91.
17. Kinoshita M, Ikeda R, Matsumoto R, *et al.* Electric stimulation on human cortex suppresses fast cortical activity and epileptic spikes. *Epilepsia* 2004; 48: 1560-67.

18. Kerrigan JF, Litt B, Fisher RS, *et al.* Electrical stimulation of the anterior nucleus of the thalamus for the treatment of intractable epilepsy. *Epilepsia* 2004; 45: 346-54.

19. Andrade DM, Zumsteg D, Hamani C, *et al.* Long-term follow-up of patients with thalamic deep brain stimulation for epilepsy. *Neurology* 2006; 66: 1571-3.

20. Gaito J, Nobrega JN, Gaito ST. Interference effect of 3Hz stimulation on kindling behavior induced by 60Hz stimulation. *Epilepsia* 1980; 21: 73-84.

21. Gaito J. The effect of variable duration one hertz interference on kindling. *Can J Neurol Sci* 1980; 7: 59-64.

22. Ullal GR, Ninchoji T, Uemura K. Low frequency stimulation induces an increase in after-discharge threshold in hippocampal and amygdaloid kindling. *Epilepsy Res* 1989; 3: 232-5.

23. Weiss SR, Eidsath A, Li XL, Heynen T, Post RMI. Quenching revisited: low level direct current inhibition inhibits amygdale-kindled seizures. *Exp Neurol* 1998; 154: 185-92.

24. Lehnertz K, Elger CE. Can epileptic seizures be predicted - evidence from nonlinear time series analysis of brain electrical activity. *Phys Rev Lett* 1998; 80: 5019-22.

25. Martinerie J, Adam C, Quyen MLV, *et al.* Epileptic seizures can be anticipated by nonlinear analysis. *Nature Med* 1998; 4: 1173-6.

26. Litt B, Esteller R, Echauz J, *et al.* Epileptic seizures may begin hours in advance of clinical onset: a report of five patients. *Neuron* 2001; 30: 51-64.

27. Litt B, Echauz J. Prediction of epileptic seizures. *Lancet Neurology* 2002; 1: 22-30.

28. Iasemidis LD, Shiau DS, Chaovalitwongse W, *et al.* Adaptive epileptic seizure prediction system. *IEEE Trans Biomed Eng* 2003; 50: 616-27.

29. Iasemidis LD, Pardalos PM, Shiau DS, *et al.* Prediction of human epileptic seizures based on optimization and phase changes of brain electrical activity. *Optimization Methods & Software* 2003; 18: 81-104.

30. Osorio I, Harrison MAF, Lai Y-C, Frei MG. Observations on the application of the correlation dimension and correlation integral to the prediction of seizures. *J Clin Neurophysiol* 2001; 18: 269-74.

31. Lai Y-C, Harrison MAF, Frei MG, Osorio I. Inability of Lyapunov exponents to predict epileptic seizures. *Phys Rev Lett* 2003; 91: 068102.

32. Lai YC, Harrison MAF, Frei MG, Osorio I. Reply to comment on 'Inability of Lyapunov exponents to predict epileptic seizures'. *Phys Rev Lett* 2005; 94: 019802.

33. Harrison MAF, Osorio I, Frei MG, Asuri S, Lai Y-C. Correlation dimension and integral do not predict epileptic seizures. *Chaos* 2005; 15: 033106.

34. Harrison MA, Frei MG, Osorio I. Accumulated energy revisited. *Clin Neurophysiol* 2005; 116: 527-31.

35. Mormann F, Andrzejak RG, Elger CE, Lehnertz K. Seizure prediction: the long and winding road. *Brain* 2007; 130(Pt 2): 314-33.

36. Saper CB. The central autonomic nervous system: conscious visceral perception and autonomic pattern generation. *Annu Rev Neurosci* 2002; 25: 433-69.

37. Leutmezer F, Schernthaner C, Lurger S, Potzelberger K, Baumgartner C. Electrocardiographic changes at the onset of epileptic seizures. *Epilepsia* 2003; 44: 348-54.

38. Zijlman M, Flanagan D, Gotman J. Heart rate changes and ECG abnormalities during epileptic seizures: prevalence and definition of an objective clinical sign. *Epilepsia* 2002; 43: 847-54.

39. Tinuper P, Bisulli F, Cerullo A, *et al.* Ictal bradycardia in partial epileptic seizures. Autonomic investigation in three cases and literature review. *Brain* 2001; 124: 2361-71.

40. Di Gennaro G, Quarato PP, Sebastiano F, *et al.* Ictal heart rate increase precedes EEG discharge in drug-resistant mesial temporal lobe seizures. *Clin Neurophysiol* 2004; 115: 1169-77.

Chapter 9

Reducing the risks of SUDEP: what do we know about risk factors and the prevention of SUDEP?

José F. Téllez Zenteno MD PhD, Associate Professor
Lizbeth Hernandez-Ronquillo MD MSc, Research Co-ordinator, Epilepsy Program
University of Saskatchewan, Division of Neurology
Department of Medicine, Royal University Hospital
Saskatoon, Canada

Introduction

Sudden unexpected death in epilepsy (SUDEP) is probably the most common direct epilepsy-related cause of death. It has long been recognized that patients with epilepsy may die suddenly and unexpectedly, often in relation to a seizure. The scientific interest in SUDEP has increased markedly during the last decade. Several suggestions have been made concerning the mechanisms behind SUDEP, most involving theories on the possible role of autonomic effects of ictal and interictal epileptiform activity, such as cardiorespiratory disturbances. Although the mechanisms remain unclear, there is a growing body of information concerning the epidemiology of SUDEP. The objective of this chapter is to review data on risk factors of SUDEP and their potential translation to prevention measures.

Overall mortality rates in people with epilepsy and risk factors

The standard mortality ratio (SMR) is the ratio of observed deaths to expected deaths in a defined population. SMR is age- and gender-adjusted to a standard population and is the most widely used method to express and measure mortality. The SMR in epilepsy ranges between 1.2 and 9.3 and depends on study methods and population [1]. Population-based studies showed a lower SMR than hospital- or clinic-based studies [1]. Although the reported range of SMRs in epilepsy is broad, some observations emerge:

- the highest SMRs are reported in children (likely reflecting the low baseline mortality rate in children) [2-5];
- the largest excess of deaths occurs in the elderly [1, 4];
- idiopathic epilepsies have lower SMRs (SMR 1.1-1.9) than symptomatic epilepsies (SMR 2.2-6.5);
- mortality is highest if there is neurological impairment since birth (SMRs 11-25) [1, 4, 6];
- acute symptomatic seizures carry a higher risk than remote symptomatic seizures [6];
- the risk of death is highest early after diagnosing epilepsy and decreases over time [1, 5, 6];
- the risk is higher in males than in females [4]. It should be noted that most data on mortality in epilepsy derive from industrialized countries. Data from developing countries are difficult to interpret because ascertaining deaths due to epilepsy and performing prospective studies is difficult in these populations [7].

The information that proves that mortality is increased in patients with epilepsy versus different types of controls is solid and comes from well-designed controlled studies (IIa/B & IIb/B).

Cause-specific mortality in epilepsy

Deaths in epilepsy may be due to the underlying cause of epilepsy, to seizures or epilepsy directly, or to factors unrelated to epilepsy [4]. The main factors contributing to epilepsy mortality relate to the causes of epilepsy, e.g. cerebrovascular disorders, degenerative disorders and cancer [1, 4, 5]. Seizure- or epilepsy-related causes include sudden unexpected death in epilepsy (SUDEP), status epilepticus, infections such as pneumonia and accidents or injuries directly related to seizures [5, 8]. This chapter analyzes the best available information on risk factors and potential prevention measures for SUDEP.

Definition of SUDEP

There are some difficulties that make the concept of a definition of SUDEP complicated. The main limitations are the lack of a pathological cause of death in the majority of cases and the unwitnessed nature of many SUDEP deaths [9]. SUDEP has been defined as "sudden, unexpected, witnessed or unwitnessed, non-traumatic, and non-drowning death of patients with epilepsy with or without evidence of a seizure, excluding documented status epilepticus, and in whom post mortem examination does not reveal a structural or toxicological cause for death" [10]. This definition is well recognized, although it is not universally used by physicians and is mainly used for clinical research studies. The definition has been criticized because it can exclude potentially life-threatening concomitant pathological processes. On the other hand when the definition is used for clinical research and the autopsy has not been done and the collection of information is retrospective it could produce biases in studies. The definition of SUDEP has been obtained from expert committee reports or opinions and/or clinical experience of respected authorities (IV/C).

Epidemiology of SUDEP

A classical population-based study from Rochester, Minnesota, reported that the rate of SUDEP was higher compared with the general population, reporting a SMR of 23.7 (95% CI, 7.7-55.0). The incidence of SUDEP is highly variable and depends on the studied population. SUDEP is the most common seizure-related cause of death in adolescents and young adults (SMR of 24) [4, 11]. SUDEP rates range between 0.09/1000 patient-years in newly diagnosed or community populations, to 10/1000 patient-years in candidates for epilepsy surgery [1, 4, 5, 6, 9, 11, 12]. SUDEP is less common in children (0.11 to 0.43 per 1000 person-years) [11, 13] and common in patients from epilepsy clinics, patients included in drug trials and patients with learning difficulties (2.0 to 4.9 per 1000 person-years) [14]. Currently the evidence regarding epidemiology of SUDEP can be categorized as grade B – well-conducted clinical studies but no randomized clinical trials on the topic of recommendations (IIa/B, IIb/B and III/B). There is a well-conducted systematic review by Téllez-Zenteno *et al* [9] **(Ia/A)** that analyzed in a comprehensive way the available evidence of the incidence of SUDEP, as well as a recent non-systematic review of the literature by Tomson *et al* [11] assessing epidemiological aspects of SUDEP.

Assessment of risk factors for SUDEP

Different types of methodologies have been used in the medical literature to explore risk factors for SUDEP. In the early years, several case reports of patients with SUDEP were published [9]. These studies helped to recognize the phenomenon of SUDEP and were useful in creating a definition over the years. Unfortunately these studies cannot provide strong evidence regarding risk factors and it is not adequate to reach conclusions with these types of studies [9]. The vast majority of the studies published in the literature of SUDEP are case-control studies. Some characteristics of SUDEP such as the low incidence of the disease with the necessity of prolonged periods of follow-up to have adequate sample sizes makes case-control studies the best strategy to asses risk factors. Most of the case-control studies on SUDEP share the same methodological problems, such as different definitions of SUDEP, different types of controls and lack of adequate analyses to express the results [9]. The retrospective nature of these studies makes difficult the ascertainment of SUDEP definitions, being one of the most consistent biases in these studies. On the other hand, the controls used in studies are not consistent, making the interpretation of data complex. Probably the strongest methodology to assess risk factors is cohort studies, although few prospective studies have been published. These types of studies can ascertain better the definition of SUDEP and the definition of case; however, they share the same biases as case-control studies regarding the type of controls and the lack of an adequate analysis to express the results [9].

Controls used in studies of SUDEP

When exploring risk factors for SUDEP, the choice of controls is important. A well-conducted systematic review identified that half of the published studies used as controls non-SUDEP deaths and the other half used living patients with epilepsy [9]. Comparisons with non-SUDEP deaths in epilepsy may best explore the circumstances surrounding death (e.g. seizures preceding death, place of death, antiepileptic drug [AED] levels at the time of death). On the other hand, comparisons with living patients with epilepsy explore best lifestyle and clinical variables that may contribute to SUDEP (e.g. frequency of seizures, number of AEDs, use of other drugs) [9]. Therefore, different risk factors uncovered by studies with different comparators are not necessarily contradictory or mutually exclusive, but rather complementary to the complex clinical profile of this condition.

Reported risk factors with non-SUDEP deaths

Epidemiological studies often point to possible causes of disease or death, which can then be subjected to further exploration. Despite their methodological limitations, studies on SUDEP provide a coherent constellation of several risk factors whose mechanisms are not yet well understood, but can help to create preventive measures for SUDEP.

Studies using non-SUDEP deaths (see Table 1) suggest that SUDEP preferentially affects patients with the following characteristics: young adults, with subtherapeutic levels of AEDs, with primary generalized epilepsy, with early epilepsy onset and short duration of epilepsy, and finally the death has been seen more frequently in bed, in the prone position and with evidence of a terminal seizure [15-20]. Some of these factors are consistent across studies and explore the circumstances surrounding the death. With these observations it is possible to put together some assumptions regarding the profile of patients that can experience SUDEP, such as patients with poor adherence to antiepileptic medications and evidence of intense generalized tonic-clonic seizures that could be in the context of epilepsy or potentially related with lack of compliance. The short duration of epilepsy is an interesting association and should bring the attention of the physician to the possible prevention of SUDEP in patients with a new diagnosis of epilepsy. Other associations such as the death happening more frequently in bed need further exploration.

Studies using living patients with epilepsy (see Table 2) suggest that SUDEP preferentially affects people with mental retardation, generalized epilepsy, use of carbamazepine, a history of frequent seizures, males, and those on polytherapy [21-30]. The information provided in cohort studies using living patients delivers a different profile of patients with risk for SUDEP. The analyzed risk factors clearly reflect the profile of patients with intractable epilepsy. This observation is important because one of the suggested measures to prevent mortality in patients with intractable epilepsy is early epilepsy surgery, as some authors have shown that epilepsy surgery reduces mortality [31].

The observation regarding idiopathic generalized epilepsy is consistent across studies with non-SUDEP deaths and living patients with epilepsy [28]. This observation is relevant because the predisposition to have generalized tonic-clonic seizures is higher in patients with idiopathic generalized epilepsy compared with focal epilepsy, being in many patients with

Table 1. Risk factors for SUDEP in studies using non-SUDEP deaths as controls.

Authors	Design	Risk factor present
Leestma [17]	Case-control	Younger age and shorter duration of epilepsy
George and Davis [15]	Case-control	Subtherapeutic level of AEDs
Opeskin [18]	Case-control	None
Opeskin [19]	Prospective	Female gender, death more commonly in bed, evidence for terminal seizure
Kloster [16]	Case-control	Young age at onset, primary generalized seizures, prone body position at death
Schnabel [20]	Case-control	Young age
Vlooswijk [32]	Prospective	Younger age at death, earlier epilepsy onset, shorter duration of epilepsy

The evidence regarding risk factors can be categorized as grade B – well-conducted clinical studies but no randomized clinical trials on the topic of recommendations (evidence levels IIa/B, IIb/B and III/B)

generalized epilepsy the only type of seizures that they experience. On the other hand some patients with partial epilepsy and a high tendency to have secondarily generalized seizures such as frontal epilepsy could have the same implication. To a clinician these associations are important, because it is possible to identify certain groups of patients with an increased risk of SUDEP and thereby design potentially preventive measures. Another association that has been consistent between studies is the increased risk of SUDEP in patients with mental retardation or learning disabilities [19]. This observation is also relevant and allows the possibility to identify some groups of patients with a higher risk of SUDEP, such as patients with Lennox-Gastaut syndrome, and other groups of patients with epilepsy and learning disabilities.

The association of carbamazepine and other antiepileptic medications such as lamotrigine with SUDEP is controversial. Carbamazepine has been shown to suppress both parasympathetic and sympathetic functions in newly diagnosed patients with epilepsy, with potential implications in SUDEP [33]. Lamotrigine has the potential to inhibit the delayed rectifier potassium ion current, a property that has been linked to increased risk of QT prolongation, cardiac arrhythmia, and sudden death for other drug classes. However,

Table 2. Risk factors for SUDEP in studies using living patients with epilepsy.

Authors	Design	Risk factor present
Jick [23]	Case-control	Mental retardation
Timmings [28]	Retrospective audit	Males, idiopathic generalized epilepsy and use of carbamazepine
Walczak [29]	Prospective	One to three generalized tonic-clonic seizures, duration of epilepsy >30 years, >2 AEDs, IQ <70
Beran [21]	Case-control study	Polytherapy
Langan [24]	Prospective	History of GTCSs, frequent GTCSs, four AEDs ever used, no use of AEDs, current use of CBZ, no supervision at night
Williams [30]	Prospective	Greater variability in AED concentrations
Hitiris [22]	Case-control study	Early onset of epilepsy <15 years, seizure within the last year
Nilsson [26]	Case-control study	Two seizures per year, polytherapy with AEDs, onset of epilepsy <15 years, two changes of AEDs per year
Nilsson [27]	Case-control study	Higher concentrations of carbamazepine
McKee [25]	Case-control study	Frequent seizures, polytherapy, non-ambulatory status

The evidence regarding risk factors can be categorized as grade B – well-conducted clinical studies but no randomized clinical trials on the topic of recommendation (evidence levels IIa/B, IIb/B and III/B)

lamotrigine use does not seem to result in prolonged QT intervals [34]. The association of SUDEP and some drugs is difficult to support with well-known pathological mechanisms, being at the moment an observation with less significance than others.

One of the main theories to explain SUDEP is the reported association between cardiorespiratory dysfunction and SUDEP [11]. Although the cardiorespiratory dysfunction theory is the main explanation of SUDEP, this risk factor has not been assessed systematically in case-control studies. The main support of this theory comes from basic research and for now the epidemiological information does not completely support this theory.

Currently the evidence regarding risk factors can be categorized as grade B – well-conducted clinical studies but no randomized clinical trials on the topic of recommendations (IIa/B, IIb/B and III/B). As we have reviewed in this chapter, all the available studies are case-control studies, retrospective cohorts and a few prospective cohorts. There is a well-conducted systematic review by Téllez-Zenteno *et al* [9] (Ia/A) that analyzed in a comprehensive way the available evidence of risk factors of SUDEP; also, there is a recent non-systematic review of the literature by Tomson *et al* [11] assessing different aspects of SUDEP, including risk factors for SUDEP.

Direct observation of SUDEP or near-SUDEP cases

Four SUDEP cases have been reported during electroencephalographic (EEG) monitoring and two cases were monitored at the time of a near-SUDEP, with successful resuscitation of cardiorespiratory arrest [35-39]. From the SUDEP cases identified during EEG monitoring, some observations could be linked with the risk factors identified in clinical studies. All cases occurred during or immediately after a partial seizure, but more commonly after a secondarily generalized seizure. This observation could support previous research where SUDEP was more commonly associated in patients with generalized seizures. In three cases, an EEG with complete suppression of brain activity was seen before any fatal cardiac or respiratory arrest, followed by cessation of brain activity. This finding could be related to the intensity of the seizure but is also the type of EEG finding commonly seen in patients with anoxia, suggesting the possibility of severe hypoxic brain injury after intense seizures. There is only one case where SUDEP was related to a seizure-triggered ventricular fibrillation followed by terminal asystole in a patient with a past history of myocardial infarction and angina. In the near-SUDEP cases, pulmonary dysfunction (apnea, either central and postictal or ictal and obstructive) was considered to be the primary dysfunction that later led to cardiac arrest [38, 39]. The information derived from these cases suggests that different seizure-induced interrelated mechanisms might contribute to SUDEP, including primary cerebral shutdown, cardiac arrhythmia, and central or obstructive apnea. The information derived from direct observation of SUDEP or near-SUDEP cases can be categorized as III/B, being based only on case reports.

Proposed mechanisms for SUDEP

Proposed mechanisms for SUDEP include cardiac, respiratory and autonomic dysfunction. In a detailed analysis, So [40] hypothesizes that these mechanisms are not independent of each other, but are rather interrelated contributors to SUDEP.

Some post mortem studies in patients with SUDEP have found fibrotic changes in the deep and subendocardial myocardium, increased lung weight, and pulmonary congestion [40]. Similarly, central or obstructive apnea or hypoxia occur commonly during or after seizures [40], postictal central apnea was documented in a case of near-SUDEP [40], and midbrain serotoninergic pathways may be implicated [40].

Reduced heart rate variability has been documented in animal seizure models and in persons with epilepsy, and it is associated with sudden death in those with myocardial infarction and heart failure [40]. Analyses of heart rate during seizures in SUDEP patients and non-SUDEP controls found that in SUDEP victims, heart rate increased more during nocturnal than during awake seizures [40].

Methodological problems of studies in SUDEP and inherent properties of SUDEP that make clinical research difficult

There are some characteristics of SUDEP that make it difficult to research. The first difficulty is the low incidence of this phenomenon. The possibility to perform prospective cohorts with a reasonable number of patients is complex due to the low rate of SUDEP in patients with epilepsy. Because of the low occurrence of SUDEP, the majority of the current published studies are case-control studies, which is the recommended methodology for these circumstances [9]. Another problem is the definition of SUDEP. The main bias in case-control studies is the ascertainment of the definition of SUDEP. The definition has changed over the years and it is difficult to assess when the review of cases is retrospective. This bias produces misclassification of cases and potential report of non-real risk factors. Another bias in the literature of SUDEP is the use of controls. As mentioned before in this chapter, the use of two types of controls gives an interesting picture of risk factors surrounding the death and regarding the profile of patients. Probably the only aspect that has not been completely explored in case-control studies is the potential use of different types of controls with epilepsy, differentiating cases with mild and severe epilepsy.

Prevention based on identified risk factors

Preventing mortality in epilepsy and specifically in SUDEP is challenging because the mechanisms are poorly understood, and because mortality is often related to the underlying cause of epilepsy. Even when the evidence is not consistent across studies, some observations can lead to recommendations as well as the design, study and implementation of prevention measures. High seizure frequency is an important risk factor for SUDEP, emphasizing the importance of complete seizure control [4]. Also, the avoidance of some known risk factors for SUDEP such as lack of adherence to AEDs and sleeping in the prone position could help to prevent this condition [11]. The only interventions subjected to rigorous analysis are epilepsy surgery and supervision. Epilepsy surgery lowers the risk of death in those who become seizure-free after surgery, but not all reports agree on this [14, 41]. The preventive aspects of supervision pertain to risk factors for SUDEP. In addition, mortality was higher in a cohort with learning disabilities when they were visiting their homes compared to when they were in a residential setting with supervision [11]. Education of physicians, caregivers, patients and, in general, people involved in the care of patients with epilepsy is a measure that can potentially prevent SUDEP, mainly by identifying populations at risk and in the modification of potential risk factors. In Table 3 we summarize some preventive measures for SUDEP. The information regarding prevention measures can be graded as IV/C, because this has been generated from expert committee reports or opinions and/or clinical experience of respected authorities [42]. We do not have guidelines regarding the prevention of SUDEP. The lack of information on this topic is also due to the fact that the full spectrum of risk factors related to SUDEP is not known.

Table 3. Potential preventive measures that may decrease SUDEP based on identified risk factors.

Measure	Risk factor addressed
Antiepileptic drugs: avoid poly-pharmacy and ensure compliance	To reduce seizure frequency
Avoidance of seizure triggers	To reduce seizure frequency
Nocturnal supervision (by sharing bedrooms or using nocturnal monitoring devices)	To ensure that nocturnal seizures are promptly identified, so that proper positioning can occur and cardiorespiratory difficulties can be promptly addressed
Communication of preventive measures to patients, caregivers and physicians	To identify groups with a high risk of SUDEP To ensure that potential risk factors for SUDEP are known by caregivers
No formal recommendations or guidelines have been published regarding prevention measures for SUDEP	

Communicating with patients, caregivers and clinicians

Discussing the risk of death with individuals with epilepsy and their families is challenging, because no definitive interventions exist to reduce mortality, and because mechanisms are not known. Clinicians should encourage patients with epilepsy to lead a normal life, but they also need to guide their patients through well-informed clinical decision-making processes in a timely manner. In some cases bringing up the topic of increased mortality can result in significant psychological distress to patients and families, and an unnecessary restriction of normal activities. After reviewing the evidence, a Joint Task Force on SUDEP of the American

Epilepsy Society and the Epilepsy Foundation [42] recommended discussing SUDEP with patients and their families and caregivers at a time when the patient is deemed to be ready to receive such information. However, they acknowledged that no information is available to guide health care professionals on how SUDEP information can best be provided. The information regarding communication of preventive measures for SUDEP for patients, caregivers and physicians can be graded as IV/C, because it has been generated from expert committee reports or opinions and/or clinical experience of respected authorities [42] given that we do not have guidelines on this topic.

Future research

Currently most of the studies have identified risk factors related to poorly controlled epilepsy. Some questions should be addressed in the future. For example, few clinical studies have explored in a comprehensive way the risk associated with individual predisposition, comorbidity of patients and lifestyles of individuals with epilepsy. Also, we need to understand what distinguishes people with chronic epilepsy who die suddenly from those who do not. In the future, studies should use other types of controls, with epilepsy probably graded by severity in order to confirm reported associations and explore other factors. Potential groups of patients with epilepsy that can be used as controls are patients with refractory epilepsy who are either surgical or not surgical candidates, patients with generalized versus focal epilepsy and patients with well-controlled epilepsy. Also, potential research evaluating the tissues of patients, including brain, heart and lungs, exploring new mechanisms of diseases such as channelopathies is advised and likely to occur in the following years. Currently, some risk factors have been identified and in the future, studies assessing prevention measures are a necessity. Probably one of the most suitable areas for clinical research in prevention of SUDEP is the educational aspect of SUDEP. With the constellation of risk factors that are currently known, potential cohort studies assessing interventions such as educating patients or physicians are interesting topics for research in the future. Considering that one of the most at-risk groups are patients with intractable epilepsy, further studies assessing epilepsy surgery and other treatments specifically focused on the prevention of SUDEP are welcome. Finally, we have to recognize that prevention of SUDEP is an important aspect but more research on risk factors is still needed in the future to understand the whole spectrum of SUDEP.

Conclusions

Although recent epidemiological studies have been helpful in identifying the patient at risk and have provided clues as to the mechanisms behind SUDEP, there is no single risk factor common to all cases, which suggests multiple mechanisms or trigger factors. Clinicians counseling patients and their families regarding SUDEP can draw on the summary evidence of incidence and risk factors in various populations. Parents of children and patients with mild, well-controlled epilepsy can be reassured. Depending on the readiness of patients, awareness should be cautiously raised in high-risk populations, emphasizing the implementation of measures that may minimize risk, such as optimization of medical and surgical therapy and adherence to AED therapy, and the importance of striving for seizure freedom.

Key points	Evidence level
◆ The information about mortality is consistent showing an increase in mortality rates in people with epilepsy compared with the general population and different types of populations without epilepsy.	IIa/B, IIb/B, & III/B
◆ The definition of SUDEP has been generated mainly from expert committee reports. There is no formal validation of the definition.	IV/C
◆ There are a fair number of studies describing the incidence of SUDEP in different types of populations. The incidence is high in some groups of patients with epilepsy, such as candidates for epilepsy surgery, patients from epilepsy clinics and participants of drug trials, and patients with learning difficulties.	IIa/B, IIb/B, & III/B
◆ Almost all the reported risk factors are derived from case-control studies. Case-control studies using non-SUDEP deaths in epilepsy may best explore the circumstances surrounding death (e.g. seizures preceding death, place of death, AED levels at the time of death). On the other hand, comparisons with living patients with epilepsy explore best lifestyle and clinical variables that may contribute to SUDEP (e.g. frequency of seizures, number of AEDs, use of other drugs).	IIa/B, IIb/B, & III/B
◆ Reported risk factors for SUDEP are the following: young adults, with subtherapeutic levels of AEDs, with primary generalized epilepsy, with early epilepsy onset and short duration of epilepsy, prone position with evidence of a terminal seizure, mental retardation, males, polytherapy, generalized epilepsy and a history of frequent seizures.	IIa/B, IIb/B, & III/B
◆ The information about preventive measures of SUDEP is very preliminary and it is supported on identified risk factors. Although we know many risk factors for SUDEP, the whole spectrum of risk factors is not known; therefore, no guidelines about prevention have been forthcoming.	IV/C
◆ Communication of preventive measures of SUDEP for patients, caregivers and physicians is currently a controversial topic due to the lack of guidelines.	IV/C

References

1. Hitiris N, Mohanraj R, Norrie J, Brodie MJ. Mortality in epilepsy. *Epilepsy Behav* 2007; 10(3): 363-76.
2. Appleton RE. Mortality in paediatric epilepsy. *Arch Dis Child* 2003; 88(12): 1091-94.
3. Berg A. Mortality in epilepsy. *Epilepsy Curr* 2001; 1(1): 28.
4. Forsgren L, Hauser WA, Olafsson E, Sander JW, Sillanpaa M, Tomson T. Mortality of epilepsy in developed countries: a review. *Epilepsia* 2005; 46 Suppl 11: 18-27.
5. Tomson T, Beghi E, Sundqvist A, Johannessen SI. Medical risks in epilepsy: a review with focus on physical injuries, mortality, traffic accidents and their prevention. *Epilepsy Res* 2004; 60(1): 1-16.
6. Beghi E, Leone M, Solari A. Mortality in patients with a first unprovoked seizure. *Epilepsia* 2005; 46 Suppl 11: 40-2.
7. Carpio A, Bharucha NE, Jallon P, *et al*. Mortality of epilepsy in developing countries. *Epilepsia* 2005; 46 Suppl 11: 28-32.
8. Lhatoo SD, Sander JW. Cause-specific mortality in epilepsy. *Epilepsia* 2005; 46 Suppl 11: 36-9.
9. Téllez-Zenteno JF, Ronquillo LH, Wiebe S. Sudden unexpected death in epilepsy: evidence-based analysis of incidence and risk factors. *Epilepsy Res* 2005; 65(1-2): 101-15.
10. Nashef L, Ryvlin P. Sudden unexpected death in epilepsy (SUDEP): update and reflections. *Neurol Clin* 2009; 27(4): 1063-74.
11. Tomson T, Nashef L, Ryvlin P. Sudden unexpected death in epilepsy: current knowledge and future directions. *Lancet Neurol* 2008; 7(11): 1021-31.
12. Logroscino G, Hesdorffer DC. Methodologic issues in studies of mortality following epilepsy: measures, types of studies, sources of cases, cohort effects, and competing risks. *Epilepsia* 2005; 46: 3-7.
13. Tomson T, Walczak T, Sillanpaa M, Sander JW. Sudden unexpected death in epilepsy: a review of incidence and risk factors. *Epilepsia* 2005; 46: 54-61.
14. Tellez-Zenteno JF, Wiebe S. Long-term seizure and psychosocial outcomes of epilepsy surgery. *Curr Treat Options Neurol* 2008; 10(4): 253-9.
15. George JR, Davis GG. Comparison of anti-epileptic drug levels in different cases of sudden death. *J Forensic Sci* 1998; 43(3): 598-603.
16. Kloster R, Engelskjon T. Sudden unexpected death in epilepsy (SUDEP): a clinical perspective and a search for risk factors. *J Neurol Neurosurg Psychiatry* 1999; 67(4): 439-44.
17. Leestma JE, Annegers JF, Brodie MJ, *et al*. Sudden unexplained death in epilepsy: observations from a large clinical development program. *Epilepsia* 1997; 38(1): 47-55.
18. Opeskin K, Burke MP, Cordner SM, Berkovic SF. Comparison of antiepileptic drug levels in sudden unexpected deaths in epilepsy with deaths from other causes. *Epilepsia* 1999; 40(12): 1795-8.
19. Opeskin K, Berkovic SF. Risk factors for sudden unexpected death in epilepsy: a controlled prospective study based on coroners' cases. *Seizure* 2003; 12(7): 456-64.
20. Schnabel R, Beblo M, May TW. Is geomagnetic activity a risk factor for sudden unexplained death in epilepsies? *Neurology* 2000; 54(4): 903-8.
21. Beran RG, Weber S, Sungaran R, Venn N, Hung A. Review of the legal obligations of the doctor to discuss sudden unexplained death in epilepsy (SUDEP) - a cohort controlled comparative cross-matched study in an outpatient epilepsy clinic. *Seizure* 2004; 13(7): 523-8.
22. Hitiris N, Suratman S, Kelly K, Stephen LJ, Sills GJ, Brodie MJ. Sudden unexpected death in epilepsy: a search for risk factors. *Epilepsy Behav* 2007; 10(1): 138-41.
23. Jick SS, Cole TB, Mesher A, Tennis PJH. Sudden unexplained death in young persons with primary epilepsy. *Pharmacoepidemiol Drug Safety* 1992; 1: 59-64.
24. Langan Y, Nashef L, Sander JW. Case-control study of SUDEP. *Neurology* 2005; 64(7): 1131-3.
25. McKee JR, Bodfish JW. Sudden unexpected death in epilepsy in adults with mental retardation. *Am J Ment Retard* 2000; 105(4): 229-35.
26. Nilsson L, Farahmand BY, Persson PG, Thiblin I, Tomson T. Risk factors for sudden unexpected death in epilepsy: a case-control study. *Lancet* 1999; 353(9156): 888-93.
27. Nilsson L, Bergman U, Diwan V, Farahmand BY, Persson PG, Tomson T. Antiepileptic drug therapy and its management in sudden unexpected death in epilepsy: a case-control study. *Epilepsia* 2001; 42(5): 667-73.
28. Timmings PL. Sudden unexpected death in epilepsy: a local audit. *Seizure* 1993; 2(4): 287-90.

29. Walczak TS, Leppik IE, D'Amelio M, *et al.* Incidence and risk factors in sudden unexpected death in epilepsy: a prospective cohort study. *Neurology* 2001; 56(4): 519-25.

30. Williams J, Lawthom C, Dunstan FD, *et al.* Variability of antiepileptic medication taking behaviour in sudden unexplained death in epilepsy: hair analysis at autopsy. *J Neurol Neurosurg Psychiatry* 2006; 77(4): 481-4.

31. Sperling MR, Feldman H, Kinman J, Liporace JD, O'Connor MJ. Seizure control and mortality in epilepsy. *Ann Neurol* 1999; 46(1): 45-50.

32. Vlooswijk MC, Majoie HJ, de Krom MC, Tan IY, Aldenkamp AP. SUDEP in the Netherlands: a retrospective study in a tertiary referral center. *Seizure* 2007; 16(2): 153-9.

33. Persson H, Ericson M, Tomson T. Carbamazepine affects autonomic cardiac control in patients with newly diagnosed epilepsy. *Epilepsy Res* 2003; 57(1): 69-75.

34. VanLandingham KE, Dixon RM. Lamotrigine in idiopathic epilepsy - increased risk of cardiac death. *Acta Neurol Scand* 2007; 116(5): 345.

35. McLean BN, Wimalaratna S. Sudden death in epilepsy recorded in ambulatory EEG. *J Neurol Neurosurg Psychiatry* 2007; 78(12): 1395-7.

36. Lee HW, Hong SB, Tae WS, Seo DW, Kim SE. Partial seizures manifesting as apnea only in an adult. *Epilepsia* 1999; 40(12): 1828-31.

37. Bird JM, Dembny AT, Sandeman D, Butler S. Sudden unexplained death in epilepsy: an intracranial monitored case. *Epilepsia* 1997; 38: S52-6.

38. So EL, Sam MC, Lagerlund TL. Postictal central apnea as a cause of SUDEP: evidence from near-SUDEP incident. *Epilepsia* 2000; 41(11): 1494-7.

39. Thomas P, Landre E, Suisse G, Breloin J, Dolisi C, Chatel M. Syncope anoxo-ischemique par dyspnee obstructive au cors d'une crise partielle complexe temporal droite. *Epilepsies* 1996; 8: 339-46.

40. So EL. What is known about the mechanisms underlying SUDEP? *Epilepsia* 2008; 49 (Suppl 9): 93-8.

41. Ryvlin P, Montavont A, Kahane P. The impact of epilepsy surgery on mortality. *Epileptic Disord* 2005; 7 Suppl 1: 39-46.

42. So EL, Bainbridge J, Buchhalter JR, *et al.* Report of the American Epilepsy Society and the Epilepsy Foundation Joint Task Force on Sudden Unexplained Death in Epilepsy. *Epilepsia* 2009; 50(4): 917-22.

Chapter 10

Behavioral therapies in the treatment of adults with epilepsy

Patricia Osborne Shafer RN MN
Epilepsy Nurse Specialist
Beth Israel Deaconess Medical Center
Boston, Massachusetts, USA

Introduction

Managing epilepsy is a complex process, involving diverse biological, psychological, and social factors. From the medical perspective, while evidence-based guidelines exist to aid in the diagnosis and treatment, the ultimate aim is to tailor the choice of treatment to the individual and the way his or her epilepsy is manifested.

When considering the use of behavioral therapies for epilepsy, a similar complexity exists and the need to tailor therapies to a range of factors is crucial. To date, research on the use of behavioral therapies for epilepsy has not taken into consideration the individual experiences of epilepsy with the many biopsychosocial factors that influence or mediate the variables involved. Outcome studies of behavioral therapies have used samples of people with epilepsy as if they are all the same; very few subgroups of people who may respond to one therapy or another have been examined. As a result, analysis of behavioral, psychological or self-management strategies have shown limited benefit in reviews of available literature [1-5]. Nevertheless, research on the diversity of behavioral therapies offers interesting data and insight into their use for adults with epilepsy as complementary therapies.

This chapter discusses the use of certain behavioral therapies with a view toward their possible indications, theory base, outcomes and relevance to clinical practice. Attempts have been made to use results of studies from randomized controlled trials; however, relevant or interesting studies or meta-analyses of some therapies are presented along with their limitations and clinical relevance.

Defining behavioral therapies

Behavioral therapies may be defined as "psychological techniques based on the premise that specific, observable, maladaptive, badly adjusted, or self-destructing behaviors can be modified by learning new, more appropriate behaviors to replace them" [6]. Theoretically, behavioral therapies focus on changing negative, inappropriate or maladaptive behaviors and promote positive healthy behaviors to achieve a specific outcome. Behavioral therapies may include those that are considered psychological therapies when changes in behavior are part of an intervention or an intended outcome.

In epilepsy, the use of the term behavioral therapies according to the definition above raises the question as to what behaviors researchers are trying to change. Many studies examined for the purpose of this review evaluate behavioral interventions to control or affect seizures. This suggests that the seizures are 'maladaptive or self-destructing behaviors' or are influenced by such behaviors. Other studies aim to increase knowledge about epilepsy, improve mood or coping, improve compliance and medication-taking behaviors, or enhance a person's self-efficacy and their ability to manage their epilepsy.

For the purpose of this chapter, behavioral therapies in epilepsy are defined as those that attempt to change a person's behavior as part of an intervention or as an intended outcome of the intervention. The goal of therapy may directly or indirectly influence the experience of epilepsy or mediating factors, by altering seizure control or severity, mood, quality of life, well-being, or a person's ability to manage their epilepsy and daily life.

Types of behavioral therapies

For years, practitioners and educators have provided information and taught strategies on how to identify and monitor seizures, medication side effects or other problems in daily life. Teaching people to monitor and identify factors that may influence their susceptibility to seizures, then teaching lifestyle and environmental modifications to manage triggers or lessen the risk of injury are commonly performed in clinical nursing practice and may be addressed by rehabilitation and mental health providers as well [7-9]. Since these strategies have been considered part of routine clinical practice or educational programs, their effectiveness has not been rigorously studied. Work by researchers such as Dahl and colleagues [10-12] and Reiter and Andrews [13, 14] have drawn attention to this area by developing specific programs that try to identify and change a person's susceptibility to and response to seizures. Mind-body techniques have also been used for many years, yet only recently can we begin drawing conclusions about their use in epilepsy. Research into different methods of delivering psychosocial, self-management, and educational programs has grown, albeit slowly, in recent years as the importance of patient-centered comprehensive care has increased.

Table 1 identifies types of behavioral therapies that are included in this chapter. Behavioral therapies for children are not included (except when older adolescents are included in an adult intervention), since the types and responses to therapy vary considerably for children and adults. Additionally, interventions to change a child's behavior or influence seizure control

Table 1. Types of behavioral therapies.
◆ Cognitive behavioral therapy (CBT): CBT alone or together with acceptance commitment therapy (ACT), mindfulness, or psycho-educational approaches
◆ Educational/psycho-educational programs
◆ Exercise: structured exercise programs, with or without other behavioral strategies
◆ Mind/body therapies: meditation, relaxation therapy, yoga
◆ Self-management interventions: motivational interviewing using telephone, web-based programs, group therapy; combined approaches for medication adherence

most likely will involve the child, parent(s), or other family members or caregivers and would need to be quite different than those aimed at adults. While some interventions may involve a form of biofeedback, studies of biofeedback as a primary intervention or that required complex EEG monitoring were not included due to the diversity of methodologies.

Articles for inclusion were chosen from extensive searches of PubMed and the common epilepsy journals using the following search terms: behavioral therapies, randomized controlled trials, yoga, relaxation therapy, exercise, educational programs, acceptance commitment therapy, psycho-eduational approaches, epilepsy self-management, compliance.

What role do educational programs have as a behavioral therapy?

Knowledge-based programs may consider that an inadequate understanding of seizures and epilepsy affects treatment of epilepsy from both the provider and patient perspectives. Fear of seizures has been identified as a major issue or barrier to managing seizures and is usually caused by misinformation about seizures [15, 16]. Effective self-management depends on people understanding their epilepsy, treatment and impact on life; being able to communicate effectively with their providers, and taking charge of their care and lives. Additionally, people must learn critical skills and find resources that help them use information appropriately [7, 17].

Individual and group educational approaches have been used in clinical practice and community forums for many years, and are recommended services of specialized epilepsy centers [18]. Program evaluations and patient/user satisfaction information has more recently given way to evaluation or outcome studies on the impact of educational initiatives. However, the question arises as to what outcomes are of interest, feasible and appropriate? While it would be optimal to say that teaching people about epilepsy by itself will improve seizure control or severity, this may be unrealistic. However, it would be very appropriate and meaningful to know the effect of teaching people about their epilepsy on their ability to manage their epilepsy. Does it improve compliance adherence or a person's ability to manage their medications or other treatments? Does understanding the disorder make a person less fearful, anxious or depressed? Are they more self-confident or do they feel less stigmatized by having epilepsy?

The use and benefits of educational programs to enhance understanding and change health behaviors will depend upon an assessment of the audience's learning needs and the ability to tailor content and methods to best meet the audience needs. Many research and program surveys have identified the needs of people with epilepsy, yet few articles have focused specifically on learning needs. Cochrane [19] explored the benefits of education from experiences of lay associations that provide epilepsy education, stressing that education should address a patient's self-efficacy, be patient-centered and involve the patient and family in decision-making processes. General guidelines or themes that should be incorporated into educational programs were recommended as well as methodological issues that coincide with much of the self-management literature of the past decade.

Couldridge *et al* [20] conducted a review of studies on counseling and information needs of people with epilepsy, and found that unmet needs for epilepsy information persist for both individual and group educational methods. Lannon [21] emphasizes that information must be taught repeatedly, as a patient's needs for information about medications or other treatments will differ at initial diagnosis than at other times. Common educational and self-management needs for people at different levels of seizure control were identified in a consensus approach including patients, family members and professionals, and included needs for knowledge and information, coping skills, and support networks or resources [17]. The difficulties evaluating educational programs have been a major factor leading to the dearth of efficacy data and problems affecting the ability to generalize results [22]. Additionally, outcomes and educational curricula vary between programs. Despite these inherent research problems, data have shown positive results of educational programs on knowledge about epilepsy, coping, misconceptions about epilepsy and seizure management, delivered individually and in groups, for certain audiences [22].

What effect does epilepsy education have on adults with seizures when offered in different formats?

Small group educational approaches

Educational information is often distributed in clinic, office visits or at community programs to improve awareness and knowledge; however, the effectiveness of this approach, particularly in people with learning disabilities, is unknown. The use of an educational package known as "Epilepsy and You", that includes a brief video geared to people with epilepsy and learning disabilities (described as "mildly intellectually disabled"), was tested in a pre/post design with 18 adults [23]. A deferred treatment and control group was used. The program was designed to be delivered in a group format; however, timing of participant recruitment led to small numbers in three treatment groups (1, 3, and 4 participants) while the delayed treatment groups had similarly small numbers (1, 3, and 6). The curriculum was delivered in 1-hour sessions for 3 weeks and included information given repeatedly in verbal and video formats, and participants were taught how to use seizure diaries. The program was found to improve knowledge about epilepsy significantly when tested by questionnaire immediately and 1 month after program completion in the treatment and delayed treatment groups [23]. The interesting feature of this study, despite its research weaknesses, is that it can be easily replicated and uses patient education principles appropriate to the target audience. (Evidence not rated due to sample size.)

Day long educational programs
Another common format for epilepsy education is to deliver a large amount of information over a 1- or 2-day program. Most voluntary lay epilepsy organizations hold these conferences on a regular basis, but research into their effectiveness is lacking. A 2-day psycho-educational treatment program, the Sepulveda Epilepsy Education program (SEE), has been conducted for many years in the United States. This program is led by one faculty person who delivers education in a group format, covering medical and psychosocial aspects of epilepsy with the goal of improving understanding and coping with epilepsy. For adults with epilepsy, the SEE program has been studied in a pre/post design with 38 participants randomized to a treatment or wait list control group [24]. Measures were evaluated pre-treatment, immediately post-treatment and at 4 months post-treatment. Improvements in the treatment group were reported in fear of death and brain damage from seizures, use of hazardous practices, and "overall level of misinformation and misconceptions about epilepsy". No changes in seizure frequency were found, but a significant improvement in psychosocial adjustment was noted using the Washington Psychosocial Seizure Inventory (WPSI). Improved compliance by increased blood levels in the treatment group was reported for the treatment group but data regarding medications or any changes during the follow-up period were not given.

Another 2-day educational program was studied in Germany, using a Modular Service Package Epilepsy (MOSES) program in 242 adults with epilepsy [25]. The MOSES program was designed to be flexible with 14-hour long lessons that could be delivered individually, in modules on a weekly basis, or in a weekend course. The objective of the program was to improve participant knowledge about epilepsy, self-esteem, coping, and empowerment. A pre/post design with randomization to a treatment (n=113) or wait list control (n=129) group was evaluated for a variety of variables at baseline, immediately after the intervention and at 6 months post-intervention. Results in the treatment group indicated significant improvement in knowledge about epilepsy and coping, as well as satisfaction with their treatment and the educational program. Generic behavioral and mood measures and epilepsy-specific factors did not show change as a result of the program. An interesting finding was that non-responders had less severe epilepsy or emotional problems and one wonders if lack of change may have been affected by less severe problems at the onset.

These two randomized controlled studies demonstrate the efficacy of educational programs using a 1- or 2-day format for knowledge and other psychosocial outcomes (Ib/A). An additional educational program conducted in Nigeria focused on self-efficacy and the reduction of psychopathology in 30 adults with epilepsy [26]. While a randomized wait list control group was used, the evidence was not rated due to limited follow-up. A decrease in depression and neurotic disorders was found in the treatment group along with an increase in knowledge about epilepsy at immediate post-test. Further testing of this intervention would be needed to determine maintenance of this impact.

Weekly educational programs

Many short-term educational programs offer a combination of education and psychological support and strategies over a period of weeks. A 6-week program developed for adolescents and their parents was included in this review as the age of the sample was older adolescents [27]. A pre/post design was used to evaluate the program which included information on medical, psychosocial, and self-management practices as well as cognitive behavioral techniques for skill-building, strategies and support. Since this was a pilot study, no control group was used and only seven participants completed the sessions. No changes in overall quality of life, depression or anxiety were seen but there were positive trends noted in this small sample. Of interest, the researchers did not focus on knowledge of epilepsy, but on psychosocial outcomes of education.

Another psycho-educational program using information giving, cognitive behavioral techniques for skill-building, and psychological support replicated part of Reiter's work [14]. Delivered over 8 weeks in seven adults with intractable epilepsy, participants were evaluated for change in seizures and psychosocial well-being [28]. Since no control group was used, within group analyses were conducted and noted decreases in seizure frequency after the intervention and at 3-month follow-up for all seven participants but no changes in psychosocial well-being or other measures.

A longer pre/post study design of 42 weeks was used to evaluate the impact of two psycho-educational strategies that could be employed as part of outpatient management of adults with epilepsy [29]. One treatment was directed to teaching participants self-control of seizures (i.e. identifying triggers, lifestyle modifications, strategies to abort seizures, relaxation strategies). The second strategy was a psychological intervention and counseling aimed at a specific concern to the participant. Seizure control improved in all 59 participants during the intervention phases, regardless of the order in which they received the treatments and even for 19 who only received the first treatment **(IIa/B – for seizure control)**. No changes on other measures of mood or behavior were noted.

Can behavioral approaches influence seizure triggers and susceptibility?

Behavioral approaches to stress, coping, and managing seizure triggers have often been called 'neurobehavioral approaches' that work on the principles of brain-behavior relationships. If people are able to identify factors that may affect brain function and ultimately their susceptibility to seizures, they may be able to learn ways of aborting or stopping the progression of a seizure, learning ways of inhibiting seizures, or modifying or avoiding triggers. These techniques, often called 'self-control' strategies or trigger management, are taught in some specialized epilepsy centers. These self-control techniques share concepts with self-management, in that they can be viewed as a process with the individual as the primary person in charge of 'guiding, directing and regulating' changes in their behavior [30]. Like self-management, personal choice and decision-making are key features and a person's locus of control and other behavioral or personal variables may influence this process [31-33]. The self-control concepts have also been linked to theories of learned resourcefulness, with experiential skill development rather than specific training [34, 35]. These theories come into play with Andrews' and Reiter's approach to managing seizures [13], ACT therapy, and mind-body approaches designed to influence seizure control.

Self-control approaches

To evaluate people with perceived high versus low control of seizures, 100 adults with intractable epilepsy were surveyed [30]. Adults who were able to identify precipitants or triggers of seizures and low-risk seizure situations were more likely to attempt self-control measures. The Andrews/Reiter approach to self-control was developed into a short-term treatment approach, whereby patients were provided treatment for 5 days. Forty-four patients with lateralized onset of complex partial seizures were tested using this approach and followed by weekly phone contact with an epilepsy counselor for 6 months following the treatment [14]. The treatment included different forms of relaxation training, two sessions of biofeedback training, and counseling. Attempts to lower medications were made in patients who presented on more than one seizure medication. Results of this study showed that 79.5% of all patients had improved seizure control for 6 months or longer. Apparently the mean reduction in seizures was greater than 90% for both the right and left hemisphere seizure onset groups. A control group was not used, thus the impact of 6 months of follow-up versus the actual effect of the 5-day intervention could not be determined.

Acceptance and commitment therapy (ACT) is aimed at teaching patients self-control techniques, which includes cognitive behavioral techniques that teach patients to 'notice' and accept their seizures and learn how to take action to avoid, inhibit or control them [11, 12, 36]. The efficacy of ACT in adults with refractory epilepsy has been evaluated in two randomized controlled trials in recent years (Ib/A – small samples). One conducted in South Africa evaluated 27 adults using a supportive therapy (ST) control group (14 ACT, 13 ST) [11], while a study in Southwest India compared ACT to yoga therapy in 18 adults (10 in ACT, 8 in yoga groups) [12]. The ACT curricula included individual and group sessions over a 5-week period with booster sessions at 6 and 12 months. Seizure control and quality-of-life outcomes were evaluated pre, post, and at 6 and 12 months following the intervention. The yoga training in the comparison study aimed to "stimulate activity in directions the participants considered meaningful" and reduce epileptic seizures [12]. While ACT was used in only 24 adults in both studies, results demonstrated significant improvements over time in seizure control and quality of life. These changes were significant when compared to the ST control group [11], and participants who received the yoga intervention also demonstrated significant changes in seizure control, though less than that obtained by those receiving ACT, as well as improved quality of life [12].

One other randomized study of 32 adults with uncontrolled epilepsy evaluated actual yoga versus control groups of sham yoga and no yoga [37] and found that seizure control improved significantly in those using the actual yoga compared to the two control groups, with four often using the actual form becoming seizure-free for the 6-month follow-up period. Despite the interesting results of these controlled trials, a Cochrane review of yoga as a treatment for epilepsy concluded that there was "no reliable evidence" concerning the use of yoga to control seizures due to the small sample sizes and other methodological factors [4].

Relaxation therapy

Other forms of mind-body techniques have been used for decades in people with epilepsy. Despite its interest as an antiepileptic treatment, the use of transcendental meditation has been limited by concern of inducing seizures in some people [38]. Relaxation therapy is easy to teach and has been used for many years to reduce stress, and enhance well-being and seizure control. A contingent relaxation therapy approach was tested in 18 adults with refractory seizures and included relaxation techniques, and how to identify and respond to seizure precipitants and high- and low-risk seizure situations [10]. This randomized study used two control groups, one receiving professional attention with supportive therapy and a wait list control maintaining seizure diaries only. While many patients in both treatment and control groups were able to identify precipitants and seizures at baseline, only the contingent relaxation group had a significant response with 66% decrease in seizures compared to baseline, while those in the attention control group had a 68% increase in seizures **(Ib/A – small sample size)**.

Progressive relaxation therapy (PRT) has demonstrated positive outcomes on seizure control in other controlled trials. Two studies of adults with refractory epilepsy used a pre/post design to evaluate PRT against a quiet sitting (QS) control group [39], and a sham wait list group [40]. Rousseau's study [40] using a sham wait list control group found that all four patients in the PRT group had a seizure reduction ranging from 38% to 100% over the treatment period; however, two of four in the sham wait list control also had seizure reductions of 39% and 51%, respectively. Puskarich et al [39] followed patients for 2 months after a PRT intervention program and found a decrease in seizures in 11 of 13 PRT patients as compared to 7 of 11 in the QS control group. The PRT group had a greater decrease in mean number of seizures, 29% versus 3%, respectively.

Some people use relaxation therapy for their emotional or social well-being rather than seizure control. A small study (n=16 adults) evaluated the use of relaxation therapy for psychosocial functioning using a pre/post design with wait list control. Of 11 in the intervention group, no significant differences were found on psychosocial function using the Washington Psychosocial Seizure Inventory (WPSI) after 6 months [41]. A limitation to this study is that both inpatients on an epilepsy unit and outpatients participated, which affected the number and delivery of training sessions for participants.

A more recent study evaluated PRT as part of a stress management program with the goal of reducing seizures by targeting stress as a potential seizure precipitant. A prospective pre/post study of a stress management program evaluated 9 adults with epilepsy receiving treatment and 9 in a control group [42]. Measures evaluated the outcomes of seizures and quality of life pre-treatment, post-treatment (14 weeks) and at 1 year. Participants were taught four different forms of relaxation in individual weekly sessions for 6 weeks, followed by individual meetings with a stress management trainer every other week for 8 weeks and additional monthly booster sessions. Incomplete results of this non-randomized study demonstrated decreased seizure frequency, improved quality of life and qualitative changes in seizures per patient report. Despite the limitations of this study, these stress management techniques are a common type of behavioral strategy that can be replicated in clinical and community settings.

Can self-management programs affect seizures and psychosocial outcomes?

In the following studies, CBT was used to address seizure control and other factors that affect seizures and quality of life, such as self-efficacy, psychosocial problems, seizure precipitants, and stress management [43-45]. While some of the outcomes are similar to those previously cited, the studies are characterized separately due to the psychosocial nature of the interventions and outcomes.

Pramuka [45] evaluated a 6-week psychosocial intervention based on an empowerment model to improve quality of life and self-efficacy, an important predictor of self-management. This randomized controlled trial of 61 adults had data on 38 participants who completed the study (19 in the treatment group, 19 in a 'treatment as usual' control group). The curricula addressed concepts and strategies of 'taking charge', setting goals, and making choices in relation to medical care issues as well as psychosocial aspects. Significant differences were noted in changes on total quality of life, role limitations and emotional scores for the treatment group. Strong trends were noted between other psychosocial factors and self-efficacy with quality of life **(Ib/A – small sample size)** [45].

In Hong Kong, CBT for cognitive restructuring and seizure control was studied using a wait list control receiving standard medical therapy and followed for 3 months [44]. Despite the small numbers (treatment group = 8; wait list = 9), significant improvements in quality of life and self-efficacy were found in the treatment group, but no significant changes in seizure frequency.

What is known about behavioral therapies in specific patient populations?

Juvenile myoclonic epilepsy
Other programs teaching patients how to identify, avoid or manage seizure precipitants (i.e. trigger management) have targeted subgroups of people with epilepsy with promising results. Martinovic [43] evaluated the effect of structured counseling for trigger management and other behavioral treatments in 22 young adults with juvenile myoclonic epilepsy (JME). If structured counseling was not effective, participants were entered into one of two groups; a stress management program or individual cognitive behavioral therapy. The treatments were offered over a 6-month period to 22 young adults, followed by 6- and 12-month follow-up evaluations to examine seizure triggers, seizure recurrence and psychological problems. All three groups showed improvements in seizure control; however, 8 or 36% of 22 with

uncontrolled seizures achieved complete control when behavioral therapy was added to structured counseling. CBT appeared to be slightly more effective, but the numbers of participants were too small to show significant results. Comorbid mental health problems were found in 20 of 22 patients and while the numbers were too small for significance, a trend towards improved seizure control and less seizure precipitants correlated with a decrease in psychological problems. Again CBT appeared more helpful, and both CBT and stress management programs were better than structured counseling alone **(III/B)** [43].

Adults with attention deficits

Behavioral strategies for cognitive function are part of neuropsychological treatment in many epilepsy centers, yet studies on their effectiveness are sparse. Engelberts *et al* [46] evaluated the effect of two methods for treating attention deficits: cognitive retraining and a compensation method. A sample of 50 adult patients with partial seizures and attention deficits on carbamazepine monotherapy were randomized to one of two treatment groups or a wait list control group. Forty-four patients completed the study and were followed for 6 months post-treatment for neuropsychological outcomes and quality of life. Both intervention groups demonstrated improvements in neuropsychological and quality-of-life outcomes more than the control group. Interestingly, the compensatory method was more helpful for those with less education, while patients with persistent seizures benefited more from either intervention than those with well-controlled seizures **(Ib/A – needs replication)**.

What is the effect of telephone and web-based self-management programs?

Many different theories underlie the use of behavioral interventions. Social cognitive theory (SCT) is the basis of a model of epilepsy self-management [31] and other behavioral strategies [47] that examine the interaction of the behavior(s) with personal and environmental factors [48]. Self-efficacy, or the belief or confidence in one's ability to manage their health has a critical role in self-management of many chronic disorders [49]. In epilepsy, self-efficacy has been found to be a main predictor of self-management, particularly for medication-taking behaviors, influence on stigma and depressive symptoms, expectations for outcomes, feelings of control, and the utilization of health resources [31, 32, 50].

Teaching patients how to manage their epilepsy and change or develop healthy behaviors can be done in a variety of ways. DiIorio and colleagues have evaluated a telephone-based self-management program and a web-based program, both of which can be implemented individually. Both mimic and support current professional practices [51-53]. Additionally, they overcome two main barriers to participation in educational programs: transportation and cost.

Telephone triage and education is conducted daily in neurology and epilepsy clinics. The telephone-based pilot study used key principles of motivational interviewing and social cognitive theory on 22 adults with epilepsy, 11 in the treatment group received one in-person meeting and four telephone sessions with a nurse trained in motivational interviewing [51]. A control group of 11 patients received courtesy calls. Treatment sessions aimed to improve social support and perceived self-efficacy in managing epilepsy, and set short-term goals for behavior change in areas of seizures, safety, information, medications, and lifestyle.

Outcomes included self-efficacy, epilepsy self-management, medication adherence, and knowledge. While no significant change in medication adherence was found as measured with MEMS caps, participants had higher self-efficacy and outcome expectancies for medication and seizure management, improved knowledge of social aspects of epilepsy, and high patient satisfaction with the treatment method. This study, while using a small sample size, demonstrated positive trends to a method of self-management that is currently practiced in many outpatient settings.

WebEase (Epilepsy Awareness Support and Education), an online self-management program, also using motivational interviewing techniques and social cognitive theory, was evaluated in a randomized controlled trial in 148 adults with epilepsy [53]. A pre/post design with a wait list control group was used. The curriculum includes modules on medication, sleep and stress management. Each interactive module assists the user to assess their readiness for change, establish goals for behavior change, learn information, develop skills, and monitor progress towards goals in their chosen area. Results indicated improved medication adherence in the treatment group but no changes in other variables when compared to the wait list control group. However, when people who completed at least one module were compared to those who did not complete the modules, completers demonstrated greater levels of self-efficacy and improvements in medication adherence, improved sleep and lower levels of stress for those completing the relevant modules **(Ib/A)**.

How can exercise affect people with seizures?

Some people have reported that exercise can exacerbate seizures and while research has confirmed this for a small number of people, it can also have an antiepileptic effect in many others. A recent review of animal studies has suggested that physical exercise may alter neurotransmitters, reduce susceptibility to seizures and the development of epilepsy, decrease the frequency of seizures in animals with chronic epilepsy, and have neuroprotective effects [54]. Additionally, it has been hypothesized that participating in exercise and sports may increase a person's ability to cope with psychological stress [55].

Exercise has also been considered a possible stressor in epilepsy. While emotional stress is most commonly reported, the role of physical stress as a trigger for seizures has been reported in up to 30% of people with epilepsy [56]. Fear of injuries during exercise or worry about what to do if seizures occur during exercise or sports are also common factors affecting participation in exercise and sports by people with epilepsy.

Can exercise improve seizures in adults with epilepsy?

A survey was conducted many years ago to examine self-reported exercise in relation to stressful life experiences, depression and psychosocial adjustment in 133 adults with epilepsy [57]. Adults who exercised regularly were noted to have fewer problems with depression and better psychosocial adjustment. Modeling of these variables noted independent effects of exercise and stress on depression, and stressful life experiences directly influencing seizure frequency, suggesting the importance of addressing all these factors, especially in people with seizures and mood disorders **(III/B)**.

Exercise programs have demonstrated small but positive physical and emotional effects in people with epilepsy. A month-long intensive physical training program in Norway was conducted in 21 adults with epilepsy on an inpatient unit [58]. The exercise program was more intense than would be used by most people in daily life, with participants exercising for three 45-minute sessions a day, 6 days a week. The exercise regimen was individualized for each participant to obtain their maximum aerobic capacity. Physiological and psychological variables were measured pre- and post-intervention and AEDs were not changed during the course of the study. No control group was used. Baseline measurements showed wide variability in fitness levels of participants, with greater fitness in women. The majority of participants from both sexes demonstrated improved fitness during the exercise program. Seizure frequency remained stable during exercise and non-exercise periods; however, individual variability was apparent. Two thirds of the sample had seizures during inactive periods, and only one third (n=6) reported seizures during the period of exercise. Seizures were not associated with timing or type of exercise or heart rate.

The impact of exercise in women was studied in a small sample with intractable epilepsy (n=15) in Norway [59]. The effects of a 15-week exercise program including aerobic dancing, strength training and stretching for 60 minutes twice a week was evaluated pre, during and 3 months post-intervention for effects on seizures, physiological and psychosocial function. No control group was available. No consistent impact on seizure control was noted. Four patients noted increased seizures while ten had fewer seizures when post-intervention data were compared to baseline data. During the exercise period, the median number of seizures weekly decreased for 13 participants, but this was not significant statistically. While self-report of seizures showed significant decline during intervention, this improvement was not sustained during the follow-up period. Additionally, the rate of subjective health problems decreased and changes were noted in plasma cholesterol ratios and maximum oxygen uptake. The authors concluded that a longer intervention period was needed to make sustained behavior changes.

A randomized controlled prospective study of a 12-week outpatient exercise program was conducted in the United States [60]. Twenty-three participants were randomized into an exercise group (n=14) which met with an exercise physiologist three times a week, and a control group (n=9) who continued their usual level of activity. Behavioral and clinical measures demonstrated no effect on seizures, but positive impact on behavior variables including overall quality of life, physical function and energy/fatigue, physical self-concept, vigor, and mood. Physiological improvements were noted in treatment versus control groups in strength, peak oxygen consumption, and endurance.

These intervention studies on the use of exercise as a behavioral treatment do not demonstrate consistent improvements in seizure control from exercise, but positive trends in behavioral and psychosocial variables that warrant further study and consideration in clinical practice **(Ib/A – small sample; other studies – III/B)**.

Can behavioral therapies be used to treat depression in people with epilepsy?

Depression can be a significant problem for many people with epilepsy, is more frequent in people with persistent seizures, and is a major factor affecting quality of life [61]. A potentially important and relevant study evaluating CBT versus counseling as usual (TAU) was conducted in adolescents with newly diagnosed epilepsy to examine if depression could be prevented in adolescents at risk [62]. Since the mean age of this study group was 17 years old, the results are noted here. Of 104 adolescents with new onset epilepsy, 28.8% were found to be at risk for depression. These 30 patients were randomized into the intervention group (CBT) or control group (TAU). The cognitive behavioral interventions were given over weekly sessions for 2 months, then monthly sessions for 4 months while the TAU group received the same number of sessions for general counseling. While no significant effect was noted in seizure frequency due to the small numbers of participants, symptoms of depressive disorders improved significantly in the 15 patients treated with CBT as compared to those with TAU. Improvements in quality of life mirrored the improvements in mood as well, stressing the importance of non-seizure outcomes for behavioral therapies [62] **(Ib/A – small sample size)**.

A home-based multimodal intervention, the PEARLS program, was evaluated in a randomized controlled trial of adults with epilepsy and comorbid depression [63]. Forty adults were randomized into the intervention and 40 into a control group of usual care. Both groups were evaluated at baseline, 6 and 12 months. The intervention consisted of collaboration among community agency therapists and team psychiatrists for problem-solving techniques, behavioral activation (i.e. exercise, social interaction, and resource referrals), and psychiatric consultation delivered via eight home-based visits over 5 months, phone call contacts with psychiatrists, and collaboration among agencies and epilepsy care providers. The PEARLS program reduced depressive symptoms and suicidal ideation by 24% in the treatment group, improved emotional well-being, but did not change seizure frequency [63], similar to the study on adolescents at risk **(Ib/A)**. Since depression is a strong predictor of quality of life and possibly a variable leading to the development of persistent epilepsy, the improvement in the main variables under study are critically important changes.

Another home-based intervention for depression in adults with epilepsy was developed to deliver mindfulness-based cognitive behavioral therapy (MCBT) by the internet or telephone [64]. The intervention consists of eight 1-hour sessions with discussions, instruction and skill building activities addressing depression, epilepsy, and the role of mindfulness and cognitive behavior change. The internet aspect of the intervention allows for discussions, viewing session materials, and posting between sessions on a secure website. A randomized controlled unblinded pilot study of Project UPLIFT tested the intervention in adults with depression and epilepsy [65]. A wait list control group was used with participants being evaluated at baseline, at 8 weeks after the first intervention group, and at 16 weeks following the wait list group's intervention. Participants were first stratified according to the use of antidepressants, then randomly assigned to the intervention (internet or phone) or treatment as usual control group. Of 53 who enrolled in the study, 32 completed at least half of the sessions and were included in the analysis. The purpose of this study was not to evaluate change in seizures; measures were used to assess changes in depression, self-efficacy, quality of life and other behavioral factors important in depression and epilepsy management. The intervention groups showed significant decline in depressive symptoms over the wait list group, but there were no differences between the phone and internet methods. However, results for the phone intervention group were slightly better than for those who used the internet method. The improvement persisted over 8 weeks while the wait list control received the intervention. Knowledge and skills increased significantly more in the intervention group than in the wait list control, and there were some other positive behavioral trends that did not reach significance (Ib/A).

Do educational or behavioral strategies enhance medication compliance?

Taking seizure medications regularly and managing the multiple factors involved in medication-taking has been studied extensively, with most research focused on assessing the extent of non-compliance or patient populations at greatest risk for adherence problems, such as those on complex medication regimes [66] or taking medications many times a day [67], and other factors, such as cost. Multiple theories have been used to understand and enhance medication adherence including the health promotion model [21, 68], which focuses on the influence of cognitive-perceptual factors as the primary motivating factors in a person's participation in health-promoting behaviors. Lannon [21] found that interpersonal influences, for example, strong family beliefs and good patient-professional relationships, are critical in patients with compliance problems and can be easily addressed in clinical practice. These and other medication management studies emphasizing the importance of patient perceptions [69], self-efficacy, and patient satisfaction [31] highlight the need to use multimodal strategies to improve medication compliance. A randomized controlled trial of 53 outpatients evaluated the efficacy of a combination of strategies to improve compliance with AEDs [70]. This pre/post design kept treating physicians blinded to those receiving the intervention, which consisted of medication counseling, med containers, self-recording of medications and seizures, and mailed reminders of appointments. Participants were evaluated at baseline and at 6 months, with measurement of AED levels, prescription refills, missed appointments, and seizure frequency. Interestingly, seizure frequency decreased an average of 50% in those who received the intervention strategies, while the control group experienced no changes (Ib/A).

A randomized controlled trial of 61 outpatients with epilepsy was conducted to evaluate the impact of a simple form for patients to monitor their intent to take their medications, using an 'if – then' plan for 1 month [71]. Adherence was monitored using the MEMS caps system and health care providers were blinded to the intervention. Results demonstrated significant improvements for the intervention group compared to controls for total doses taken, days correct doses taken, and doses taken on schedule. While the monitoring period was relatively short (1 month) and no baseline or post-intervention data were collected, this randomized trial suggests another simple behavioral strategy to enhance medication management.

What are the difficulties evaluating behavioral therapies for epilepsy?

The major factors affecting research on the use of behavioral therapies for epilepsy are the wide diversity of methods and outcomes, small sample sizes, and the lack of replication of interventions in different populations. Recent studies have involved control groups and randomization, though data about randomization techniques are often not detailed. Unfortunately, only two blinded studies were available to review for this chapter. Engelberts and colleagues expressed similar concerns after evaluating seven studies on psychological interventions for adults with well-controlled epilepsy [72]. The ability to draw conclusions was limited by small sample sizes, different methodologies, and inconsistent use of control groups. However, interesting positive trends were noted with many interventions. The Cochrane Collaboration found similar limitations in evaluations of psychological therapies, self-management, yoga and educational programs [1-4].

Another factor limiting the use of behavioral therapies is that different studies examined similar behaviors, for example, seizure precipitants or mood, but with different methodologies or interventions. Rarely were studies replicated in different populations, thus limiting the ability to generalize study findings. However, some of the studies on meditation or relaxation therapy were conducted in a similar manner, enhancing the ability to generalize these findings.

Recruiting people for research trials is inherently difficult, but likely moreso for research on behavioral therapy. These studies may have strict inclusion criteria and require participants to hold medications or other medical therapies stable for the testing period. Interventions may be complex or require multiple visits and follow-up strategies at home. These factors lead to small sample sizes which can influence the statistical analysis of the intervention, as well as the ability to generalize findings.

Clinical implications

Important changes were noted by educational programs offered in different formats. Many of the cognitive behavioral interventions were of interest as they addressed similar aspects of seizure management but from slightly different perspectives or theories. The use of CBT appeared to enhance educational programs by adding the important dimension of teaching skills to change thoughts and behaviors that affect seizure management. One- or 2-day educational programs appeared to demonstrate changes in knowledge, coping or other psychosocial factors, while programs conducted over time showed trends towards changes in seizures. Programs that incorporated psychosocial interventions were more likely to influence mood and behavioral variables such as self-efficacy, especially when using patient-centered strategies such as goal setting, assessing readiness and motivation, tailoring content and strategies to patient needs, and incorporating different methods of enhancing support networks.

To fully evaluate the impact and usefulness of behavioral therapies for epilepsy, clinicians must consider the ability to use these therapies in clinical practice or in community settings. Complicated interventions that require the use of many different providers or therapies, or frequent visits, may not be feasible or reimbursable in many countries. While interventions conducted over time may offer the best hope of influencing seizure control, changing complicated behaviors or maintaining changes will likely require motivated and dedicated patients with resources to help them with the practical aspects of long-term therapies, for example, transportation, cost and support. The self-management programs testing the use of different methodologies (telephone or internet for mood and seizure management) offer ways to extend the reach of behavioral therapies in a low cost manner. Additional research will be needed to examine the effect of these therapies, as well as others cited, on the maintenance of behavior change over time.

Future research

The importance of and popularity of patient-centered care emphasizes the need for additional research into behavioral therapies. Non-drug measures have gained popularity in wellness programs and many treatment programs for chronic illness. People with chronic health problems such as epilepsy have greater access to information now and many want, and benefit from, an active role in the management of their health.

Future research into behavioral therapies for epilepsy must consider and evaluate the following areas:

- test simpler interventions that can be implemented in different settings;
- evaluate the impact of different strategies when multimodal interventions are used;
- identify groups who may benefit from different interventions;
- replicate studies to obtain larger sample sizes;
- conduct multicenter studies for larger sample sizes and to eliminate unintended bias of researchers and people performing the interventions;
- conduct studies with treating providers blinded to the intervention and control groups;
- use standardized outcome measures appropriate to the goals of the study and intervention;
- use standardized ways of collecting seizure information, considering electronic seizure diaries for real-time recording of seizures, symptoms, and interventions.

Conclusions

While nearly two-thirds of the people with epilepsy in the United States may have seizures controlled with medical therapy, many do not or experience unacceptable side effects of medical therapy. Additionally, people must learn how to manage seizures, medical therapies and the many consequences that epilepsy may have on individuals and families. This chapter evaluated behavioral therapies for their impact on adults with epilepsy, and evaluated outcomes in addition to seizure control. While some research studies have methodological weaknesses, there is evidence suggesting the benefits of some behavioral therapies when targeted to appropriate outcomes. Researchers and clinicians are encouraged to take a new interest in these approaches; more rigorous studies are needed, yet many of these therapies should be incorporated into multidisciplinary care right now.

Key points	Evidence level
◆ Randomized controlled trials of educational programs delivered over 1 or 2 days may enhance knowledge, coping and psychosocial function.	Ib/A
◆ Psycho-educational programs using educational and behavioral strategies delivered weekly over a period of time may influence seizure control.	IIa/B
◆ Strategies to enhance a person's self-control over seizures and identify seizure precipitants may improve seizure control in some people:	
o neurobehavioral approaches;	III/B
o acceptance and commitment therapy;	Ib/A
o relaxation therapy, yoga.	Ib/A
◆ Behavioral therapies with a combination of cognitive behavioral techniques and information giving have shown positive benefits for the treatment of adults with epilepsy and older adolescents at risk for depression in terms of decreased depressive symptoms and improved well-being or quality of life, but no change in seizure control.	Ib/A
◆ Structured exercise programs have shown positive benefits on physical health and well-being in adults with epilepsy, but no consistent impact on seizure control.	Ib/A & III/B
◆ Medication adherence in adults with epilepsy is improved with the use of multiple strategies to aid medication-taking.	Ib/A
◆ Psychosocial interventions that teach self-management strategies using motivational interviewing by phone and/or internet can improve knowledge, skills, medication adherence, and self-efficacy, while overcoming barriers of cost and transportation.	Ib/A
◆ Cognitive behavioral therapy combined with other stress management techniques may be more helpful than structured counseling alone in patients with juvenile myoclonic epilepsy.	III/B
◆ Outcomes of behavioral therapies for adults with epilepsy that have shown positive results or trends include seizure control, self-efficacy, psychosocial function, mood, physical function, medication adherence, skills for managing mood and seizures, and some aspects of quality of life.	Ib/A

References

1. Ramaratnam S, Baker GA, Goldstein LH. Psychological treatments for epilepsy. The Cochrane Library. *Cochrane Database Syst Rev* 2008; 3: CD002029.
2. Bradley PM, Lindsay B. Care delivery and self-management strategies for adults with epilepsy. The Cochrane Library. *Cochrane Database Syst Rev* 2008; 1: CD006244.
3. Shaw EJ, Stokes T, Camosso-Stefinovic J, Baker R, Baker GA, Jacoby A. Self-management education for adults with epilepsy. The Cochrane Library. *Cochrane Database Syst Rev* 2010; 10: CD004723.
4. Ramaratnam S, Sridharan K. Yoga for epilepsy. The Cochrane Library. *Cochrane Database Syst Rev* 1999; 2: CD001524.
5. Mittan RJ. Psychosocial treatment programs in epilepsy: a review. *Epilepsy Behav* 2009; 16: 371-80.
6. Behavioral Therapy. HealthLine. http://www.healthline.com/galecontent/behavioral-therapy. Accessed 2/27/2011.
7. Shafer PO, DiIorio C. Managing life issues in epilepsy. *Continuum: Lifelong Learning in Neurology – Epilepsy* 2004; 10(4): 138-56.
8. Legion V. Health education for self-management by people with epilepsy. *J Neurosci Nurs* 1991; 23(5): 300-5.
9. Kwan I, Ridsdale L, Robins D. An epilepsy care package: the nurse specialist's role. *J Neurosci Nurs* 2000; 32(3): 145-52.
10. Dahl J, Melin L, Lund L. Effects of a contingent relaxation treatment program on adults with refractory epileptic seizures. *Epilepsia* 1987; 28(2): 125-32.
11. Lundgren T, Dahl J, Melin L, Kies B. Evaluation of acceptance and commitment therapy for drug refractory epilepsy: a randomized controlled trial in South Africa - a pilot study. *Epilepsia* 2006; 47(12): 2173-9.
12. Lundgren T, Dahl J, Yardi N, Melin L. Acceptance and commitment therapy and yoga for drug-refractory epilepsy: a randomized controlled trial. *Epilepsy Behav* 2008; 13(1): 102-8.
13. Richard A, Reiter J. *Epilepsy - A New Approach*. New York, USA: Prentice Hall Press, 1990.
14. Andrews DJ, Reiter JM, Schonfeld W, Kastl A, Denning P. A neurobehavioral treatment for unilateral complex partial seizure disorders: a comparison of right- and left-hemisphere patients. *Seizure* 2000; 9: 189-97.
15. Mittan RJ. Fear of seizures. In: *Psychopathology in epilepsy: social dimensions*. Whitman S, Hermann BP, Eds. New York, USA: Oxford University Press, 1986: 90-121.
16. Fisher RS, Vickrey BG, Gibson P, *et al*. The impact of epilepsy from the patient's perspective. I: Descriptions and subjective perceptions. *Epilepsy Res* 2000; 41: 39-51.
17. Living Well with Epilepsy II. A report of the 2003 National Conference on Public Health and Epilepsy. Epilepsy Foundation. (http://www.epilepsyfoundation.org.)
18. Labiner DM, Bagic AI, Herman ST, Fountain NB, Walczak TS, Gumnit RJ. Essential services, personnel, and facilities in specialized epilepsy centers- revised 2010 guidelines. *Epilepsia* 2010; 51(11): 2322-33.
19. Cochrane J. Patient education: lessons from epilepsy. *Patient Education and Counseling* 1995; 26: 25-31.
20. Couldridge L, Kendall S, March A. 'A systematic overview - a decade of research'. The information and counseling needs of people with epilepsy. *Seizure* 2001; 10: 605-14.
21. Lannon SL. Using a health promotion model to enhance medication compliance. *J Neurosci Nurs* 1997; 29(3): 170-8.
22. May TW, Pfafflin M. Psychoeducational programs for patients with epilepsy. *Disease Management & Health Outcomes* 2005; 13(3): 185-99.
23. Clark AJ, Espie CA, Paul A. Adults with learning disabilities and epilepsy: knowledge about epilepsy before and after an educational package. *Seizure* 2001; 10: 492-9.
24. Helgeson DC, Mittan R, Siang-Yang T, Chayasirisobhon S. Sepulveda Epilepsy Education: the efficacy of a psychoeducational treatment program in treating medical and psychosocial aspects of epilepsy. *Epilepsia* 1990; 31(1); 75-82.
25. May TW, Pfafflin M. The efficacy of an educational treatment program for patients with epilepsy (MOSES): results of a controlled randomized study. *Epilepsia* 2002; 43(5): 539-49.
26. Olley BO, Osinowo HO, Brieger WR. Psycho-educational therapy among Nigerian adult patients with epilepsy: a controlled outcome study. *Patient Education and Counseling* 2001; 42(1): 25-33.

27. Snead K, Ackerson J, Bailey K, Schmitt MM, Madan-Swain A, Martin RC. Taking charge of epilepsy: the development of a structured psychoeducational group intervention for adolescents with epilepsy and their parents. *Epilepsy Behav* 2004; 5: 547-56.

28. Spector S, Tranah A, Cull C, Goldstein LH. Reduction in seizure frequency following a short-term group intervention for adults with epilepsy. *Seizure* 1999; 8: 297-303.

29. Gillham RA. Refractory epilepsy: an evaluation of psychological methods in outpatient management. *Epilepsia* 1990; 31(4): 427-32.

30. Spector S, Cull C, Goldstein LH. High and low perceived self-control of epileptic seizures. *Epilepsia* 2001; 42(4): 556-64.

31. DiIorio C, Shafer PO, Letz R, Henry T, Schomer DL, Yeager K. Project EASE: a study to test a psychosocial model of epilepsy medication management. *Epilepsy Behav* 2004; 5: 926-36.

32. DiIorio C, Shafer PO, Letz R, Henry TR, Schomer DS, Yeager K. Behavioral, social and affective factors associated with self-efficacy for self-management among people with epilepsy. *Epilepsy Behav* 2006; 9: 158-63.

33. Goldfried MR, Merbaum M. A perspective on self-control. In: *Behavior Change through Self-control*. Goldfried MR, Merbaum M, Eds. New York, USA: Holt, Rinehart & Winston, 1973: 3-34.

34. Rosenbaum M. The role of learned resourcefulness in the self-control of health behavior. In: *Learned Resourcefulness: on Coping Skills, Self-control, and Adaptive Behavior*. Rosenbaum M, Ed. New York, USA: Springer Publishing, 1990: 3-30.

35. Meichenbaum D. *Cognitive-behavior Modification: an Integrative Approach*. New York, USA: Plenum Press, 1977.

36. Acceptance and commitment therapy. Wikipedia. http://en.wikipedia.org/wiki/Acceptance_and_Commitment_Therapy. Accessed 2/27/2011.

37. Panjwani U, Selvamurthy W, Singh SH, Gupta HL, Thakur L, Rai UC. Effect of Sahaja yoga practice on seizure control and EEG changes in patients of epilepsy. *Indian Journal of Medical Research* 1996; 103: 165-72.

38. Lansky, EP, St. Louis, EK. Transcendental meditation: a double-edged sword in epilepsy? *Epilepsy Behav* 2006; 9: 394-400.

39. Puskarich CA, Whitman S, Dell J, Hughes JR, Rosen AJ, Hermann BP. Controlled examination of effects of progressive relaxation training on seizure reduction. *Epilepsia* 1992; 33(4): 675-80.

40. Rousseau A, Hermann B, Whitman S. Effects of progressive relaxation on epilepsy: analysis of a series of cases. *Psychological Reports* 1985; 57: 1203-12.

41. Snyder M. Effect of relaxation on psychosocial functioning in persons with epilepsy. *J Neurosci Nurs* 1983; 15(4): 250-4.

42. Berger NM. The effect of a stress-management training program on epilepsy. AES Proceedings. *Epilepsia* 2001; 42(Suppl 7): 245.

43. Martinovic Z. Adjunctive behavioural treatment in adolescents and young adults with juvenile myoclonic epilepsy. *Seizure* 2001; 10: 42-7.

44. Au A, Chan F, Li K, Leung P, Li P, Chan J. Cognitive-behavioral group treatment program for adults with epilepsy in Hong Kong. *Epilepsy Behav* 2003; 4: 441-6.

45. Pramuka M, Hendrickson R, Zinski A, Van Cott AC. A psychosocial self-management program for epilepsy: a randomized pilot study in adults. *Epilepsy Behav* 2007; 11: 533-45.

46. Engelberts NHJ, Klein M, Ader HJ, Heimans JJ, Kasteleijn-Nolst Trenite DGA, van der Ploeg HM. The effectiveness of cognitive rehabilitation for attention deficits in focal seizures: a randomized controlled study. *Epilepsia* 2002; 43(6): 587-95.

47. Robinson E, DiIorio C, DePadilla L, *et al*. Psychosocial predictors of lifestyle management in adults with epilepsy. *Epilepsy Behav* 2008; 13: 523-8.

48. Bandura A. *Self-efficacy: The Exercise of Control*. New York, USA: Freeman, 1997.

49. Lorig KR, Holman HR. Self-management education: history, definition, outcomes, and mechanisms. *Annals of Behavioral Medicine* 2003; 26(1): 1-7.

50. Kobau R, DiIorio C. Epilepsy self-management: a comparison of self-efficacy and outcome expectancy for medication adherence and lifestyle behaviors among people with epilepsy. *Epilepsy Behav* 2003; 4: 217-25.

51. DiIorio C, Reisinger EL, Yeager KA, McCarty F. A telephone-based self-management program for people with epilepsy. *Epilepsy Behav* 2009; 14: 232-6.

52. DiIorio C, Escoffery C, Yeager KA, et al. WebEase: development of a web-based epilepsy self-management intervention. *Preventing Chronic Disease: Public Health Research, Practice, and Policy* 2009; 6(1): 1-7.

53. DiIorio C, Walker ER, Bamps Y. Results of a randomized controlled trial: evaluating WebEase, an online epilepsy self-management program. Abstract No. 2.358, 2010, American Epilepsy Society Annual Meeting, www.aesnet.org.

54. Arida RM, Scorza FA, Cavalheiro EA. Favorable effects of physical activity for recovery in temporal lobe epilepsy. *Epilepsia* 2010; 51(Suppl. 3): 76-9.

55. Arida RM, Scorza FA, Gomes da Silva S, Schachter SC. The potential role of physical exercise in the treatment of epilepsy. *Epilepsy Behav* 2010; 17: 432-5.

56. Frucht MM, Quigg M, Schwaner C, Fountain NB. Distribution of seizure precipitants among epilepsy syndromes. *Epilepsia* 2000; 41: 1534-9.

57. Roth DL, Goode KT, Williams VL, Faught E. Physical exercise, stressful life experience, and depression in adults with epilepsy. *Epilepsia* 1994; 35(6): 1248-55.

58. Nakken KO, Bjorholt PG, Johannessen SI, Loyning T, Lind E. Effect of physical training on aerobic capacity, seizure occurrence, and serum level of antiepileptic drugs in adults with epilepsy. *Epilepsia* 1990; 31(1): 88-94.

59. Eriksen HR, Ellertsen B, Gronningsaeter H, Nakken KO, Loyning Y, Ursin H. Physical exercise in women with intractable epilepsy. *Epilepsia* 1994; 35(6): 1256-64.

60. McAuley JW, Long L, Heise J, et al. A prospective evaluation of the effects of a 12-week outpatient exercise program on clinical and behavioral outcomes in patients with epilepsy. *Epilepsy Behav* 2001; 2: 592-600.

61. Loring DW, Meador KJ, Lee GP. Determinants of quality of life in epilepsy. *Epilepsy Behav* 2004; 5: 976-80.

62. Martinovic Z, Simonovic P, Djokic R. Preventing depression in adolescents with epilepsy. *Epilepsy Behav* 2006; 9: 619-24.

63. Ciechanowski P, Chaytor N, Miller J, et al. PEARLS depression treatment for individuals with epilepsy: a randomized controlled trial. *Epilepsy Behav* 2010; 19: 225-31.

64. Walker ER, Obolensky N, Dini S, Thompson NJ. Formative and process evaluations of a cognitive-behavioral therapy and mindfulness intervention for people with epilepsy and depression. *Epilepsy Behav* 2010; 19: 239-46.

65. Thompson NJ, Walker ER, Obolensky N, et al. Distance delivery of mindfulness-based cognitive therapy for depression: Project UPLIFT. *Epilepsy Behav* 2010; 19: 247-54.

66. Yeager KA, DiIorio C, Shafer PO, et al. The complexity of treatments for people with epilepsy. *Epilepsy Behav* 2005; 7(4): 679-86.

67. Cramer JA, Mattson RH, Prevey ML, Scheyer RD, Ouellette VL. How often is medication taken as prescribed? A novel assessment technique. *JAMA* 1989; 261: 3273-7.

68. Pender NJ. *Health Promotion in Nursing Practice*, 2nd ed. Appleton and Lange, 1987: 58.

69. Buelow JM, Smith MC. Medication management by the person with epilepsy: perception versus reality. *Epilepsy Behav* 2004; 5: 401-6.

70. Peterson GM, Mclean S, Millingen KS. A randomized trial of strategies to improve patient compliance with anticonvulsant therapy. *Epilepsia* 1984; 25(4): 412-7.

71. Brown I, Sheeran P, Reuber M. Enhancing antiepileptic drug adherence: a randomized controlled trial. *Epilepsy Behav* 2009; 16: 634-9.

72. Engelberts NHJ, Klein M, Kasteleijn-Nolst Trenite DGA, Heimans JJ, van der Ploeg HM. The effectiveness of psychological interventions for patients with relatively well-controlled epilepsy. *Epilepsy Behav* 2002; 3: 420-6.

Chapter 11

Herbal remedies in epilepsy

Dana Ekstein MD, Senior Neurologist
Head, Epilepsy Center, Department of Neurology
Hadassah University Medical Center, Jerusalem, Israel

Introduction

Approximately one third of people with epilepsy (PWE) have drug-resistant seizures [1, 2]. Surgery is highly effective and safe for selected patients with treatment-resistant focal epilepsy [3, 4], but is still underused, even in high-income countries [5]. Many PWE may not be candidates for surgery because a single site of origin of their seizures cannot be localized or exists within eloquent regions of the cortex. Other treatment strategies are primarily palliative (vagal nerve stimulation) or still under investigation (closed loop cortical stimulation) [6]. Although the newer antiepileptic drugs (AEDs) may offer a better adverse events profile in comparison to the older generation AEDs, they may still have significant undesired CNS effects such as decreased cognitive abilities and psychiatric complications [7]. Notwithstanding these limitations, the ease of use and ready availability of medications, as well as the prompt reversibility of dose-related side effects, will keep AEDs as the mainstay of epilepsy treatment for the foreseeable future. Therefore, new drug therapies with efficacy against drug-resistant seizures, favorable adverse events profiles, especially in regard to neurological and psychiatric effects, and, if possible, low costs to patients and high worldwide availability are clearly needed.

Complementary and alternative medicine (CAM) is defined by the National Center for Complementary and Alternative Medicine (NCCAM) as a group of diverse medical and health care systems, practices, and products that are not generally considered part of conventional medicine as practiced in the west (e.g. the United States) [8]. Four domains of practices are recognized: mind-body medicine (meditation, prayer, mental healing, art, music, dance), biologically-based practices (use of substances found in nature such as herbs, foods, vitamins, animal compounds), manipulative and body-based practices (chiropractic or osteopathic manipulation, massage), and energy medicine (biofield and bioelectromagnetic therapies). Separately recognized are whole medical systems, such as homeopathy, naturopathy, Ayurveda and traditional Chinese medicine (TCM), each of them characterized by a complex and unique system of diagnostics and therapeutics. For example, the practitioners of TCM use herbal medicine, acupuncture and moxibustion as therapeutic methods. The efficacy of different CAM interventions for epilepsy has not been adequately proved in clinical trials. For example, three Cochrane reviews evaluated the published data on the use of acupuncture [9], yoga [10], and TCM [11] for epilepsy and none found sufficient evidence of efficacy of any of these techniques (see also Chapters 7 and 10).

Herbal medicines are any crude or chemically extracted plant materials or their combinations used as therapeutic products. This chapter focuses on the available evidence on the efficacy and safety for use of herbal medicines in people with epilepsy.

Treatment of epilepsy with herbal medicines in traditional medical systems

Ayurveda and TCM are among the best known systems of traditional medicine. Ayurveda originated thousands of years ago and continues to be widely practiced in South Asia, especially in India. TCM is widely practiced and carefully regulated by the Chinese government. The Kampo system in Japan, as well as Korean Oriental Medicine (KOM), are derived from TCM and remain broadly similar. The vast clinical experience with the use of herbal remedies in these medical systems represents level IV of evidence (IV/C) for their efficacy in epilepsy.

Ayurveda

This is the oldest known system of medicine, developed by the ancient Hindus, and based on balancing the three elements (vata, pitta, kapha) in the human body. Epilepsy (*Apasmara*) is considered a mental disease and classified into four types, three with predominant involvement of each of the three elements and a fourth characterized by combined involvement of all three. Although some characteristics of seizures as defined in western medicine also appear in Ayurvedic writings, there are differences in how seizures are recognized between these two systems. Treatment usually starts with drastic cleansing of the body through emesis, enemas and purgatives, followed by different Ayurvedic drug formulations. Additional Ayurvedic drugs are then recommended for use and are administered by various ways: orally, by nasal or ocular application, anointing the body or by fumigation [12].

Ayurvedic practitioners prescribe PWE mixtures of natural products, containing herbal extracts, as well as animal ghee, honey and milk. The most widely used herbal extracts are prepared from *Acacia arabica*, *Acorus calamus*, *Bacoppa monnieri*, *Clitorea turuatea*, *Celastrus paniculata*, *Convolvulus pluricaulis*, *Emblica officinalis*, *Mukta pishti*, *Withania somnifera*, and *Vaca brahmi yoga* [13].

TCM

This medical system concerns the study of human physiology and pathology, and the prevention, diagnosis and treatment of human diseases, and dates back more than 2500 years. The theory of TCM for PWE is difficult to understand from a western perspective because of the TCM approach to diagnosis and treatment, and the related principles of holism and differentiation. Four subtypes of epilepsy are recognized, but, as is the case with the classification of seizures in Ayurveda, they do not match directly to the ILAE classification of seizures and epilepsies. Treatments typically involve mixtures of different herbal extracts (each containing many active compounds), some to directly treat the seizure disorder and others to maintain the general well-being of the host. The treatment may be applied in three phases. First, seizures are treated by herbs and acupuncture; then, herbs, acupuncture and moxibustion are used for tonic strengthening of organs; and finally, daily life guidelines are recommended to prevent relapse [14].

The most frequently used herbal medicines in the published clinical epilepsy literature from the Far East are *Pinella ternate*, *Arisaema japonicum*, *Acorus calamus*, *Gastrodia elata*, *Buthus martensii*, *Poria cocos*, *Bombyx batryticatus*, *Citrus reticulata*, *Uncaria rhynchophylla*, *Glycyrrhiza glabra*, *Salviae miltiorrhizae*, *Scolopendra subspinipes*, *Bupleurum falcatum*, *Succinum*, *Paeonia albiflora*, *Panax ginseng*, *Perichaeta communissma* and *Curcuma longa* [13]. However, as mentioned earlier, there is insufficient evidence at the present time to recommend the use of TCM for treatment of epilepsy [11]. Nevertheless, extracts used for seizure control in TCM, as well as single compounds derived from these extracts, are being tested alone and in combinations for anticonvulsant effects in animal models of epilepsy.

Efficacy of herbal medicines in monotherapy

There are no English-language publications of randomized clinical trials (RCTs) of herbal medicines for treatment of epilepsy. The authors of a Cochrane review on TCM for epilepsy found seven Chinese trials of herbal products compared with AEDs for treatment of epilepsy, diagnosed according to the International League Against Epilepsy (ILAE) classifications (Table 1) [11]. Two of the studies (both by Ma *et al*) were excluded from the formal review due to unclear design and an unusual allocation of 6:1 between the study and control arms. The other five studies were of single center, parallel design and had a control group. Randomization was mentioned, but the randomization procedures were unclear. None of the studies were blinded and their duration ranged from 2 months to 3 years. Only limited descriptions on baseline and follow-up data were provided. Variation of the baseline patients' characteristics, the herbal formulations, and the AEDs between the studies precluded meta-analysis of the results. Although the studies did report some benefit, no reliable conclusion

Table 1. Trials of herbal medicines in monotherapy [11].

Study	Baseline data	Treatment (Tx)	Control	Subjects (Tx:control)	Duration of follow-up	TCM AE	Outcome (Tx:control)
Liu 1994	Primary GTCS. 0.5-20 years after first seizure (sz)	Xaxingci granule 4g tid; 3 courses of 4 weeks each	PHT 10mg/kg/day tid; 3 courses of 4 weeks each	20:20 4-53 years old	12 weeks to 1 year	No AE on routine blood tests, hepatic and renal function	1) SF-RR 1.00; 95% CI, 0.07-14.90, p=1.00 2) ≥75% reduction in sz frequency - RR1.50; 95% CI, 0.28-8.04, p=0.64 3) ≥25% reduction in sz frequency - RR1.00; 95% CI, 0.81-1.23, p=1.00 4) EEG improvement - 15% vs. 10%
Song 2001	Epilepsy (ILAE 1989) - GTCS, absence, SPS, CPS, myoclonus, atonic. 1-30 years after first sz	Dianxianning tid for 90 days; adults 4g/day, children 2.5g/day	VPA tid for 90 days; adults 0.4g/day, children 0.2g/day	100:50 2-45 years old	90 days to 1 year	No AE	1) SF-RR 13.00; 95% CI, 0.74-227.72, p=0.08 2) ≥80% reduction in sz frequency - RR 2.73; 95% CI, 2.00-3.74, p <0.00001 3) ≥60% reduction in sz. frequency - RR 0.98; 95% CI, 0.92-1.04, p=0.52 4) EEG improvement - 100%: 40% obviously, 36% improved, 24% unchanged
Tian 2006	Epilepsy (ILAE 1989) - GTCS, absence, SPS, CPS. History of treatment with AEDs, such as VPA, CBZ, TPM	Tianmadingxian tid for 90 days, <8y - 1.05g; 8-12y - 1.4g; >13y - 2.1g; at least 1 month after AED	PHT tid for 90 days; adults 0.15g, children 8mg/kg/day	178:156 4-70 years old	90 days	Not mentioned	1) ≥75% reduction in sz frequency - RR 2.38; 95% CI, 1.83-3.09, p <0.00001 2) ≥50% reduction in sz frequency - RR 1.37; 95% CI, 1.23-1.53, p <0.00001 3) ≥25% reduction in sz frequency - RR 1.19; 95% CI, 1.10-1.28, p <0.00001
Xiang 1998	Primary GTCS. 0.3-25 years after first sz. At least 1 sz per month, more than 3 sz in total	Zhixian I bid for 60 days	PHT 0.2-0.8g bid-tid for 60 days	100:100 8-61 years old	60 days to 3 years	Slight GI discomfort (32%), no effects on routine blood, hepatic and renal function	1) ≥75% reduction in sz frequency - RR 1.42; 95% CI, 1.20-1.68, p<0.0001 2) ≥50% reduction in sz frequency - RR 1.31; 95% CI, 1.16-1.48, p <0.0001 3) ≥25% reduction in sz frequency - RR 1.10; 95% CI, 1.03-1.18, p=0.006 4) EEG improvement - 55% became normal and 14% improved:10% became normal, 25% improved, 2% aggravated 5) Relapse rate - 1y - 13.4%:39.8%; 2y - 20.6%:20.6%; 3y - 25.8%:68.9%
Xin 1999	Primary GTCS, partial STCS. 1-2 sz per month 3 months before inclusion, more than 3 sz in total	Antiepilepsy cap. tid for 90 days. 3-6y - 2.5g, > 6y - 4g.	PB 1.5-2mg/kg tid for 90 days	301:100 3-13 years old	90 days	Slight GI discomfort	1) ≥75% reduction in sz frequency - RR 1.46; 95% CI, 1.13-1.88, p=0.003 2) ≥50% reduction in sz frequency - RR 1.21; 95% CI, 1.02-1.43, p=0.03 3) ≥75% reduction in sz duration - RR 1.29; 95% CI, 0.98-1.69, p=0.07 4) ≥50% reduction in sz duration - RR 1.25; 95% CI, 1.05-1.48, p=0.01 5) EEG improvement - 51% improved: 45% improved

Table 1 _continued_. Trials of herbal medicines in monotherapy [11].

Study	Baseline data	Treatment (Tx)	Control	Subjects (Tx:control)	Duration of follow-up	TCM AE	Outcome (Tx:control)
Ma 2003a	Primary GTCS. Up to 14 years after first sz. Up to 3 sz per month.	Xifeng cap. and antiepilepsy cap. - each tid <1y - 1; 1-3y - 2; 3-7y - 5; >7y - 8	PB 2mg/kg tid for 180 days	200:100:100 2-14 years old	180 days	Not mentioned	1) SF for ≥1y 25%: 8%: 3% 2) ≥75% reduction in sz frequency - 57%: 56%: 38% 3) ≥50% reduction in sz frequency - 8%: 24%: 42%
Ma 2003b	Epilepsy (ILAE 1981). More than 6 sz in 6 months before study	Antiepilepsy cap. tid for 180 days: 1-5y - 1-5 cap; 6-10y - 7; 11-14y - 8	PB 1.5-2mg/kg tid for 180 days	930:160 1-14 years old	180 days	Not mentioned	1) ≥75% reduction in sz frequency - 57%:40% 2) 51-75% reduction in sz frequency - 26%:12% 3) 25-50% reduction in sz frequency - 10%:24% 4) No reduction in sz frequency - 1%:6%

AE = adverse effects; TCM = Traditional Chinese Medicine; SF = seizure free; GTCS = generalized tonic-clonic seizure; ILAE = International League Against Epilepsy; SPS = simple partial seizure; CPS = complex partial seizure; STCS = secondary tonic-clonic seizure; AED = antiepileptic drug; VPA = valproic acid; CBZ = carbamazepine; TPM = topiramate; PHT = phenytoin; PB = phenobarbital; tid = three times a day; bid = two times a day

on the effect of TCM for epilepsy could be drawn, due to a high probability of selection, detection and performance bias [11]. The methodological limitations of these trials do not allow their consideration as Ib level of evidence.

Efficacy of herbal medicines as add-on to AEDs

There are no English-language RCTs testing the efficacy of herbal medicines as add-on to AEDs. The authors of the Cochrane review reporting on TCM for treatment of epilepsy were able to find three Chinese articles where botanicals were used in conjunction with AEDs and they will be included in the update of the review [11]. Three different herbal products were assessed in these trials: alkaline extract of _Euphorbia fischeriana_ (in 72 patients with epilepsy), Ningxian capsules (in 180 patients with epilepsy) and ginkgo biloba [11].

Search of planned clinical trials for herbal remedies for epilepsy revealed one study initiated by Dr. Siegward Elsas, from Oregon Health and Science University, and aimed to be completed in 2011. This phase II randomized, placebo-controlled, double-blind, cross-over clinical trial will test the safety and potential anticonvulsant efficacy of a botanical extract from _Passiflora incarnata_, in patients with partial onset epilepsy [15]. The investigators of this study intend to randomize approximately 25 people with active focal onset epilepsy who take one or two conventional AEDs for two crossover arms of treatment and placebo (11 weeks for each). The primary outcome measure will be seizure frequency and the secondary outcome measures – anxiety, cognitive function and quality of life. Screening for adverse effects will be performed. Upon completion, this trial will provide Ib level of evidence for the efficacy of _Passiflora_ in the treatment of epilepsy.

Efficacy of herbal medicines for treatment of common comorbidities of epilepsy

Over the past few decades, the use of natural products by patients in western countries has significantly increased. According to the 2007 American National Health Interview Survey of 23,393 adults and 9417 children, 38.3% of adults and 11.8% of children reported using CAM therapies, with the most commonly utilized form of CAM being natural products, which were used by 17.7% of the surveyed adults [16]. According to available studies among patients with epilepsy, between 24% and 56% of the adults and 12% to 32% of children have used CAM therapies at some time and many of them do not report the use of CAM to their physicians [17]. Although only 2% to 44% of these patients reported using these products specifically for control of seizures, the reasons noted by many patients may be relevant to known comorbidities of epilepsy such as depression or to common AED adverse events such as impaired memory. Indeed, current evidence supports the use of St. John's wort in treating mild to moderate depression [18], and the use of kava in treatment of generalized anxiety [18, 19] (Ia/A). Rosenroot was found to improve attention in cognitive function in fatigue (Ia/A), to have an anti-fatigue effect in physical, emotional and mental exhaustion (Ib/A), to treat mild depression (III/B) and to improve mental performance (III/B) [20]. There is not yet enough evidence for the use of other herbal remedies in psychiatric disorders [21] or insomnia [22] or as adjuvants to conventional antidepressants, mood stabilizers or benzodiazepines [23].

No publication has specifically studied the efficacy of herbal medicines for comorbidities in the epilepsy patient population. However, search of planned clinical trials of herbal products in patients with epilepsy revealed a trial intended to be completed in 2011, whose primary investigator is Wang Xin, from China [24]. This study will evaluate the efficacy and safety of add-on therapy of the wuling capsule in epilepsy patients with depression. It is a multi-center, randomized, double-blinded, placebo-controlled superiority clinical trial, taking place in eight centers from four different cities in China, aiming to enroll 230 patients with epilepsy and depression, and randomize to either treatment or placebo for 3 months. The primary outcome is improvement in depression and the secondary outcomes are frequency and severity of seizures, sleeping condition and quality of life.

Safety of herbal medicines in people with epilepsy

As is the case with publications that study the efficacy of herbal medicines for epilepsy, there are very few reports that address safety issues for use of botanicals in people with epilepsy. In general, herbal medicines are considered as relatively safe and indeed only minimal GI discomfort was reported in the available clinical trials of herbal products for treatment of epilepsy (Table 1) [11]. One study (by Xin) reported the incidence of adverse effects both in the 'antiepilepsy capsule' and phenobarbital group and the Peto odds ratio was 0.04 (99% CI, 0.01-0.12; p <0.00001), favoring the antiepilepsy capsule [11].

While many botanicals are known to affect the central nervous system, only case reports of association between use of herbal products and the occurrence of seizures have been published in humans and involved mainly ephedra, caffeine, gingko biloba seeds, star anise,

Table 2. Human studies of interactions between herbal medicines and AEDs.

Study	Subjects	Outcome
Pattanaik 2006 [30]	20 patients with uncontrolled epilepsy	Piperine increased concentration of PHT at steady state
Velpandian 2001[31]	6 healthy volunteers	Piperine increased concentration of coadministered PHT
Garg 1998 [32]	10 patients with epilepsy	Grapefruit juice increased concentration of CBZ at steady state
Ozdemir 1998 [33]	8 healthy volunteers	Grapefruit juice increased concentration of coadministered diazepam
Wang 2001 [36]	Healthy volunteers	St. John's wort taken for 14 days decreased concentration of oral midazolam
Kawaguchi 2004 [35]	13 healthy volunteers	St. John's wort taken for 14 days decreased concentration of quazepam, but did not change its pharmacodynamic effects
Dresser 2003 [34]	Healthy volunteers	St. John's wort taken for 12 days decreased concentration of oral midazolam
Etman 1995 [38]	4 healthy volunteers	Psyllium decreased concentration of coadministered CBZ
Kupiec 2005 [37]	One case report	Ginkgo biloba decreased concentration of PHT and VPA

PHT = phenytoin; CBZ = carbamazepine; VPA = valproic acid

star fruit and evening primrose [25, 26]. A review of the 65 cases of dietary supplement-associated seizures reported to the FDA between 1993 and 1999 concluded that 20 seizures were probably related to the dietary supplement (19 of them involved ephedra consumption and 14 – caffeine), 13 – possibly related (7 involved ephedra, 5 – caffeine, and creatine, St. John's wort, and ginkgo biloba were also implicated), and 10 – unrelated [27]. Five cases were not seizures, and 17 cases contained insufficient information.

Although multiple interactions between botanicals and AEDs may be assumed from the knowledge on the effects of herbal products on motility of the intestines, absorption and liver enzymes, and from animal trials, very few works directly studied these interactions in humans (Table 2) [25, 26, 28, 29]. The best available evidence for interaction between an herbal medicine and AEDs was provided by a study which showed that piperine coadministration significantly increased the mean plasma concentration of two different doses of phenytoin at steady state in 20 patients with uncontrolled epilepsy [30]. This finding was further supported by a trial that showed a similarly significant rise in the concentration of phenytoin after its coadministration with piperine in six healthy volunteers [31]. Similarly, grapefruit juice increased the bioavailability of carbamazepine at steady state in patients with epilepsy [32] and increased the concentration of diazepam in healthy subjects [33]. Chronic treatment with St. John's wort was found to decrease the bioavailability of benzodiazepines in healthy subjects, presumably through its effects on the cytochrome P450 system [34-36]. Interestingly, this decrease in the plasma concentration did not induce pharmacodynamic effects in one of the studies [35]. In one case report of fatal seizures accompanied by low plasma concentrations of phenytoin and valproic acid in an epilepsy patient who had been using herbal supplements that contained gingko biloba, it was assumed that gingko may decrease the bioavailability of these AEDs [37]. Many herbal remedies that contain high fiber concentrations may theoretically interfere with the absorption of concomitantly ingested drugs, including AEDs. However, this theory has only been tested in humans in regard to psyllium, which was found to decrease the plasma concentration of carbamazepine when taken together by four healthy subjects [38].

Methodology challenges

Publications of CAM clinical trials for the treatment of epilepsy that have encouraging results generally use inadequate methodologies. Many do not adequately randomize study subjects or use proper controls, while others are not blinded or do not rigorously monitor the results of the interventions. While the requirements of evidence-based medicine have become familiar to conventional/western practitioners, implementing these principles into trials of other medical systems is problematic because these systems may involve a holistic, personalized approach to treating patients rather than one that is disease-focused and therefore applied in the same way to all patients characterized by a specific disease. In addition, there are cultural differences between western and traditional populations that raise ethical issues which make the incorporation of evidence-based principles for RCTs even harder [39].

The Consolidated Standards of Reporting Trials (CONSORT) statement, based on a 22-item checklist, guides authors, readers, reviewers and editors on the essential information required in reports of two-group parallel RCTs [40, 41]. In 2006, specific recommendations for reporting RCTs of herbal medicines were issued by a group of individuals with international expertise in clinical trial methodology, pharmacognosy and herbal products [42]. Nine items of the CONSORT statement were elaborated for relevance to RCTs of herbal medicines. Specific attention was given to the precise description of the intervention to include all the details of the name, manufacturer, plant part used, type of preparation, source and authentication of the herbal material, pharmaceutical quality, dosage regimen and purity testing. Further and even more elaborated recommendations for reporting of RCTs of TCM interventions [43], outcomes [44] and adverse events [45] were then proposed by Chinese researchers. A follow-up work that looked at the implementation of the herbal medicines CONSORT recommendations in 406 RCTs up to the end of 2007 found that although only

38% of the required information was reported, the reports were better in the more recent years [46].

Conclusions

There is no evidence from well-designed clinical trials to support efficacy of herbal medicines in the treatment of epilepsy. Although no trials studied specific treatment of comorbid conditions in patients with epilepsy, there is good evidence for the use of St. John's wort in depression, kava in anxiety and rosenroot in fatigue and depression. There are case reports of association between the use of certain herbal remedies and seizures. Herbal products may interact with AEDs. Better designed clinical studies for herbal therapies in patients with epilepsy are needed.

Key points	Evidence level
◆ There is vast clinical experience with use of herbal remedies in traditional medical systems, such as Ayurveda and TCM.	IV/C
◆ There are no good quality RCTs or well-conducted clinical studies on the efficacy of herbal remedies in monotherapy for epilepsy.	
◆ There are no RCTs or well-conducted clinical studies on the efficacy of herbal remedies as add-on to AEDs for epilepsy.	
◆ St. John's wort is effective for treatment of depression (not specifically tested in patients with epilepsy).	Ia/A
◆ Kava is effective for treatment of anxiety (not specifically tested in patients with epilepsy).	Ia/A
◆ Rosenroot improves attention in cognitive function in patients with fatigue (not specifically tested in patients with epilepsy).	Ia/A
◆ Rosenroot has an anti-fatigue effect in physical, emotional and mental exhaustion (not specifically tested in patients with epilepsy).	Ib/A
◆ Rosenroot is effective for treatment of mild depression (not specifically tested in patients with epilepsy).	III/B
◆ Use of herbal remedies has been rarely associated with seizures, but no RCTs or well-conducted clinical studies have tested this association.	
◆ Piperine increases plasma concentration of phenytoin at steady state in patients with epilepsy.	III/B
◆ Grapefruit juice increases plasma concentration of carbamazepine at steady state in patients with epilepsy.	III/B
◆ Additional interactions between herbal remedies and AEDs have been reported, but no well-conducted studies have tested these interactions.	

References

1. Kwan P, Arzimanoglou A, Berg AT, *et al.* Definition of drug resistant epilepsy: consensus proposal by the ad hoc Task Force of the ILAE Commission on Therapeutic Strategies. *Epilepsia* 2010; 51(6): 1069-77.
2. Kwan P, Brodie MJ. Early identification of refractory epilepsy. *N Engl J Med* 2000; 342(5): 314-9.
3. Choi H, Sell RL, Lenert L, *et al.* Epilepsy surgery for pharmacoresistant temporal lobe epilepsy: a decision analysis. *JAMA* 2008; 300(21): 2497-505.
4. Engel J, Jr., Wiebe S, French J, *et al.* Practice parameter: temporal lobe and localized neocortical resections for epilepsy: report of the Quality Standards Subcommittee of the American Academy of Neurology, in association with the American Epilepsy Society and the American Association of Neurological Surgeons. *Neurology* 2003; 60(4): 538-47.
5. Engel J, Jr. Surgical treatment for epilepsy: too little, too late? *JAMA* 2008; 300(21): 2548-50.
6. Boon P, Raedt R, de Herdt V, Wyckhuys T, Vonck K. Electrical stimulation for the treatment of epilepsy. *Neurotherapeutics* 2009; 6(2): 218-27.
7. Schmidt D. Drug treatment of epilepsy: options and limitations. *Epilepsy Behav* 2009; 15(1): 56-65.
8. National Institutes of Health in National Center for Complementary and Alternative Medicine Home Page. http://nccam.nih.gov/.
9. Cheuk DK, Wong V. Acupuncture for epilepsy. *Cochrane Database Syst Rev* 2008; 4: CD005062.
10. Ramaratnam S, Sridharan K. Yoga for epilepsy. *Cochrane Database Syst Rev* 2000; 2: CD001524.
11. Li Q, Chen X, He L, Zhou D. Traditional Chinese medicine for epilepsy. *Cochrane Database Syst Rev* 2009; 3: CD006454.
12. Jain S. Ayurveda: the ancient Indian system of medicine. In: *Complementary and Alternative Therapies for Epilepsy.* Devinsky O, Schachter SC, Pacia S, Eds. New York, USA: Demos Medical, 2005: 123-8.
13. Schachter SC, Acevedo C, Acevedo KA, Lai C, Diop AG. Complementary and alternative medical therapies. In: *Epilepsy: A Comprehensive Textbook*, 2nd ed. Engel J, Pedley TA, Eds. Philadelphia, USA: Wolters Kluwer/Lippincott Williams & Wilkins, 2008: 1407-14.
14. Wang S, Li Y. Traditional Chinese medicine. In: *Complementary and Alternative Therapies for Epilepsy.* Devinsky O, Schachter SC, Pacia S, Eds. New York, USA: Demos Medical, 2005: 177-82.
15. http://clinicaltrials.gov/ct2/show/NCT00982787?term=epilepsy&rank=85.
16. Barnes PM, Bloom B, Nahin RL. Complementary and alternative medicine use among adults and children: United States, 2007. *Natl Health Stat Report* 2008; 10(12): 1-23.
17. Ekstein D, Schachter SC. Natural products in epilepsy - the present situation and perspectives for the future. *Pharmaceuticals* 2010; 3(5): 1426-45.
18. Sarris J, Kavanagh DJ. Kava and St. John's wort: current evidence for use in mood and anxiety disorders. *J Altern Complement Med* 2009; 15(8): 827-36.
19. Sarris J, LaPorte E, Schweitzer I. Kava: a comprehensive review of efficacy, safety, and psychopharmacology. *Aust N Z J Psychiatry* 2011; 45(1): 27-35.
20. Panossian A, Wikman G, Sarris J. Rosenroot (*Rhodiola rosea*): traditional use, chemical composition, pharmacology and clinical efficacy. *Phytomedicine* 2010; 17(7): 481-93.
21. Sarris J. Herbal medicines in the treatment of psychiatric disorders: a systematic review. *Phytother Res* 2007; 21(8): 703-16.
22. Sarris J, Byrne GJ. A systematic review of insomnia and complementary medicine. *Sleep Med Rev* 2011; 15(2): 99-106.
23. Sarris J, Kavanagh DJ, Byrne G. Adjuvant use of nutritional and herbal medicines with antidepressants, mood stabilizers and benzodiazepines. *J Psychiatr Res* 2010; 44(1): 32-41.
24. http://clinicaltrials.gov/ct2/show/NCT01125241?term=epilepsy&rank=96.
25. Samuels N, Finkelstein Y, Singer SR, Oberbaum M. Herbal medicine and epilepsy: proconvulsive effects and interactions with antiepileptic drugs. *Epilepsia* 2008; 49(3): 373-80.
26. Ulbricht C, Basch E, Weissner W, Hackman D. An evidence-based systematic review of herb and supplement interactions by the Natural Standard Research Collaboration. *Expert Opin Drug Saf* 2006; 5(5): 719-28.
27. Haller CA, Meier KH, Olson KR. Seizures reported in association with use of dietary supplements. *Clin Toxicol (Phila)* 2005; 43(1): 23-30.

28. Izzo AA, Ernst E. Interactions between herbal medicines and prescribed drugs: an updated systematic review. *Drugs* 2009; 69(13): 1777-98.

29. Ulbricht C, Chao W, Costa D, Rusie-Seamon E, Weissner W, Woods J. Clinical evidence of herb-drug interactions: a systematic review by the natural standard research collaboration. *Curr Drug Metab* 2008; 9(10): 1063-120.

30. Pattanaik S, Hota D, Prabhakar S, Kharbanda P, Pandhi P. Effect of piperine on the steady-state pharmacokinetics of phenytoin in patients with epilepsy. *Phytother Res* 2006; 20(8): 683-6.

31. Velpandian T, Jasuja R, Bhardwaj RK, Jaiswal J, Gupta SK. Piperine in food: interference in the pharmacokinetics of phenytoin. *Eur J Drug Metab Pharmacokinet* 2001; 26(4): 241-7.

32. Garg SK, Kumar N, Bhargava VK, Prabhakar SK. Effect of grapefruit juice on carbamazepine bioavailability in patients with epilepsy. *Clin Pharmacol Ther* 1998; 64(3): 286-8.

33. Ozdemir M, Aktan Y, Boydag BS, Cingi MI, Musmul A. Interaction between grapefruit juice and diazepam in humans. *Eur J Drug Metab Pharmacokinet* 1998; 23(1): 55-9.

34. Dresser GK, Schwarz UI, Wilkinson GR, Kim RB. Coordinate induction of both cytochrome P4503A and MDR1 by St John's wort in healthy subjects. *Clin Pharmacol Ther* 2003; 73(1): 41-50.

35. Kawaguchi A, Ohmori M, Tsuruoka S, *et al*. Drug interaction between St John's wort and quazepam. *Br J Clin Pharmacol* 2004; 58(4): 403-10.

36. Wang Z, Gorski JC, Hamman MA, Huang SM, Lesko LJ, Hall SD. The effects of St John's wort (*Hypericum perforatum*) on human cytochrome P450 activity. *Clin Pharmacol Ther* 2001; 70(4): 317-26.

37. Kupiec T, Raj V. Fatal seizures due to potential herb-drug interactions with ginkgo biloba. *J Anal Toxicol* 2005; 29(7): 755-8.

38. Etman MA. Effect of a bulk forming laxative on the bioavailability of carbamazepine in man. *Drug Development and Industrial Pharmacy* 1995; 21(16): 1901-6.

39. Zaslawski C. Ethical considerations for acupuncture and Chinese herbal medicine clinical trials: a cross-cultural perspective. *Evid Based Complement Alternat Med* 2010; 7(3): 295-301.

40. Begg C, Cho M, Eastwood S, *et al*. Improving the quality of reporting of randomized controlled trials. The CONSORT statement. *JAMA* 1996; 276(8): 637-9.

41. Moher D, Schulz KF, Altman D. The CONSORT statement: revised recommendations for improving the quality of reports of parallel-group randomized trials. *JAMA* 2001; 285(15): 1987-91.

42. Gagnier JJ, Boon H, Rochon P, Moher D, Barnes J, Bombardier C. Reporting randomized, controlled trials of herbal interventions: an elaborated CONSORT statement. *Ann Intern Med* 2006; 144(5): 364-7.

43. Bian Z, Moher D, Li Y, *et al*. Precise reporting of traditional Chinese medicine interventions in randomized controlled trials. *J Chinese Integrative Med* 2008; 6(7): 661-7.

44. Bian Z, Moher D, Li Y, *et al*. Appropriately selecting and concisely reporting the outcome measures of randomized controlled trials of traditional Chinese medicine. *J Chinese Integrative Med* 2008; 6(8): 771-5.

45. Cheng C, Bian Z, Li Y, *et al*. Transparently reporting adverse effects of traditional Chinese medicine interventions in randomized controlled trial. *J Chinese Integrative Med* 2008; 6(9): 881-6.

46. Gagnier JJ, Moher D, Boon H, Beyene J, Bombardier C. Randomized controlled trials of herbal interventions underreport important details of the intervention. *J Clin Epidemiol* 2011; Jan 3: epub ahead of print.

Chapter 12

Treatment of epilepsy and related comorbidities in patients with intellectual disabilities

Mike Kerr FRCPsych, Professor
Learning Disability Psychiatry, Cardiff University, Cardiff, UK

Ivana Dojcinov MRCPsych, Specialist Trainee in Psychiatry of Learning Disability
ABMU NHS Trust, Cardiff, UK

Introduction

People with an intellectual disability form a significant proportion of the prevalent active epilepsy population. This is in the main due to the fact that epilepsy is often pediatric in onset and more refractory to treatment [1]. Whilst patients with an intellectual disability benefit from the full range of investigations and interventions covered in this book, certain areas of epilepsy care pose specific challenges for the neurologist or epileptologist. To meet these challenges clinicians need knowledge of the data and of approaches to certain key clinical issues: the diagnosis of epilepsy, identifying the impact of epilepsy, the use of interventions and the treatment of related behavioral and other psychological comorbidity. Comorbidities, physical and psychological, are commonly associated with intellectual disability. Whilst all are important to health, some of these, in particular associated challenging behavior, can have a significant impact on the clinical management of epilepsy [2].

The focus of this chapter will be on issues relating to the care of adults, although in many cases the data pertaining to adults involve mixed child and adult research populations. There are specific challenges in providing an evidence base in this population due to the complexity of designing studies, as the population is heterogeneous, and an increased complexity in ethical issues. For this reason the evidence base is often limited with a tendency to interpretation of data from the general epilepsy population rather than intellectual disability specific data. We will, where possible, focus on data derived from people with an intellectual disability and epilepsy.

Misdiagnosis of epilepsy

Certain characteristics of people with an intellectual disability may increase the likelihood of diagnostic error. These include: communication difficulties, associated stereotypies, comorbidity such as autism and challenging behavior and the high prevalence of epilepsy. Put together the clinician is challenged by reduced access to investigations, as patients may not tolerate these, and potential diagnostic overshadowing from an expectation that epilepsy is a likely diagnostic explanation of episodic behavioral disturbance.

A recent systematic review [3] addressed the issue of misdiagnosis in this population. A total of eight studies met the author's strict criteria for study population, methodology, data collection, findings and follow-up. These included six cohort and two case studies; the majority were performed in children or adolescents. Across these studies, which included specific syndromes such as Rett and individuals from tertiary clinics, the prevalence ranged from 15-43% (III/B). A range of differential diagnosis was identified as highlighted in Table 1. Unfortunately such studies cannot identify the appropriate evidence-based approach to ensure accurate diagnosis. However, consensus statements on diagnosis do exist for this population [4] (IV/C). Table 2 summarizes the key recommendations.

Table 1. Reasons for misdiagnosis in people with an intellectual disability [3].

Syndrome-related	Rett vacant spells
	Sandifer syndrome
Medication-related	Personality change related to AED withdrawal
	Decreased daytime alertness due to AEDs
Psychological	Conversion disorder
Behavioral	Stereotypy
	Self-stimulatory
	Staring spells
	Simulation
	Spontaneous smiling
Physiological	Buccolingual movements
	Hypnic jerks
	Dystonic limb posturing

Table 2. Recommendations for the diagnostic process in people with an intellectual disability [4].

- An eyewitness account of the seizure, with an accurate description of the whole process, is needed in every case. This description should be recorded soon after the event; however, an exact description may often be too challenging for even an experienced observer when simultaneously satisfying the immediate requirements of the patient. A simple video recording of seizures (increasingly possible with modern mobile phones) can be a valuable tool and particularly succeeds in cases with frequent seizures.

- A careful assessment of potential seizure-provoking factors should be made: fever, infection, hypoglycemia, stress, excessive waking, alcohol withdrawal, hyperventilation, some medications, sudden discontinuation of sedative drugs, and specific activities should be taken into account.

- Non-convulsive epileptic phenomena and even partial seizures may be difficult to diagnose in people with intellectual disability (PWID). This may lead to an under-diagnosis of these particular seizure types (grade C). Attention should be paid to physiological and motor changes that may be associated with epileptic phenomena; these may include skin color, cardiac rhythm, eye movements, sucking and lip smacking.

- Successful electroencephalogram (EEG) recording needs the patient to co-operate and possibly sleep during the investigation. It is helpful, if possible, for prior acquaintance with the facilities to be made, in order for the patient to be less anxious and to maximize the opportunity of each appointment. Some patients may need melatonin or chloral hydrate, and these do not affect the EEG findings (grade C).

- During the recording clinicians should be sensitive to the patient's reactions and proceed gently. Prolonged video-EEG monitoring is of use in order to distinguish between epileptic and non-epileptic seizures and in selecting candidates for epilepsy surgery. If this investigation is not available, portable cassette recording of the EEG may also be of considerable value.

- Sleep disorders are often present in PWID who have difficult-to-treat epilepsy and behavioral problems. It is important to understand the sleep disorder, categorize the problem, investigate appropriately and then come to a diagnosis. It is important that treatment of sleep disorders should be available for this group as it is a significant quality-of-life issue.

- Magnetic resonance image (MRI) scanning is important in the diagnosis of conditions such as: neoplasm, dysplasia, heterotopia, or diseases in the brainstem and/or posterior fossa. If MRI is not available, computed tomography (CT) is recommended. Criteria for investigation should be agreed locally for people with epilepsy. These criteria should be followed for PWID who should not be excluded from MRI on the basis of their disability. This may mean anesthesia for MRI scanning may be required; this bears another set of risks that should be noted but should not mean exclusion from investigation. Brain CT, with contrast, is particularly useful in emergency situations.

To treat or not to treat?

For all patients with epilepsy, our decision to treat, or to change treatment, is based on an assessment of the impact of epilepsy and on informed patient choice. For people with an intellectual disability this still holds true. However, certain adjustments need to be made due to special circumstances, often overlapping, that apply to this group. These include: communication impairment, chronicity of epilepsy and the presence of associated behavioral problems.

Communication challenges

In many situations the individual themselves will not be their own advocate and decisions will be made in the individual's best interest through another family member or advocate. This 'management by proxy' is central to the care of this population but has clear challenges when assessing the impact of seizure. Professionals will need to focus on the collection of objective measures of severity including direct seizure pathology such as seizure rate, type, injury and hospitalization, or measures of general ill health such as weight and alertness. There should be a high index of suspicion for seizure-related psychopathology, either peri-ictal or interictal. Depression and anxiety should be monitored. In many cases this will be through biological features such as sleep and appetite. Good clinical practice focuses on supporting carers to provide appropriate information using diaries, education and scales such as the Epilepsy Outcome Scale **(IV/C)** [5, 6].

The impact of chronicity

For any individual with a chronic illness there is likely to be some attenuation to its impact and some resignation to the value of treatment change. However, for the general epilepsy population, a treatment decision remains an individual choice, or at least it should. An individual with an intellectual disability may face the double challenge of determination (the disease will inevitably be resistant to treatment) and valued judgment (the gaining of seizure change is of less value for such an individual). Both these scenarios need to be countered by objective clinical decision-making.

Associated behavioral problems

Behavioral problems associated with epilepsy will be addressed later in this chapter. Their presence is a barrier across the modalities of epilepsy management. The individual with such problems may have difficulty accessing investigations and interpretation of treatment side effects can be complicated.

These three areas notwithstanding, evidence exists **(III/B)** that people with an intellectual disability have a reduced life expectancy [7], greater hospitalization [1], and psychological disturbance [8]. As it is likely that these relate to seizure frequency, treatments aimed at seizure reduction should be considered in individuals with continued seizures **(IV/C)**.

The use of antiepileptic medication

Antiepileptic medication remains the mainstay of treatment options for people with epilepsy and this is also the case for those with an associated intellectual disability. The higher seizure frequency and greater seizure-related pathology, including sudden unexpected death in epilepsy (SUDEP), should make a vigorous evidence-based approach to treatment essential.

Ideally our approach would be backed up by high-quality evidence-based data on drug efficacy and associated safety parameters. Unfortunately, as we have already mentioned, whilst there is an intellectual disability-based evidence base, which will be discussed later, it is relatively small and cannot guide many treatment decisions. The reasons for this may largely relate to difficulties in organizing trials in those without capacity but may well be compounded by a lack of prioritizing this most needy of populations.

The clearest data on AED efficacy come from a recent Cochrane review [9]. The Cochrane review involves a systematic assessment of all papers in the field. The key outcome indicators used are the same as for the general epilepsy population: seizure and side effect variables. Unfortunately the quality of side effect assessment is very variable in these studies. This in the main relates to the use of non-validated measures to measure significant side effects such as behavioral or cognitive change. These factors notwithstanding, the data from studies in intellectual disability are valuable to clinical practice.

The review identified several relevant randomized controlled trials (RCTs). Of these, some were for drugs that are no longer in routine clinical usage, such as cinromide [10] and flunarizine [11]. The remaining studies were, in general, performed on mixed adolescent and adult samples or on a population of individuals with Lennox-Gastaut syndrome. Table 3 shows the key findings in these clinical trials **(Ib/A)**.

It is unfortunate that outside of the trial of rufinamide [12] **(Ib/A)**, there are no RCTs for other significant new AEDs. These include tiagabine, levetiracetam, pregabalin, zonisamide, eslicarbazepine and lacosamide. The lack of RCT evidence does not preclude the usage of these drugs **(III/B)**. Alternative data to guide practice can be found in various case series performed in samples of adults with an intellectual disability. We will not describe these studies in this chapter; they exist for most new AEDs and provide useful data on retention in the main; however, the data provided are not placebo-controlled or comparative, so whilst they can inform practice, the evidence level is low **(III/B)**.

In summary, strong evidence exists that AEDs have a significant impact on seizure reduction and seizure freedom in adults with an intellectual disability **(Ib/A)**. Evidence for a significant impact on behavior is rare in those studies that have explored it, and in essence the side effect profile is similar to that seen in the general epilepsy population, particularly for

Table 3. Randomized controlled trials in people with an intellectual disability and epilepsy. *Adapted from Beavis J, et al [9].*

Study population	Side effect data	Efficacy data
Child and adolescent study of lamotrigine vs. placebo in refractory generalized epilepsy [30]	No adverse effects were reported during the lamotrigine phase in the double-blind period. When receiving placebo during the double-blind phase, 10 patients complained of fatigue and four had more intense seizures. No withdrawals were reported due to adverse events.	One patient was seizure-free during the lamotrigine treatment phase. Nine of 15 children who completed the double-blind phase achieved a greater than 50% seizure reduction. The authors noted in their study a clear difference in behavior and alertness between the lamotrigine-treated patients and the placebo-treated patients, even without concomitant seizure reduction.
Lamotrigine vs. placebo in patients with Lennox-Gastaut syndrome [31]	There were no significant differences between the groups in the incidence of adverse events except for colds or viral illnesses, which were more common in the lamotrigine group (p=0.05), compared to the placebo group. Three patients in the lamotrigine group and seven in the placebo group withdrew from the study due to adverse events. The adverse event most frequently responsible for withdrawal was clinical deterioration of seizure control (one in the lamotrigine group, six in the placebo group). Seven patients in the lamotrigine group (9%) and six in the placebo group (7%) reported a rash which led to the withdrawal of two lamotrigine-treated patients and one placebo-treated patient, all of whom were also receiving valproate.	33% of lamotrigine-treated patients and 16% of placebo-treated patients had a reduction of at least 50% in the frequency of all types of major seizures (p=0.01). Significantly more lamotrigine-treated patients than placebo-treated patients had a reduction of at least 50% in the frequency of drop attacks and tonic-clonic seizures (p=0.04 and p=0.007). Median reduction from baseline for all major seizures in the lamotrigine-treated group was 32% and in the placebo-treated group was 9% (p=0.002) during a 16-week treatment period. The results were similar when drop attacks and tonic-clonic attacks were examined separately.

Table 3 continued. Randomized controlled trials in people with an intellectual disability and epilepsy. *Adapted from Beavis J, et al [9].*

Study population	Side effect data	Efficacy data
Adult learning disability comparison of gabapentin vs. lamotrigine in partial seizures [28]	The overall incidence of adverse events was similar in both treatment groups (62% with gabapentin and 50% with lamotrigine). Approximately 10% reported serious adverse events on gabapentin and 11% on lamotrigine. Drug-related adverse events were 33% (13) in the gabapentin group and 25% (11) in the lamotrigine group. 8% (three) and 9% (four) of patients were withdrawn due to adverse events in the gabapentin and lamotrigine groups, respectively. One patient on gabapentin was withdrawn due to vomiting (considered probably drug-related); three patients on lamotrigine were withdrawn due to rash and peripheral edema. One patient treated with gabapentin died due to myocardial infarction but this was not considered to be study drug-related.	The percentage of patients achieving a greater than or equal to 50% reduction in seizure frequency on gabapentin was 50% and on lamotrigine was 48.6%, showing no significant difference. Mean percentage reduction in seizure frequency of 50.6% in the gabapentin group and 50.8% reduction in the lamotrigine group. Three (7.7%) patients on gabapentin and five (11.4%) patients on lamotrigine were seizure-free during a 10-week minimum evaluation phase. The key carer rating scale showed significant improvement in seizure severity in the gabapentin-treated patients and also in the lamotrigine comparator treated patients. The physician's rating scale showed significant improvement in seizure severity in the gabapentin-treated group. Behavioral outcomes: Crawford reported data using the Crichton Royal Behaviour Rating Scale, which showed significant improvement in co-operation and restlessness in the gabapentin-treated patients, compared to baseline. Significant differences between the gabapentin and lamotrigine groups were seen in communication, co-operation and restlessness on the Crichton Royal Behaviour Scale. Total score also improved significantly (p=0.01) in the gabapentin group but not in lamotrigine patients. The Whelan and Speake Rating Scale measuring challenging behavior showed gabapentin was similar to lamotrigine with both drugs reducing the level of challenging behavior as a total score over the duration of the trial.

Table 3 *continued*. Randomized controlled trials in people with an intellectual disability and epilepsy. *Adapted from Beavis J, et al* [9].

Study population	Side effect data	Efficacy data
Adult learning disability placebo-controlled trial of topiramate in focal seizures [29]	92% of patients in the topiramate group and 84% in the placebo group reported adverse events. Sixteen percent of the topiramate group reported serious adverse events, possibly drug-related in four cases and 11% in the placebo group. The number of patients reporting at least one adverse event leading to a permanent stop in study medication was 18.9% (n=7) in the topiramate group and 16.2% (n=6) in the placebo group. One patient died in the active group following hospitalization with increasing drowsiness and confusion. This was reported as likely to be associated with the drug by the investigator.	No significant difference (p=0.099) in the reduction in mean total seizure frequency between the topiramate-treated group (32.43 ± 46.59% reduction) and the placebo group (1.08 ± 80.63% reduction) during a 12-week treatment period. No statistical difference between the topiramate- and placebo-treated groups in the number of responders: 29.7% and 25.7%, respectively. There was no significant difference between the topiramate- and placebo-treated groups in the mean total EOS (Epilepsy Outcome Scale) scores, mean total ABC (Aberrant Behaviour Checklist) or mean total ELDQOL (Epilepsy and Learning Disabilities Quality of Life) scores. There was, however, a trend toward significance for improvement of the mean ELDQOL behavior subscale score for patients treated with topiramate.
Topiramate in patients with Lennox-Gastaut syndrome [32]	23% of topiramate-treated patients had severe adverse events, compared with 10% of the placebo-treated patients. Three patients in the placebo group and nine in the topiramate-treated group experienced at least one adverse event that required either a dosage reduction or temporary discontinuation of treatment. These adverse events included nervousness, personality disorder, nausea, arthrosis, rash and urinary incontinence in the placebo group and gait abnormality, fatigue, pallor, aggressive reaction, personality disorder, somnolence and agitation in the topiramate group. However, no patient discontinued the study due to an adverse event.	The percentage of patients with a 50% or greater reduction from baseline in major seizures (drop attacks and tonic-clonic seizures) during the double-blind phase was significantly greater in the topiramate group compared to placebo (33% versus 8%, p=0.002). There was no significant difference between the treatment group and the placebo group with respect to all seizures in the 50% or greater responder group. Eight topiramate-treated (17%) versus two (4%) placebo-treated patients had a 75% or greater reduction in major seizure rates and one patient in the topiramate group was free of major seizures during the double-blind phase. During the double-blind phase, 28% (13/46) of the topiramate-treated patients achieved a 50% or greater reduction in drop attacks compared to 14% (7/49) of the placebo-treated patients.

Table 3 continued. Randomized controlled trials in people with an intellectual disability and epilepsy. *Adapted from Beavis J, et al* [9].

Study population	Side effect data	Efficacy data
		A 75% or greater reduction in the frequency of drop attacks was achieved in 17% (8/46) of the topiramate group and 6% (3/49) of the placebo group. Median percentage reduction from baseline in the average monthly seizure rate for generalized and partial seizures was 20.6% for the topiramate group and 8.8% for the placebo group, which was not significant. However, the median percentage reduction from baseline in the average monthly seizure rate of drop attacks was significantly greater for the topiramate group (14.8%) compared to the placebo-treated group, a 5.1% increase (p=0.041) during a treatment period of 11 weeks. The median percentage reduction from baseline in the average monthly rate of major seizures (drop attacks and tonic-clonic seizures) in the topiramate group was 25.8% as compared to a 5.2% increase in the placebo group (p=0.015).
Placebo-controlled study of rufinamide in Lennox-Gastaut [12]	41 patients (55.4%) in the rufinamide group and 28 (43.8%) in the placebo group had at least one adverse event believed to be drug-related. Common adverse events seen in at least 10% of the rufinamide group were somnolence (24.3% with rufinamide versus 12.5% with placebo) and vomiting (21.6% versus 6.3%). 6 patients (all on rufinamide) withdrew from the study due to side effects (vomiting [n=3], rash [n=2]).	There was a significant reduction in the median percentage of total seizure frequency between the rufinamide therapy group compared to the placebo group (32.7% versus 11.7%, p=0.0015). There was also a highly significant reduction in tonic-atonic ('drop attack') seizure frequency between the rufinamide group (42.5% median percentage reduction) and placebo (1.4% increase) (p <0.0001). There was a higher 50% responder rate in the rufinamide group compared with placebo for total seizures (p=0.0045) and tonic-atonic seizures (p=0.002), indicating similar rates of adverse effects between the group treated with rufinamide and placebo (81.1% and 81.3%, respectively).

identifiable effects such as weight loss. Drug choice should therefore be based on similar criteria to that for the general epilepsy population: gender, seizure type and syndrome classification (Ib/A). In addition to this, further consideration can be given to the availability of different formulations of the drugs, the potential for drug interaction and specific side effects such as weight loss in those with feeding difficulty (IV/C).

Epilepsy surgery

As described elsewhere in this book, resective and/or disconnection surgery provides for some individuals a potential cure for their seizure disorder; other surgical interventions can add further amelioration of seizure severity and/or frequency. There had been an historical concern [13] that the presence of a low IQ would in some way increase unsatisfactory outcomes from surgery. The reasons for this concern included the possibility that low IQ predicts more widespread brain damage and fears of a poor reaction to the postoperative process. However, a range of recent studies has come out in strong support of the inclusion of individuals with an intellectual disability in surgical programs (III/B). The evidence base does to some degree somewhat mirror the problems seen in pharmacological studies, in that there is an even greater absence of RCT data. Davis and colleagues [14] performed an audit on the 953 surgical evaluation cases seen between 1988 and 2007. The authors identified 69 patients with a verbal IQ of 70 or less; a trend to increasing assessment from 3% of the sample in the years 1988-1999 to 10% from 2000 to 2007 was noted. Individuals were still less likely to go through to surgery from the assessment process and in the main this was due to poorly localized seizures. The outcome in the 17 patients undergoing surgery was 10/15 (66%) Engel class 1A (seizure-free) at 1 year. This was comparable to the 68% seen in those with an IQ >70. Liang and colleagues [15] compared surgical technique in patients with intellectual disability and temporal lobe epilepsy. Anterior temporal lobectomy was compared with anterior temporal lobectomy and anterior corpus callosotomy. The authors suggested an improvement in outcome for those with the combined procedure over the pure temporal lobectomy (III/B).

Malmgren and colleagues [16] explored outcome from resective procedures identified in the Swedish National Epilepsy Surgery Register. The authors identified individuals who achieved sustained seizure freedom with or without aura at 2-year follow-up as a function of pre-operative IQ level categorized as IQ <50, IQ 50-69 and IQ >70. Important associated factors such as age at epilepsy onset, age at surgery and histopathological diagnosis were adjusted for. Resective epilepsy surgery meeting the follow-up requirements occurred in 448 individuals: 72 (16%) had an IQ <70 (18 with an IQ <50 and 54 with an IQ 50-69) and 376 an IQ >70. Three hundred and twenty-five patients underwent temporal lobe resections (TLR) and 123 underwent various extratemporal resections (XTLR). At the 2-year follow-up, 56% (252/448) of the patients were seizure-free: 22% (4/18) in the IQ <50 group, 37% (20/54) in the IQ 50-69 group and 61% (228/376) in the IQ >70 group. There was a significant relation between IQ category and seizure freedom (odds ratio [OR] 0.41, 95% confidence interval [CI], 0.27-0.62) and this held also when adjusting for clinical variables (OR 0.58 [95% CI, 0.35-0.95]). In this population-based epilepsy surgery series, IQ level was shown to be an independent predictor of seizure freedom at the 2-year follow-up. The authors concluded that low IQ should not exclude patients from resective epilepsy surgery, but should be recognized as an important prognostic factor (III/B).

Other groups have looked at surgery in specific populations associated with intellectual disability, in particular tuberous sclerosis. A review of epilepsy surgery in tuberous sclerosis [17] highlighted 25 articles pertaining to 177 patients. It is not clear from the review but none of these studies appear to have included randomization or controls. Seizure freedom was seen in 101 patients (57%) at a mean follow-up of 3.7 years and a large improvement seen in a further 32 (18%) of patients (III/B). Whilst extremely encouraging, the absence of a control group and the presence of potential reporting bias, i.e. only successful series reported, must be recognized.

Vagal nerve stimulation

A recent Cochrane review on non-pharmacological interventions for adults with an intellectual disability [18] failed to find RCT evidence for vagal nerve stimulation (VNS) (III/B), although its use is widespread in people with an intellectual disability. Clinicians must instead rely on case studies or on information from case series. The authors of a recent such case series of the use of VNS in individuals who had failed surgery [19] concluded that in this refractory population the impact of VNS is minimal on seizures but can be positive in terms of quality of life (III/B). This is of course an extremely refractory population. Other case series data, without control, such as that by Huf and colleagues [20], showed in their sample of 40 individuals undergoing VNS a 50% reduction in 11/40 subjects. A further pediatric study in children with autism and epilepsy [21] studied a small sample of eight children. The authors used a baseline control and a 2-year follow-up, and assessed outcome beyond seizure change to include autistic syndromes. No patients had a decrease in their seizures; minor improvements in general functioning were seen in three patients.

The conclusion of the authors should be noted that prospective studies are needed to prevent false expectations of improvement in the severely disabled group (IV/C).

Treating related comorbidity in the epilepsy clinic

The combination of epilepsy and an intellectual disability is in itself a comorbidity commonly compounded by further health conditions to such a degree that most treatment decisions and treatment outcomes will be affected by their presence (IV/C). The reason for this high rate of comorbidity is multifactorial with, most probably, very strong genetic factors. The dominant fact is the bidirectional link between epilepsy and lower levels of IQ and between the level of IQ and an increased prevalence of comorbidity. Many studies have identified the range of comorbidities experienced in people with an intellectual disability. Oeseburg identified comorbidities in a Dutch sample of adolescents with an intellectual disability [22]. Only 37% had no comorbidity with 28.9% having one comorbidity and 16.4% two comorbidities.

The distribution of these were somatic (21.6%), mental (22.6%) and a combination of somatic and mental (18.6%). It is beyond the scope of this chapter to address all these conditions and how they impact on epilepsy care, but the importance of behavioral and psychological comorbidity is explored briefly as an exemplar.

Challenging behavior and psychopathology

The high prevalence of challenging behavior in particular has an impact on the management of epilepsy (IV/C). As many as 30% [23] of adults may be on major tranquilizers with an associated risk of seizure worsening [24]. Whilst several studies have attempted to identify a link between epilepsy and challenging behavior in both adult and childhood populations [8, 25], in general, when studies have controlled with a gender and level of ability matched cohort, no such association is seen (III/B). Matthews and colleagues explored the presence of challenging behavior and psychopathology in a population of adults with an intellectual disability and when matching the epilepsy and non-epilepsy populations, this showed no difference in either psychopathology or challenging behavior. This is counterintuitive to clinical practice where a link between seizures and AEDs and behavior is often made (III/B). A recent paper [26] has thrown more light on the situation. This study prospectively compared an age, gender and level of ability matched cohort of patients with active epilepsy and intellectual disability. The study was the first to address the impact of active epilepsy and showed that continued seizures led to a seven-fold increased incidence of mental illness, often an organic disorder, but no increase in challenging behavior (IIa/B). Espie and colleagues [27] examined a large database of individuals with an intellectual disability and using a cross-sectional analysis showed that again psychopathology had some association with seizure variables but that challenging behavior was more closely linked to disability-related variables such as intellectual or motor disability (III/B).

Guidance does exist for the assessment of behavioral problems in adults with epilepsy and intellectual disability. The evidence base appears to show us that the epileptologist should focus on assessment for concurrent psychopathology in those with ongoing seizures, and where challenging behavior is present, ensure that appropriate care provision and support are available for the individual before attribution to epilepsy-related variables (IV/C).

Conclusions

The evidence-based management of epilepsy in people with an intellectual disability is crucial to the outcomes of this vulnerable population. Evidence for intervention is most strong for pharmacotherapy but even this remains weak in terms of newer medication and in particular for behavioral side effect profiles. Other interventions exist; resective surgery in particular seems promising. The presence of comorbidity has a major impact on management and clinicians need to be aware of this.

Key points	Evidence level
◆ Misdiagnosis of epilepsy in people with an intellectual disability is common; the prevalence ranges from 15-43%.	III/B
◆ Good clinical practice in assessing seizure impact focuses on supporting carers to provide appropriate information using diaries, education and scales such as the Epilepsy Outcome Scale.	IV/C
◆ Due to the impact of seizures, treatments aimed at seizure reduction should be considered in individuals with continued seizures.	IV/C
◆ Evidence exists for AED treatment in Lennox-Gastaut syndrome for lamotrigine, topiramate and rufinamide.	Ib/A
◆ Evidence exists for the use of AEDs in adults with an intellectual disability for lamotrigine, gabapentin and topiramate.	Ib/A
◆ For tiagabine, levetiracetam, pregabalin, zonisamide, eslicarbazepine and lacosamide, the lack of RCT evidence in people with an intellectual disability does not preclude the usage of these drugs.	III/B
◆ There is strong support for the inclusion of individuals with an intellectual disability in epilepsy surgical programs.	III/B
◆ The high prevalence of challenging behavior in particular has an impact on the management of epilepsy.	IV/C
◆ Continued seizures lead to an increased incidence of mental illness, often organic disorder, but no increase in challenging behavior.	IIa/B

References

1. Morgan CL, Baxter H, Kerr MP. Prevalence of epilepsy and associated health service utilization and mortality among patients with intellectual disability. *American Journal on Mental Retardation* 2003; 108(5): 293-300.
2. Kerr M. Behavioral assessment in mentally retarded and developmentally disabled patients with epilepsy. *Epilepsy Behav* 2003; 3: S14-7.
3. Chapman M, Iddon P, Atkinson K, *et al*. The misdiagnosis of epilepsy in people with intellectual disabilities: a systematic review. *Seizure* 2011; 20: 101-6.
4. Kerr M, Guidelines Working Group, Scheepers M, Arvio M, *et al*. Consensus guidelines into the management of epilepsy in adults with an intellectual disability. *J Intellect Disabil Res* 2009; 53: 687-94.
5. Watkins J, Espie CA, Curtice L, Mantala K, Corp A, Foley J. Development of a measure to assess the impact of epilepsy on people with an intellectual disability: the Glasgow Epilepsy Outcome Scale - Client version (GEOS-C). *J Intellect Disabil Res* 2006; 50(Pt 3): 161-71.
6. Kerr M, Espie C. Learning disability and epilepsy. 1, towards common outcome measures. *Seizure* 1997; 6(5): 331-6.
7. Opeskin K, Berkovic SF. Risk factors for sudden unexpected death in epilepsy: a controlled prospective study based on coroners cases. *Seizure* 2003; 12(7): 456-64.
8. Matthews T, Weston N, Baxter H, Felce D, Kerr M. A general practice-based prevalence study of epilepsy among adults with intellectual disabilities and of its association with psychiatric disorder, behaviour disturbance and carer stress. *J Intellectual Disability Research* 2008; 52: 163-73.

9.   Beavis J, Kerr M, Marson AG, Dojcinov I. Pharmacological interventions for epilepsy in people with intellectual disabilities. *Cochrane Database Syst Rev* 2011; 3: CD005399.

10. The Group for the Evaluation of Cinromide in the Lennox-Gastaut Syndrome. Double-blind, placebo-controlled evaluation of cinromide in patients with the Lennox-Gastaut Syndrome. *Epilepsia* 1989; 30: 422-9.

11. Battaglia A, Ferrari AR, Guerrini R. Double-blind placebo-controlled trial of flunarizine as add-on therapy in refractory childhood epilepsy. *Brain Dev* 1991; 13: 217-22.

12. Glauser T, Kluger G, Sachdeo R, Krauss G, Perdomo C, Arroyo S. Rufinamide for generalized seizures associated with Lennox-Gastaut syndrome. *Neurology* 2008; 70: 1950-8.

13. Levisohn PM. Epilepsy surgery in children with developmental disabilities. *Semin Pediatr Neurol* 2000; 7: 194-203.

14. Davies R, Baxendale S, Thompson P, Duncan JS. Epilepsy surgery for people with a low IQ. *Seizure* 2009; 18: 150-2.

15. Liang S, Li A, Zhao M, Jiang H, Meng X, Sun Y. Anterior temporal lobectomy combined with anterior corpus callosotomy in patients with temporal lobe epilepsy and mental retardation. *Seizure* 2010; 19(6): 330-4.

16. Malmgren K, Olsson I, Engman E, Flink R, Rydenhag B. Seizure outcome after resective epilepsy surgery in patients with low IQ. *Brain* 2008; 131(Pt 2): 535-42.

17. Jansen FE, van Huffelen AC, Algra A, van Nieuwenhuizen O. Epilepsy surgery in tuberous sclerosis: a systematic review. *Epilepsia* 2007; 48: 1477-84.

18. Beavis J, Kerr M, Marson AG, Dojcinov I. Non-pharmacological interventions for epilepsy in people with intellectual disabilities. *Cochrane Database Syst Rev* 2011; 4: CD005502.

19. Vale FL, Ahmadian A, Youssef AS, Tatum WO, Benbadis SR. Long-term outcome of vagus nerve stimulation therapy after failed epilepsy surgery. *Seizure* 2011; 20(3): 244-8.

20. Huf RL, Mamelak A, Kneedy-Cayem K. Vagus nerve stimulation therapy: 2-year prospective open-label study of 40 subjects with refractory epilepsy and low IQ who are living in long-term care facilities. *Epilepsy Behav* 2005; 6: 417-23.

21. Danielssona S, Viggedala G, Gillberg C, Olssona I. Lack of effects of vagus nerve stimulation on drug-resistant epilepsy in eight pediatric patients with autism spectrum disorders: a prospective 2-year follow-up study. *Epilepsy Behav* 2008; 12: 298-304.

22. Oeseburg B, Jansen DE, Dijkstra GJ, Groothoff JW, Reijneveld SA. Prevalence of chronic diseases in adolescents with intellectual disability. *Res Dev Disabil* 2010; 31: 698-704.

23. de Kuijper G, Hoekstra P, Visser F, Scholte FA, Penning C, Evenhuis H. Use of antipsychotic drugs in individuals with intellectual disability (ID) in the Netherlands: prevalence and reasons for prescription. *J Intellect Disabil Res* 2010; 54(7): 659-67.

24. Alper K, Schwartz KA, Kolts RL, Khan A. Seizure incidence in psychopharmacological clinical trials: an analysis of Food and Drug Administration (FDA) summary basis of approval reports. *Biol Psychiatry* 2007; 62(4): 345-54.

25. Lewis JN, Tonge BJ, Mowat DR, Einfeld SL, Siddons HM, Rees VW. Epilepsy and associated psychopathology in young people with intellectual disability. *J Paediatr Child Health* 2000; 36(2): 172-5.

26. Turky A, Felce D, Jones G, Kerr M. A prospective case control study of psychiatric disorders in adults with epilepsy and intellectual disability. *Epilepsia* 2011; in press.

27. Espie CA, Watkins J, Curtice L, *et al.* Psychopathology in people with epilepsy and intellectual disability; an investigation of potential explanatory variables. *J Neurol Neurosurg Psychiatry* 2003; 74: 1485-92.

28. Crawford P, Brown S, Kerr M; Parke Davis Clinical Trials Group. A randomized open-label study of gabapentin and lamotrigine in adults with learning disability and resistant epilepsy. *Seizure* 2001; 10: 107-15.

29. Kerr M, Baker G, Brodie MD. A randomized double-blind, placebo controlled trial of topiramate in adults with epilepsy and intellectual disability: impact on seizures, severity and quality of life. *Epilepsy Behav* 2005; 7: 472-80.

30. Eriksson A-S, Nergårdh A, Hoppu K. The efficacy of lamotrigine in children and adolescents with refractory generalized epilepsy: a randomized, double-blind, crossover study. *Epilepsia* 1998; 39: 495-501.

31. Motte J, Trevathan E, Arvidsson JFV, Barrera MN, Mullens EL, Manasco P, the Lamictal Lennox-Gastaut Study Group. Lamotrigine for generalized seizures associated with the Lennox-Gastaut syndrome. *N Engl J Med* 1997; 337: 1807-12.

32. Sachdeo RC, Glauser TA, Ritter F, Reife R, Lim P, Pledger G, the Topiramate YL Study Group. A double-blind, randomized trial of topiramate in Lennox-Gastaut syndrome. *Neurology* 1999; 52: 1882-7.

Chapter 13

Treatment of psychogenic non-epileptic seizures

Danielle G. Koby PhD, Staff Psychologist
Department of Psychiatry, Division of Behavioral Medicine
The Miriam Hospital, Providence, Rhode Island, USA

Introduction

Psychogenic non-epileptic seizures (PNES) have been defined as paroxysmal alterations in motor, sensory, autonomic, emotional, or conscious functioning, in the absence of epileptiform brain activity [1] and assumedly 'of psychological etiology' [2]. The incidence of PNES has been estimated at 1.4 [3] to 4.6 per 100,000 [4] in two population-based studies, or approximately 4% that of epilepsy. The documented prevalence of comorbid epilepsy among patients with PNES ranges from 5% to 50% depending on factors including precise diagnostic criteria and the duration of monitoring [5-7]. Video EEG is the widely accepted gold standard for diagnosis, although this should always be combined with clinical history given limits to interrater reliability on EEG alone [8]. The prevalence of PNES among patients admitted for epilepsy monitoring is estimated at 30% in tertiary care referral centers [9, 10]. The average diagnostic delay among patients with PNES has been estimated at 7.2 years (SD = 9.3 years) [11], during which the majority receive treatment with antiepileptic drugs (AEDs) [12, 13]. Symptom onset is typically in adulthood between the ages of 20 and 40 while PNES are also observed in childhood [14] and among older adults [15], and the majority of patients with PNES are female.

Patients with PNES comprise a frequently distressed as well as distressing population with poor health-related quality of life and significant symptom-related disability. The majority of comparisons have been made to patients with epilepsy, where patients with

PNES report more frequent seizures [16], worse health-related quality of life [17, 18], and more seizure-related impairment [16, 19]. Psychological distress has been linked to reduced quality of life over and above the contribution of seizure frequency [20] and psychiatric comorbidity is indeed common. While patients with PNES constitute an extremely heterogeneous group, certain clinical themes [21] are observed to recur including:

♦ recent or remote adversity or trauma [22, 23];
♦ clinically significant anxiety including post-traumatic stress disorder [24, 25];
♦ clinically significant depression [26, 27];
♦ persistent somatization [17, 28-30]; and
♦ a personality style characterized by dramatic, erratic, or unpredictable behavior [31, 32].

The need for treatment

On the whole, clinical outcomes for patients with PNES have been regarded as poor [33], particularly in the long term (Figure 1).

McKenzie et al [13] recently conducted a short-term assessment of 187 patients with PNES within 12 months of diagnosis. While 38% were seizure-free and an additional 23% reported at least a 50% reduction in seizure frequency, a concerning 18.7% reported a significant increase in the frequency of events. Such findings echo those of Arain et al [34] where 35% of patients were seizure-free 3 months after diagnosis yet only 50% of those with seizure remission had resumed working.

Jones et al [18] recently conducted a retrospective, longer-term follow-up study among 221 patients with PNES including 71 with at least some evidence of comorbid epilepsy. Sixty-one patients returned questionnaires an average of 4.1 (SD=2.7) years after diagnosis where patients were admitted for monitoring between 1995-2004 and follow-up was conducted between 2005-2006. Those returning questionnaires were more likely to have been monitored more recently, between 2001-2005 (77%; 47 patients). The majority (87%) of patients returning follow-up materials continued to have seizures during the preceding 12 months and greater than 50% reported two or more seizures per month; only 13% reported seizure freedom. Thirty-five point six percent (35.6%) reported subsequent PNES-related hospital stays while 39% continued to take AEDs. Nearly 66% were judged likely to have a psychiatric illness based on responses to a standardized measure of symptomatology*. Eleven point five percent (11.5%) of patients had what the authors classified as a 'good' outcome (seizure-free and employed/not on disability), while 47.5% had intermediate (seizure-free and unemployed/disabled, or independent with seizures) and poor (ongoing seizures and unemployed/disabled; 36.1%) outcomes, respectively. While the authors acknowledge the potential for bias given a low response rate (27%), similarly poor findings by Reuber et al [12] underscore the longstanding need for more effective, more accessible

* Symptom Checklist - 90.

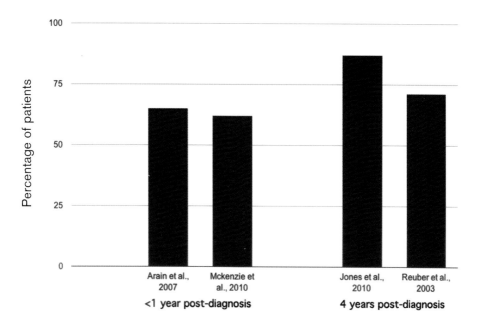

Figure 1. Patients with ongoing seizures after diagnosis.

treatments. In that early study, outcomes among 164 of 329 patients diagnosed with PNES (or PNES and epilepsy) were also recorded an average of 4.1 years after diagnosis. While a substantial proportion (41.5%) received inpatient psychiatric treatment during the follow-up period, as many as 71.2% continued to have seizures and 56.4% were dependent upon disability benefits.

Predictors of positive treatment outcome

Several studies have examined predictors of positive outcome following a diagnosis of PNES. As might be expected, Arain et al [34] identified higher education and being accompanied to the initial visit (a marker of social support) among predictors of seizure remission in the 35% of 48 patients surveyed 3 months after diagnosis. Interestingly, patients with less observably dramatic, e.g. motionless, seizures were also more likely to have achieved remission than were patients with motor seizures (p=0.01). Selwa et al [35] also documented greater rates of seizure remission among patients with motionless, e.g. 'catatonic', seizures (53%) compared to those with motor or 'thrashing' episodes (21% seizure-free) among 57 patients surveyed between 19 months and 4 years post-diagnosis.

Selwa and colleagues [35] further identified a shorter duration of illness among positive predictors of seizure remission such that 47% of seizure-free patients reported the onset of events within the last 1 year (mean 7 years, median 2 years). Put another way, 84% of patients whose events began in the last year reported at least a 90% reduction in the frequency of events at follow-up. Only 12% of those patients with no reduction in seizure frequency reported onset of events within the last year (mean duration 15 years, median 14 years). Reuber et al [12] (discussed above) similarly found patients with a younger age of onset, with less dramatic seizures, and with higher education to demonstrate better outcomes in regards to seizure frequency and employment.

The current state of treatment

In 2008, LaFrance [36] queried then current members of the American Epilepsy Society as to practices and 'treatment as usual' for PNES, finding that among 317 responding clinicians the majority referred patients to a psychiatrist (75%) or to a clinical psychologist or therapist (50%). More than two thirds (69%) continued to follow patients after a diagnosis had been rendered where treatment included withdrawal of anticonvulsant medications (83%) and prescriptions for psychotropic medications (47%). Psychotherapy and psycho-education were considered most efficacious treatments for PNES among nearly equal numbers of respondents (81% and 80%, respectively), while approximately one third endorsed pharmacotherapy.

Existing studies do suggest some benefit from psychological intervention in typical delivery settings. For example, Aboukasm and colleagues [37] retrospectively examined the outcome of psychotherapy or no intervention among 61 patients diagnosed with PNES across a 4-year period. Follow-up data were gathered an average of 22 months (range 6-30 months) after diagnosis. Comparisons were made between groups having received treatment including psychotherapy in various settings: within a comprehensive epilepsy treatment center (CEP;

n=16), community psychotherapy (n=25), or care from a CEP neurologist (n=15). A small no-treatment comparison group was also identified (n=5). Rates of seizure cessation at follow-up were 43.8%, 53.3%, 40%, and 0%, respectively, with no statistically significant differences detected between the three treatment groups. Improvements in quality of life were also uniform across the three treatment groups with no change reported among those receiving no intervention.

Consistent with Aboukasm and colleagues [37], Selwa *et al* [35] interviewed 57 patients between 19 months and 4 years post-diagnosis, finding that among those receiving mental health treatment at the time of follow-up (n=22), approximately half reported seizure freedom (27%) or a greater-than-90% reduction in seizure frequency (23%). Across the entire group of 57 patients, however, a similar 56% also reported substantial improvement, including 23 who were seizure-free and another nine patients with substantial (90%) reductions in seizure frequency. While study comparisons are complicated by numerous factors, findings nonetheless suggest potentially different needs for and responses to treatment among subgroups of patients, with corresponding uncertainties around how to identify these and deliver treatment.

Several thorough reviews of the available treatment literature have been conducted [38-40] including a Cochrane database review [41]. While the preponderance of available papers describes case studies or small case series, more recent investigations reflect increasingly sound experimental designs. In every case, conclusions have centered on a lack of sufficient evidence to support treatment efficacy and a corresponding call for further large-scale, well-designed treatment trials.

Methodology

A review of the literature was performed with the Scopus (from 1960) and PsychINFO (from 1806) databases. Keywords included: nonepileptic; non-epileptic; pseudoseizures; dissociative seizures; functional seizures; hysterical seizures; psychogenic seizures. The words 'attacks' and 'convulsions' were substituted for 'seizures' to ensure retrieval of all relevant studies. Prospective experimental or quasi-experimental studies providing clear descriptions of methods and results and published in English language journals were included in the current review. Case reports, case series, service reviews, conference presentations, and academic works, e.g. dissertations, were not included.

Results are displayed in Table 1 and discussed in the text in the context of seminal background and supporting research. The rationale for each category of intervention is briefly presented while investigations providing strong empirical support are highlighted.

Table 1. Summary of prospective treatment trials for PNES.

Reference	N	Design	Intervention	Classification
Diagnostic and psycho-educational interventions				
Zaroff *et al*, 2004 [42]	N=10	Open, uncontrolled, non-randomized	Psycho-educational group therapy	IIb/B
Hall-Patch *et al*, 2010 [43]	N=50	Open, uncontrolled, non-randomized	Patient education	IIb/B
Cognitive behavioral interventions				
Ataoglu *et al*, 2003 [44]	T=15 C=15	Randomized controlled trial	Inpatient paradoxical vs. outpatient BZ	Ib/A
Goldstein *et al*, 2004 [45]	N=20	Open, uncontrolled, non-randomized	CBT	IIb/B
LaFrance *et al*, 2009 [25]	N=21	Open, uncontrolled, non-randomized	CBT	IIb/B
Goldstein *et al*, 2010 [46]	T=33 C=31	Randomized controlled trial	CBT vs. SMC	Ib/A
Psychodynamic and hypnosis-based interventions				
Moene *et al*, 2002 [47]	T=26 C=23	Randomized controlled trial	Inpatient hypnosis	Ib/A
Moene *et al*, 2003 [48]	T=24 C=25	Randomized controlled trial	Inpatient hypnosis	Ib/A
Barry *et al*, 2008 [49]	N=12	Open, uncontrolled, non-randomized	Group psychodynamic	IIb/B
Pharmacologic interventions				
LaFrance *et al*, 2010 [2]	T=19 P=19	Double-blind, randomized, placebo-controlled	Sertraline 50-200mg	Ib/A
Pintor *et al*, 2010 [50]	N=19	Open-label, non-randomized, uncontrolled	Venlafaxine 75-300mg	IIb/B
Oto *et al*, 2010 [51]	T=14 DT=11	Randomized controlled trial	Immediate vs. delayed AED withdrawal	Ib/A

T = treatment; DT = delayed treatment; C = control; P = placebo; CBT = cognitive-behavioral therapy; SMC = standard medical care; BZ = benzodiazepine

Evidence-based treatment modalities

Delivering the diagnosis

In an effort to maintain patients' engagement in care following the recognition of PNES, Shen and colleagues [52] developed a seven-step standardized protocol for presenting the diagnosis (Figure 2):

- A. The patient and family are engaged in discussion of one or more captured events and video of the event may be presented. Patients and family members are encouraged to verify that such events are representative of typical seizures and are given an opportunity to provide additional details such as memory for the events, subjective experience, etc.
- B. The "Good News" includes informing the patient and family that epilepsy is not present and thus a potentially lifelong regimen of anticonvulsant medications, possible surgeries, and ongoing seizure activity is not forecast.
- C. The "Bad News" includes an acknowledgement that "at this time we cannot tell you exactly what these spells are," yet with emphasis on preserving the patient-provider relationship, e.g. however, "we can continue to work together".
- D. Psychiatric care is recommended as "upsetting emotions of which the patient is not aware," have been implicated in the majority of cases. The authors note that at this point patients may become defensive or distressed.

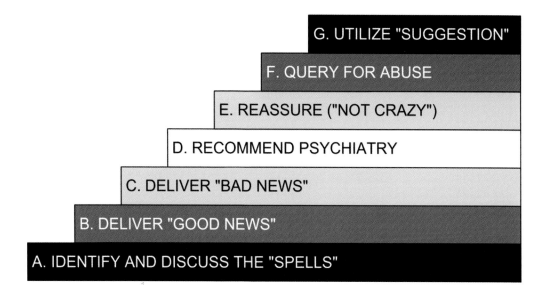

Figure 2. Components of the Shen et al protocol for presenting the diagnosis of PNES.

♦ E. It is explicitly stated that the patient is "not crazy," and is not deliberately producing the symptoms. Rather, symptoms are explained as occurring outside of awareness on a "subconscious" level. Reassurance is provided that counseling typically leads to improved control over the events.

♦ F. Clinicians are encouraged to gently broach the topic of sexual abuse and inquire as to whether this is a particular aspect of the patient's history as it has been found in many cases.

♦ G. Capitalizing on the "power of suggestion," patients are informed, "Spells may spontaneously resolve on their own with time". Emphasis is placed upon maintaining a positive outlook and attitude, identifying triggers, and initiating behavior change, e.g. slow breathing when seizure "warning signs" are detected.

The authors repeatedly stress that negative findings, e.g. no evidence for epilepsy, should be treated as a positive step forward in diagnosis and management as knowing what it is not is just as important as knowing what it is (particularly from the standpoint of avoiding potentially harmful treatments).

Beyond engaging patients in treatment as the authors had intended, several uncontrolled and non-randomized investigations suggest the effectiveness of the diagnostic protocol alone for reducing the frequency of non-epileptic events. In a comparative study, Berkhoff and colleagues [53] utilized the Shen *et al* protocol following placebo infusion to precipitate non-epileptic events. Among 10 patients with PNES, eight were seizure-free within 6 months, while the remaining two patients experienced at least a 50% reduction in seizure frequency. Farias *et al* [54] retrospectively examined the frequency of non-epileptic seizures on an epilepsy monitoring unit in the 24 hours immediately following diagnosis, where routine practice included utilization of the Shen protocol. Twenty-two patients with PNES were identified while 10 consecutively admitted patients with epilepsy served as a control comparison group. In each group patients continued to undergo video-EEG recording for 24 hours post-diagnosis (while doses of anticonvulsant medications were held constant). Patients with PNES displayed significantly fewer seizures after diagnosis (p=0.001) including no events among 18 (82%) patients and a greater than 50% reduction in seizure frequency among three additional patients with continuing yet less frequent events. Similar declines in seizure frequency were not observed among patients with epilepsy. Between-group comparisons revealed significant differences after (0.27 versus 1.1, p=0.008) but not before (1.6 versus 1.2, p=0.09) between patients with PNES and epilepsy, respectively.

Thompson and colleagues [55] later modified the Shen protocol such that video of any recorded events was presented only upon patient request, and inquiries were restricted to the broad experience of past trauma rather than sexual abuse specifically. Remaining elements of the original protocol included presenting the diagnosis with the "Good News" and the "Bad News", recommendations for psychotherapy, reassurance, and emphasis on the power of suggestion and hope for seizure remission with stress management and psychotherapy. In their naturalistic study of outcomes among 50 patients diagnosed with PNES, 48 patients completed follow-up at 2 years. Seizure remission was reported in 24 (50%) patients while 19 additional patients reported less intense or less frequent seizures.

Five patients reported no change in the frequency of their events including one ultimately diagnosed with a movement disorder and four failing to continue in psychotherapy; all patients attended at least one (range 1-8) psychotherapy session.

Recognizing persistent patient and provider confusion around the diagnosis of PNES, Hall-Patch et al [43] developed and evaluated a new strategy for communicating the diagnosis using a comprehensive patient education booklet (Figures 3 and 4). Treating neurologists in this investigation were provided with empirically supported guidelines for presenting the diagnosis as well as a checklist to aid in the presentation of key points.

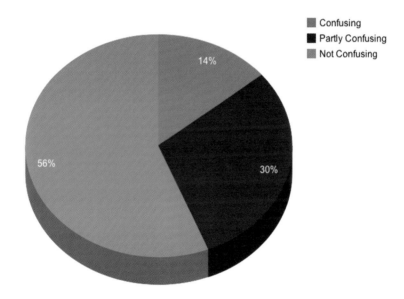

■ Confusing
■ Partly Confusing
■ Not Confusing

14%

56%

30%

Figure 3. Patient reported confusion after diagnosis. *Adapted from Hall-Patch L, et al, 2010* [43].

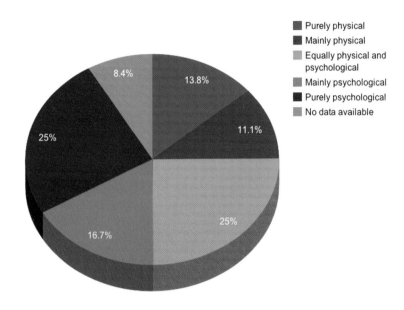

Figure 4. Attribution for symptoms after diagnosis. *Adapted from Hall-Patch L, et al, 2010* [43].

Fifty newly diagnosed patients participated in follow-up telephone interviews after 2 weeks. The majority of patients (70%) were satisfied with their consultation and more than half (56%) denied any confusion associated with their visit or the information presented. Notably, only 13% of patients attributed their symptoms to purely physical causes after receiving the education materials. Four of the six most common attributions for seizures were psychosocial in nature, e.g. stress, worry, family problems, attitude, etc. Seizure freedom was reported among 6% and 14% of patients at 2 and 11 weeks, respectively, while 63% reported a greater than 50% reduction in seizure frequency. Results from this well-designed uncontrolled prospective study provide preliminary evidence for the efficacy of a diagnostic communication strategy involving provider training and patient education materials.

Psycho-educational interventions

Psycho-education often involves the provision of contextual information, e.g. basic physiology, introductory psychological concepts, such that patients have a framework for understanding and approaching their symptoms. Moving beyond presenting the diagnosis as in Shen and others, Zaroff *et al* [42] conducted a 10-week psycho-educational group intervention among 10 patients with PNES. A different topic related to PNES symptomatology and self-management was presented each week including the potential roles of trauma and abuse, emotional distress, typical patterns of somatization, and ways of coping with stress. Among seven patients completing the majority of sessions, four were seizure-free at the conclusion of treatment. Notably, this seizure-free group included three who reported no weekly seizures at the time of treatment onset, reflecting the potential impact of diagnosis alone. An additional two patients experienced a decrease in seizure frequency over the course of the study. Significant improvements were further observed on standardized measures of dissociative and post-traumatic symptoms, likely stemming from the emphasis placed on discussion of motor symptoms arising as a function of dissociation. This small, non-controlled, group-based intervention suggests that discussion of psychological concepts in non-epileptic events may have beneficial effects on seizure frequency as well as frequently observed patterns of affective distress, e.g. post-traumatic responding.

Despite increasingly widespread knowledge of PNES and attention to best practices in delivering the diagnosis, patient comprehension and acceptance remains incomplete. As Jones and colleagues [18] recently found, 19% of 61 patients responding to questionnaires a mean 4.1 years after diagnosis continued to believe they had epilepsy while a similar percentage were unclear on the diagnosis. Approximately 56% acknowledged the diagnosis of PNES or another psychological or stress-related condition while 5% maintained comorbid epilepsy. As these data were collected at follow-up it was not possible to evaluate patient understanding at the time of diagnosis as a predictor of outcome. Incomplete acceptance and understanding of the diagnosis may also play a significant role in compliance with ongoing care. As discussed in Arain and colleagues [34], only 29% of 165 patients with a diagnosis of PNES returned for neurology follow-up at 3 months despite extensive discussion of the diagnosis. Follow-through on referrals to neuropsychology (18%) and psychiatry (12%) were also limited although the study design did not allow for assessment of understanding as a predictor of treatment outcome.

While seemingly obvious, understanding and acceptance of the diagnosis and awareness of psychological factors perpetuating PNES may be critical to the cessation of events. Carton and colleagues [56] specifically examined the roles of understanding and of patients' reaction to the diagnosis of PNES among factors in outcome between 6 months and 7 years post-diagnosis. Among 84 newly diagnosed patients, approximately two thirds voiced no awareness or acceptance of psychological factors playing a causal role in their experience of seizures. The most frequently reported reaction to diagnosis was confusion among 38% of the sample while nearly 20% of patients cited anger and appeared to harbor particular discontent around previous misdiagnoses of epilepsy. The majority (65%) of the 72 participants receiving a recommendation for psychotherapy did follow through although the median number of sessions attended was two (2; range 1-36). Twenty-eight percent of those surveyed reported cessation of PNES while the 48% continuing to experience events reported at least a 50% decrease in event frequency. Between-group comparisons revealed more frequent confused ($x^2 = 0.6$, p <0.001) and angry ($x^2 = 9.1$, p <0.002) reactions to diagnosis among those continuing to experience seizures.

Evidence from numerous studies thus raises questions as to interactions between patient understanding, acceptance, participation in follow-up care, and clinical improvement. An example may be found in Aboukasm et al [37], where significantly fewer or no seizures were reported among 70% of patients receiving psychotherapy within a comprehensive epilepsy center. An informal measure of patients' understanding of their diagnosis was greatest among those receiving CEP-based psychotherapy and significantly greater than those receiving physician intervention (p <0.001) and no treatment (p <0.001). Understanding of diagnosis was also better with community-based psychotherapy than with no treatment although no relationship was described between patients' understanding per se and the likelihood of seizure remission or quality of life. The authors do, however, assert that 68.8% and 73.3% of patients in the CEP therapy and physician intervention groups were either seizure-free or had experienced a "significant reduction" in the frequency of events, respectively. This was compared to 48% among patients receiving community psychotherapy from providers not necessarily familiar with the diagnosis and unlikely to utilize aspects of the Shen protocol. They make the point that intervention by clinicians unfamiliar with the diagnosis yielded outcomes consistent with previous literature (cessation among 40% of patients and "significant reduction" among another 8%).

Sophisticated research designs are needed to reveal the active and critical elements of treatment, and interactions between such. Without systematically assessing patient understanding and acceptance of the diagnosis (modeled after the Shen protocol with presentation of videotaped events), we are unable to evaluate this as a predictor of compliance with treatment recommendations (all patients attended at least five psychotherapy sessions).

Psychodynamic and hypnosis-based interventions

The use of hypnosis to effect change in somatoform and conversion disorders is based upon early theoretical conceptualizations of physical symptoms as dissociative phenomena, displayed by highly suggestible or highly hypnotizable individuals. French neurologist Jean-Martin Charcot was a developer and strong proponent of this treatment approach during his tenure at the Salpêtrière. Within this context non-epileptic events and conversion disorders more broadly formally became the subject of psychiatric intervention.

The preponderance of literature examining hypnosis in the treatment of PNES is limited to anecdotal reports and case studies, yet a recent Cochrane database review [41] highlighted two investigations of adequate methodological rigor conducted by Moene and colleagues. In the first of these [47], researchers examined the incremental benefit of hypnosis above existing treatment for patients with conversion symptoms, with particular attention to the predictive value of hypnotizability on response to treatment. Forty-nine (49) patients were randomized and 45 completed treatment, including hypnosis plus standard care (n=24) and attention control (n=21). Standard care included a multidisciplinary approach of nursing, psychiatry, physical therapy, and individual and group psychotherapy. Hypnosis was conducted across eight weekly 1-hour sessions with suggestions for physical movement incompatible with symptoms as well as expression of presumed "pent-up or dissociated emotions." The control condition included eight sessions with a therapist in which patients considered the role of recent and remote stressors in their current experience of symptoms.

At the conclusion of treatment and at an 8-month follow-up point, all patients reported less emotional distress and less symptom-related disability while displaying fewer physical symptoms on videotape assessment. There was no added improvement among patients receiving hypnosis, however, and hypnotizability did not predict treatment outcome or changes in pre- to post-treatment or follow-up values on any measure. The majority of gains on outcome measures were detected at post- rather than at mid-treatment, leading the authors to conclude 4 weeks may generally be too short a window within which to observe and expect change in this patient population.

In 2003, Moene and colleagues [48] randomized patients to hypnosis (n=20) or wait list control (n=24). Treatment consisted of 10 weekly sessions of hypnosis emphasizing direct symptom alleviation with conditioned cues or emotional insight and affective expression. Videotaped assessment of symptoms and pre- and post-treatment (6 months after the 10th session) was conducted while there was no follow-up in the wait list control. At follow-up patients receiving hypnosis were significantly improved on observable behavioral symptoms and reported less symptom-related disability compared to their own functioning at baseline and compared to patients in the wait list control condition. There were no between-group differences on a measure of overall psychiatric symptom severity and while hypnotizability was a stronger predictor of outcome than patient expectations, it did not independently predict response to treatment with any significance.

As noted in a recent Cochrane database review of treatments for non-epileptic attack disorder (PNES), each of the studies by Moene *et al* included patients with conversion symptoms other than those mimicking epilepsy, e.g. gait disturbance, tremor, while the minority appeared to have had seizures or other seizure-like events. While randomization was adequate, intervention guided by training and adherence to a manual, and assessors blinded to treatment condition, outcome measures did not include pre- or post-treatment estimates of seizure frequency nor was concurrent use of medications clearly documented (although these were largely held constant by the authors' report).

Barry *et al* [49] more recently conducted a pilot trial of psychodynamic group therapy among 11 patients with PNES, seven of whom completed at least 75% of the 32 90-minute weekly group sessions. Treatment was focused on discussion of PNES "as an expression of hidden/unconscious emotions," promoting constructive verbal expression of distress. At the conclusion of treatment, 4/7 (57%) of patients were seizure-free while an additional two patients reported a decrease in seizure frequency. Mean values on a standardized measure of depressive symptoms* were also significantly decreased at the conclusion of treatment from 16.6 (SD=10.1) to 13.3 (SD=7.9), p <0.01, with additional significant reductions on the majority (10/12) subscales on a widely-used measure of psychiatric symptomatology **.

Isolating the effect of this intervention is complicated by the likely significant contribution of outside sources of support. Specifically, participants were encouraged to seek out concurrent individual therapy and in fact five patients did so with one of the primary authors while another patient intermittently saw a former therapist. Additionally, "outside of the group, the members created a support network to discuss events that occurred between sessions," and these issues and developments were also brought into the group for discussion in session.

Taken together, results of the described studies speak to the aforementioned need for additional, more rigorous and controlled treatment research of this type within this patient population. Owing to a host of historical and sociological factors there is at least the perception of less standardized research involving psychodynamic and hypnosis-based interventions [57]. As with all psychological methods the central tasks of operationally defining change and achieving methodological specificity may be complicated by what are often subjective, largely unobservable experiences of the patient, and this may be particularly true in the case of dynamic therapies. Across all treatment indications psychodynamic psychotherapies generally appear favorable to no treatment although further randomized controlled trials are needed to assess their contribution relative to active, empirically supported interventions [58].

Cognitive behavioral therapy

Cognitive behavioral therapy (CBT) includes a wide array of problem-focused interventions broadly targeting patients' beliefs, corresponding actions (or inaction) toward the goal of alleviating affective distress. Therapeutic interventions falling under the rubric of cognitive and behavioral therapies constitute first-line treatments for symptoms commonly observed in PNES, including anxiety [59, 60], depression [61, 62], and post-traumatic stress disorder [63, 64]. There is also consistent evidence for the effectiveness of CBT in the treatment of most somatoform disorders [65-67] with the notable exception of conversion disorders for which further research is needed [68].

Paradoxical intervention, or "prescribing the symptom," may broadly be categorized as a cognitive behavioral intervention in which patients confront and test beliefs about how much control they are able to exert over symptoms. During paradoxical interventions patients are also exposed to internal (mental, physical) and external (environmental) triggers for symptoms, as they are asked to recreate and re-experience situations in which symptom attacks first occurred. Ataoglu and colleagues [44] conducted a randomized intervention study

---

* Beck Depression Inventory-II.
** Symptom Checklist - 90.

comparing inpatient paradoxical therapy to outpatient pharmacotherapy for patients with conversion disorder symptoms resembling PNES. Fifteen patients randomized to receive paradoxical intervention were hospitalized for approximately 3 weeks with twice-daily treatment sessions. A randomly assigned comparison group of 15 outpatients were treated with diazepam 5-15mg daily with biweekly follow-up; between-group comparisons were made after 6 weeks. Patients treated with paradoxical and exposure-based interventions demonstrated greater reductions (p=.015) on a standardized clinician-administered measure of anxiety* (27.60, SD=5.00 vs. 14.47, SD=5.36). While patients treated with diazepam also displayed significant reductions in anxiety (mean=25.60, SD=4.27 vs. 18.20, SD=3.47), those receiving paradoxical therapy were more likely to be seizure-free (14/15 compared with 9/15) at the end of 6 weeks.

In an open-label pilot study, Goldstein et al [45] evaluated the efficacy of a cognitive behavioral intervention primarily targeting fear and avoidance. In this model seizures were seen as "dissociative responses to arousal arising when the patient is confronted with intolerable or fearful circumstances," ultimately maintained by anxious and avoidant cognitions and behaviors. Twenty tertiary care outpatients with PNES and no EEG evidence of epilepsy were invited to participate in 12-weekly outpatient sessions with concurrent withdrawal of AEDs. Among 16 patients completing treatment, 25% were seizure-free at the end of treatment and 43.8% were seizure-free at a 6-month follow-up point. Seizure remission was associated with shorter duration of illness (15.5 months [range 3-168] versus 29.5 months [range 12-90]). The majority (81.3%) of treatment completers reported a 50% or greater reduction in seizure frequency at 6 months. Additionally, treatment completers demonstrated significant reductions in anxiety, depression, fear, and avoidance behavior on standardized measures **, and reported improvement in work status with six individuals working fulltime after 6 months versus only one at the outset of treatment.

Based upon their previous work, Goldstein and colleagues then conducted the only randomized controlled trial [46] of (the same) cognitive behavioral therapy among 66 patients with PNES without current or past epilepsy. Thirty-one patients were randomized to standard medical care (SMC) including supportive care as needed with a neuropsychiatrist, psycho-education, and supervised withdrawal of AEDs. Participants in the intervention group (n=33) were offered 12 sessions of CBT across 4 months in addition to SMC. Patients receiving cognitive behavioral intervention displayed significantly reduced median seizure frequency from pre- (12.0, IQR=22.50) to post-treatment (2.0, IQR=6.00) versus reductions from a median of 8.75, IQR=29.25 to 6.75 (IQR=38.63) with SMC. Non-significant trends were also reported for ongoing reductions in seizure frequency and for seizure freedom at 6 months with CBT as well as for participants to have achieved at least 3 months of seizure freedom. There were no changes in anxious or depressive symptoms or employment status between groups as a function of treatment. Despite conducting a well-designed trial, the authors reported several protocol violations, the majority necessitated by clinical need, that complicate interpretation of findings. They further cited low pre-treatment levels of anxious and depressive symptoms and thus less opportunity for change among likely contributors to negative findings.

* Hamilton Rating Scale for Anxiety.
** Hospital Anxiety and Depression Scale; Fear Questionnaire.

LaFrance and colleagues [25] also conducted an open trial of manualized cognitive behavioral therapy for patients with PNES consisting of 12 weekly sessions. The authors described their intervention as "Beckian-based CBT with reattribution of symptoms," indicating a strong cognitive component and emphasis upon identifying maladaptive, e.g. catastrophic, thoughts about symptoms. The authors also adapted their manual from a well-known manual for improving quality of life and functioning among patients with epilepsy, *Taking Control of your Epilepsy: a Workbook for Patients and Professionals* [69]. Significant improvement was noted in seizure frequency such that 76% of participants achieved a 50% or greater reduction in seizure frequency and 65% of participants were seizure-free by week 12. The median seizure frequency was reduced from eight to zero events per week throughout the course of treatment. Standardized measures* of depression, post-traumatic symptoms, quality of life, and overall psychiatric symptom severity were also improved as a function of treatment, including numerous reductions below the clinically significant range. There were no improvements, however, on a measure of dissociation** where scores remained suggestive of psychopathology.

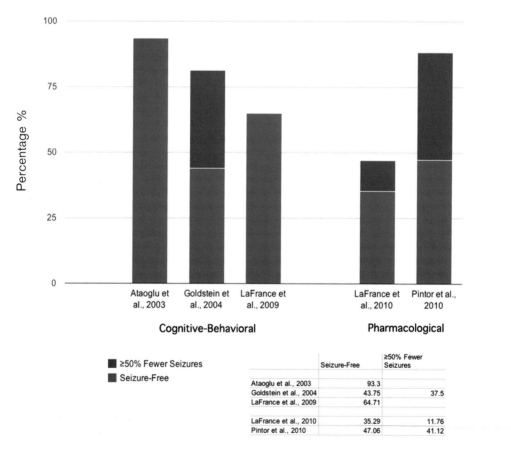

Figure 5. Seizure-related outcomes of well-designed cognitive behavioral and pharmacological interventions.

	Seizure-Free	≥50% Fewer Seizures
Ataoglu et al., 2003	93.3	
Goldstein et al., 2004	43.75	37.5
LaFrance et al., 2009	64.71	
LaFrance et al., 2010	35.29	11.76
Pintor et al., 2010	47.06	41.12

* Beck Depression Inventory-II; Davidson Trauma Scale; Quality of Life in Epilepsy - 31; Clinical Global Impressions.
** Dissociative Experiences Scale.

The work of Goldstein and of LaFrance and colleagues constitutes the strongest evidence (Ib/A) to date for the effectiveness of behavioral interventions – specifically cognitive behavioral – for PNES. While promising, significant replication of these studies is necessary before an adequate evidence base is considered established. Current and future work will compare the outcomes of distinct behavioral interventions and will likely examine the contribution of variables such as comorbid epilepsy and other psychiatric disorders, and will include assessment of longer-term clinical outcomes.

Pharmacotherapy

Psychotropic medications are often used to treat symptoms of anxiety and depression in PNES [36]. Given the role of accepted serotonergic dysfunction in such co-occurring affective disorders it has been hypothesized that compounds targeting this class of receptor may produce beneficial effects in patients with PNES. More broadly there is also some evidence to support the use of psychotropic medications in the treatment of somatoform symptoms [70-72].

Based upon their own initial pilot feasibility study [73], LaFrance and colleagues recently conducted the first double-blind, randomized, placebo-controlled trial of pharmacotherapy for PNES, utilizing flexible-dose sertraline. Participants randomly assigned to receive sertraline (n=19) or placebo (n=19) attended six bi-weekly visits with a neuropsychiatrist blinded to group assignment. All participants were started on 25mg (medication or placebo) following a 2-week baseline period and thereafter titrated up by 25 and then 50mg as tolerated without side effects. Ten patients tolerated the full 200mg daily dose of sertraline while 16 of 19 received at least 100mg. While considerable variability within the data obscured between-group reductions in mean seizure frequency, within-group analyses revealed a 45% reduction in weekly seizure counts among patients receiving sertraline compared to 8% with placebo. Three of 16 placebo treatment completers experienced a greater than 50% reduction in seizures compared with 8/17 sertraline treatment completers including six who were seizure-free. There were no between-group differences on standardized measures of depression, post-traumatic symptoms, dissociation, global psychopathology, quality of life, family functioning, or symptom-related disability, however, from baseline to the end of treatment.

Citing the apparent benefit of dual antidepressants over SSRIs in at least one previous investigation [74], Pintor and colleagues undertook a 5-month open-label trial of venlafaxine with the aim of evaluating reductions in depressive and anxious symptoms regardless of change in seizure frequency [50]. Participants initially received venlafaxine 75mg with individual doses adjusted up to 300mg based on clinical response and across five monthly visits with a study psychiatrist. Average daily doses increased from 157.9mg (SD=34.4) to 189.71 (SD=59.9) between follow-up months two through five. Participants' scores of standardized measures of anxiety and depression* revealed significant reductions in these symptoms throughout treatment. Specifically, group means on clinician-administered measures in the severe range at baseline were mild after 5 months with greater than 50% reductions in anxiety and

---

* Hamilton Anxiety and Depression Rating Scales; Hospital Anxiety and Depression Scale.

depression among 41.2% and 64.7% of participants, respectively. Additionally, 15/17 treatment completers (88.2%) experienced a 50% or greater reduction in seizure frequency including eight patients who were seizure-free.

Taken together, there is moderately strong (Ib/A) emerging evidence for the efficacy of pharmacotherapy to reduce PNES frequency and associated symptoms of anxiety and depression. Given the extremely small number of investigations to date, however, replication is necessary before prescriptions for psychotropics become a component of standard medical care. The existing studies are designed to address symptoms of affective distress and thus there remains the question of psychotropic effectiveness or appropriateness of this intervention among patients denying indications of anxiety, depression, or impulsivity. Behavioral and other intervention studies suggest that substantial numbers of patients with PNES receive pharmacotherapy during the course of the prolonged diagnostic and treatment processes [25, 75]. As Pintor and colleagues note in their discussion, previous research suggests that such patients receive higher doses of psychotropics for longer periods of time when compared to other patient populations. It therefore remains to be determined what components of the two described interventions differ from otherwise routine care. Given the current uncertainties around the choice of therapeutic agents and appropriate dosages, patients should be referred to a psychiatrist or neuropsychiatrist familiar with the treatment of non-epileptic seizures and other functional neurological symptoms.

Interpreting meaningful outcomes

As in treatment for epilepsy seizure, remission (rather reductions in the frequency of events) is frequently the goal of intervention for PNES as it has been associated with better quality of life. Indeed, among 30 patients with PNES interviewed approximately 18 months post-diagnosis, those with complete seizure remission (n=10) displayed significantly better quality of life as measured with the QOLIE-10 compared to those with ongoing seizure activity [76]. Notably, while another 17 patients (56%) achieved a 50% or greater reduction in seizure frequency there was no corresponding, proportional improvement in quality of life.

Debate exists, however, as to the contribution of seizure remission to other clinically significant outcomes, namely employment. Reuber *et al* [33] have utilized a designation system for outcomes in this patient group including the following:

- ongoing events;
- events stopped yet patient "unproductive"; and
- events stopped and patient "productive."

In this classification "unproductive" referred to the receipt of health-related government benefits whereas "productive" implied participation in gainful employment, education, or retirement due to old age rather than symptom-related disability.

In their assessment of 147 patients with PNES an average of 4.2 years after diagnosis, the vast majority (105 patients) continued to report seizure activity. This sample was composed of 86 patients with PNES only and 61 patients with comorbid events. For the total group, roughly equivalent numbers of patients reported cessation of seizures for greater than one year with and without productivity (n=24 and n=18, respectively). Notably, no significant difference was observed between the percentages of unproductive patients with ongoing (60%) or remitted (42.7%) seizures. Furthermore, the presence of seizures was not found to distinguish between patients receiving state disability benefits versus those who were not, leading the authors to conclude, "seizure control is not a major factor in the self-assessment and third-party assessment of disability in this patient group."

"Productive" patients in whom seizures had remitted displayed the lowest overall psychiatric symptom severity, while measures of affective distress did not distinguish patients with ongoing seizures from those who were seizure-free yet unproductive. Among all seizure-free patients productivity was associated with lower scores on measures of depression, overall psychiatric severity, and somatization, e.g. a tendency to experience physical symptoms in the context of emotional upset.

Subgroup analyses revealed contrasting patterns for patients with and without comorbid epilepsy. Among the 61 patients with epilepsy and PNES, productivity status was associated with overall psychiatric symptom severity in those patients who continued to have seizures. Among the 86 patients with exclusively non-epileptic events, ongoing seizure activity (rather than productivity) was associated with greater anxiety, depression, and global psychiatric symptom severity.

Clearly the pattern of relationships between seizure activity, productivity, and affective distress is complex. As nearly half of patients in whom PNES had ceased remained unproductive with psychiatric symptoms, Reuber et al suggest additional endpoints (beyond seizure remission or reduced seizure frequency) to better illustrate potentially significant consequences of intervention. They cite, for example, findings from the epilepsy literature in which quality of life has been independently correlated with measures of affective distress, e.g. depression, anxiety, seizure worry [77, 78] beyond indices of seizure control.

Additional issues in management

Withdrawal of anticonvulsant medications

Following a diagnosis of PNES, perhaps the most immediate question in the minds of patients and providers alike centers on continued use of anticonvulsant medications. While LaFrance [36] found that 83% of clinicians surveyed report tapering AEDs, questions are likely to surface around safety, timing, benefits and risks, and any ways to maximize the therapeutic impact of this intervention.

In 2005, Oto *et al* [79] conducted what was then the largest observational study of AED withdrawal among 78 patients with PNES, with the stated primary aim of assessing safety. The risk of undetected comorbid epilepsy was ostensibly lowered with exclusion criteria including clear description and observation of all current event types, no current or past events suspicious for epilepsy, no events in childhood (as vague descriptions frequently raised suspicions of epilepsy), and no interictal epileptiform abnormalities on EEG. Patients were those seeking treatment at a regional (secondary) referral center with an average age of 39.6 (SD=14.35), age of onset 32.4 years (SD=15.35), and thus apparent duration of events consistent with previous estimates (7.1 years) [11]. Six-month and 12-month follow-up data were collected and available for the majority (100% and 91%, respectively) at each time point. AEDs were initially prescribed by a neurologist or GP among 49% of patients while the median number of prescriptions was two (range 1-3; mean 1.4). Side effects were retrospectively reported by 20 patients (28%) while four patients (5%) reported increased attack frequency after starting AED therapy. Consistent with the assumed ineffectiveness of AEDs for PNES, only six patients (8%) initially experienced sustained improvements with medications while 27 (35%) reported temporary, unsustained improvement.

Following a standardized protocol specific to the compound prescribed (the reader is directed to this article for further detail), the authors accomplished withdrawal on an outpatient basis in 64 of 78 (82%) of patients. The majority followed the titration schedule as planned (57/64; 89%) while eight patients abruptly stopped medications after diagnosis of their own volition (n=5) or per their general practitioner (GP) (n=2). Fourteen patients were admitted for supervised withdrawal. While clearly written instructions were provided to GPs as well as to patients and families, two patients were re-started on AEDs by an emergency department physician in one case and by a non-compliant GP in another. These patients were subsequently withdrawn with no adverse consequences.

New types of attacks were observed in three patients including two with no apparent risk factors and one with a previously resected brain tumor (whose seizures started approximately 1 year after withdrawal, indicating a potentially new set of events). AED monotherapy was successful for seizure control in all three patients and at lower doses than what was previously utilized. As patients were closely monitored there were no adverse events. While 29% of patients reported at least one episode of PNES status (defined as prolonged events thought to be epilepsy and treated with AEDs) prior to withdrawal, only four patients had similar episodes upon discontinuation of anticonvulsants. There were no other ensuing events of any significance or negative valence.

The frequency of PNES decreased significantly between the point of referral (mean = 22.33 [SD=30.78]; median = 15) and 6-month follow-up (mean = 13.01 [SD= 38.46]; median = 2). There was a further significant decrease in seizure frequency at 12 months (9.01; SD=32.51; median 0), at which point 49% of patients (35/71) had been seizure-free for more than 2 months. Eight patients (10%) reported a temporary increase in seizure frequency immediately following withdrawal although this resolved in all cases. Approximately one quarter of patients voiced new medical or psychological complaints while 10 patients (13%) were started on new alternate medications, most often antidepressants (6/10). No acute psychiatric intervention was warranted in any case. The authors emphasize confidence in the exclusion of epilepsy as well as closely controlled monitoring to ensure safety.

Oto *et al* [51] subsequently conducted a randomized controlled trial of AED withdrawal among patients with PNES to determine any corresponding improvement in outcomes. Twenty-five patients were randomized to immediate (n=14) or delayed (n=11) withdrawal from anticonvulsant medications across two consecutive 9-month periods. Patients immediately tapered off AEDs showed a significant reduction in seizure frequency at 9 months from 20 (range = 5-720) to 2 (range 0-290), p=0.028. Rates of remission at 18 months were not statistically different, however, including 7/14 (50%) among those immediately tapered and 3/11 (27%) in those tapered after 9 months. Patients immediately withdrawn from AEDs showed significantly less use of rescue medication (0/14 versus 4/11, p=0.026) and patients in the immediate withdrawal group were more likely to endorse psychological causes for their seizures and to harbor positive beliefs about their ability to control symptoms. Notably, patients in each group were offered and participated in up to six sessions of CBT with a mean of four sessions attended in each group. Study limitations included small sample size and inadequate power as well as significant attention from staff perhaps obscuring the true effect of medication withdrawal.

Comorbid epilepsy and non-epileptic seizures

In the context of evidence-based treatment of epilepsy and related disorders, it is worth noting a small number of studies document the emergence of non-epileptic seizures following epilepsy surgery. The prevalence of PNES in post-surgical populations has been estimated at 1.8% to 3.6% in two original studies [80, 81]. Among 228 surgical patients with intractable epilepsy, Davies *et al* [82] also found de novo PNES in 3.5% (eight) patients between 6 weeks and 6 years after surgery (mean = 23 months).

As a caveat, several papers [83, 84] have anecdotally noted the development of non-epileptic seizures after head trauma or cranial surgery unrelated to epilepsy. Reuber *et al* [85] later reported on 17 patients for whom non-epileptic events began after intracranial surgery and 12 of whom also developed epileptic seizures confirmed by video EEG. Hudak [86] and colleagues highlighted the frequent finding of remote head injury among patients with NES referred for video-EEG monitoring; in their study, 33% had non-epileptic events following moderate-to-severe brain injury. Such reports, combined with the growing body of literature suggesting abnormal EEG in patients with PNES, may carry treatment implications in the future. At present it would seem prudent to recognize brain abnormalities among potential risk factors for the development of PNES.

The observance of PNES after surgery may variably represent a continuation of previously detected or undetected events, or the development of new events. Krahn [87] documented ongoing non-epileptic seizures in three patients after epilepsy surgery and new events among another three patients. The clinical significance of each is not yet known, nor has a link to successful or limited surgical outcomes been identified. Parra *et al* [80] described the later development of PNES among three patients with otherwise good surgical outcomes including two who were ultimately seizure-free with medications and one who experienced only monthly seizures. While there was a suspicion of comorbid non-epileptic events in one patient prior to surgery, the new seizures did not resemble previous epileptic events in any of the three. In a detailed case report, Montenegro et al [88] also highlighted non-epileptic events after surgery when ictal semiology is different than that previously observed.

Regarding predictors for developing non-epileptic events after surgery, Ney et al [81] recognized low full-scale IQ, significant postoperative psychopathology, and significant surgical complications. Davies et al [82] also noted post-surgical complications and pre-operative epilepsy-related psychiatric symptoms among patients developing de novo PNES. Glosser et al [89] did not find evidence of low IQ potentially related to the later development of epileptic events (after adolescence) among patients with new-onset PNES after surgery. They did observe a greater number of additional psychiatric problems in this group however, and suggest de novo PNES as one component of overall post-surgical "instability".

Prior to epilepsy surgery, rates of comorbid non-epileptic events among surgical candidates have been observed to be under 10% (8% [90]).

Castro and colleagues have outlined the evaluation and surgical management of patients with comorbid epilepsy and non-epileptic seizures [91], noting that epilepsy surgery may reduce the overall burden of disease if such seizures are the primary source of disability. They emphasize patient and family education around both types of events and encourage recognition of the two types of events. Reuber et al [92] examined outcomes following epilepsy surgery in 13 patients with comorbid epilepsy and PNES, seven of whom were seizure-free while the remainder demonstrated mixed outcomes.

There have been no published treatment studies specifically targeting NES among post-surgical patients with epilepsy and the majority of prospective treatment studies have excluded participants with comorbid events. A notable exception is the open trial conducted by LaFrance et al [25] in which three (of 21) enrolled PNES patients with comorbid epilepsy were able to clearly distinguish between their seizure types. While outcomes for this small subgroup were not separately reported it is logical to assume that cognitive and behavioral strategies targeting elements of a fear-avoidance model, e.g. "fear of the next seizure," might be beneficial in the management of epileptic as well as non-epileptic seizures. Additionally, as LaFrance and colleagues based their manualized treatment on adaptations from a workbook for managing epilepsy and improving quality of life, benefits would expectably extend to patients with comorbid events as well as those with PNES alone. Finally, LaFrance and colleagues also included two patients with comorbid events in their pharmacologic treatment trial yet complexities such as medication interactions necessitate significant future research.

Follow-up care

In a recent editorial, Kanner [93] advocated for the continued involvement of neurologists in the care of patients with PNES post-diagnosis. Central to his position is the prevention of harm – as may occur when patients unaccepting or not understanding of their diagnosis present for and receive inappropriate, potentially dangerous treatment. Additional benefits of follow-up care may include the recognition and diagnosis of other pseudoneurological complaints likely to accompany PNES, e.g. pain syndromes, the supervision of anticonvulsant tapers, clarification of the diagnosis in other medical settings, e.g. emergency, and communication and coordination of care with mental health providers. Carton *et al* [56] also stressed how the role of communication with other healthcare providers may be a critical component of care. They found that among 84 general practitioners contacted about the ongoing care of their PNES patients, 10 disagreed with the diagnosis and continued to prescribe anticonvulsant medications. In each case the corresponding patient reported ongoing seizures and five of the 10 had not accepted their events as non-epileptic in nature. The necessity of disseminating diagnostic and treatment information to patients' other providers is inadvertently underscored by the work of Arain *et al* [34] as well, in which only 29% of 165 patients with PNES returned to their treating neurologist for 3-month follow-up.

Throughout the process of diagnosis and treatment, LaFrance and Devinsky [94] do, however, caution against querying for "more affect and underlying issues than the neurologist/epileptologist was trained to deal with." They cite Harden and Ferrando's [95] discussion of the difficulties likely to arise in the management of patients with PNES, many of whom present with challenging psychiatric and characterological symptoms. Negative reactions, e.g. frustration, anger, disbelief, to the diagnosis may be elicited for both patient and physician, complicating the doctor-patient relationship and threatening the prospect of follow-up care. As such, Ferrando advised the early inclusion of psychiatry as a member of the treatment team, supporting and extending the established therapeutic relationship with the treating neurologist. Over time then a patient's gradual transition from neurologic to primary psychiatric care may feel less like abandonment and more like continued treatment with trusted providers.

Conclusions

While psychogenic non-epileptic seizures continue to present diagnostic and treatment challenges, the last decade has given rise to increasingly rigorous intervention research. Perhaps more so than in most areas of medicine, the process of treating PNES begins with a thorough evaluation and clear statement of what the symptoms are and are not. The importance of engaging patients, families, and existing treatment providers in a clear discussion of the diagnosis cannot be understated, first and foremost as it concerns minimizing the risk of inappropriate and unnecessary interventions. Consistent with clinical experience the literature offers sound evidence that anticonvulsant medications can be safely withdrawn under close supervision and with good communication between all treating providers. There is also recent evidence to suggest patient benefit from immediate rather than delayed withdrawal of AEDs.

Presenting the diagnosis in a clear, consistent, and patient-centered fashion may provide the necessary foundation for patients to engage in treatment. In some cases, making the diagnosis may in fact comprise the majority of clinical intervention while in others it may serve as a starting point for longer-term collaborative care. Given the growing body of literature on PNES we have an opportunity to transform what has been a diagnosis of exclusion, e.g. not epilepsy, into an increasingly approachable, identifiable, and treatable constellation of symptoms. The use and dissemination of patient (and provider) education materials, by increasing understanding of this disorder, may promote patient involvement in treatment while reducing the likelihood of inappropriate care.

Intervention research has also advanced to include two randomized controlled trials supporting the efficacy of:

- cognitive behavioral therapy over standard medical care; and
- psychopharmacologic treatment with sertraline over placebo.

Each of these trials demonstrated primary decreases in seizure frequency while preliminary open-label studies also revealed improvement on indices of mood and quality of life. While patients with PNES remain a heterogeneous population with multiple symptom etiologies, interventions targeting final common pathways, e.g. behavior, coping, or underlying biologic mechanisms, e.g. serotonergic dysfunction, may offer relief to the largest number of individuals. Future investigations will include replication and side-by-side comparisons of behavioral and pharmacological interventions compared to standard medical care.

Increased understanding of PNES has revealed targets for intervention beyond seizure remission, including decreased healthcare utilization, lower symptom-related disability, better health-related quality of life, and return to independent psychosocial, e.g. work, family, functioning. A central figure in the identification and early treatment of such patients, the neurologist has a unique opportunity to begin to illuminate a path back to health, optimally with the support and collaboration of a multidisciplinary team.

Key points	Evidence level
◆ Engage the patient in a clear, standardized discussion of diagnosis following the Shen or similar protocol.	IIb/B
◆ Initiate and closely supervise the withdrawal of anticonvulsant medications with clear communication to other treating providers.	Ib/A
◆ Develop and disseminate patient education materials to aid in the process of diagnosis, increase patient engagement, increase understanding among family members, and facilitate treatment.	IIb/B
◆ Refer the patient for psycho-educational intervention.	IIb/B
◆ Refer the patient for cognitive behavioral therapy.	Ib/A-IIb/B
◆ Refer the patient to a psychiatrist for pharmacotherapy with SSRIs or SNRIs.	Ib/A-IIb/B

References

1. Gumnit RJ, Gates JR. Psychogenic seizures. *Epilepsia* 1986; 27 Suppl 2: S124-9.
2. LaFrance WC, Jr., Keitner GI, Papandonatos GD, *et al.* Pilot pharmacologic randomized controlled trial for psychogenic nonepileptic seizures. *Neurology* 2010; 75: 1166-73.
3. Sigurdardottir KR, Olafsson E. Incidence of psychogenic seizures in adults: a population-based study in Iceland. *Epilepsia* 1998; 39: 749-52.
4. Szaflarski JP, Ficker DM, Cahill WT, *et al.* Four-year incidence of psychogenic nonepileptic seizures in adults in Hamilton County, OH. *Neurology* 2000; 55: 1561-3.
5. Martin RC, Burneo JG, Prasad A, *et al.* Frequency of epilepsy in patients with psychogenic seizures monitored by video-EEG. *Neurology* 2003; 61: 1791-2.
6. Mari F, Di Bonaventura C, Vanacore N, *et al.* Video-EEG study of psychogenic nonepileptic seizures: differential characteristics in patients with and without epilepsy. *Epilepsia* 2006; 47: 64-7.
7. Marchetti RL, Kurcgant D, Gallucci-Neto J, *et al.* Epilepsy in patients with psychogenic non-epileptic seizures. *Arq Neuropsiquiatr* 2010; 68: 168-73.
8. Benbadis SR, LaFrance WC, Papandonatos GD, *et al.* Interrater reliability of EEG-video monitoring. *Neurology* 2009; 73: 843-6.
9. Benbadis SR, Allen Hauser W. An estimate of the prevalence of psychogenic non-epileptic seizures. *Seizure* 2000; 9: 280-1.
10. Koby DG, Zirakzadeh A, Staab JP, *et al.* Questioning the role of abuse in behavioral spells and epilepsy. *Epilepsy Behav* 2010; 19: 584-90.
11. Reuber M, Fernandez G, Bauer J, *et al.* Diagnostic delay in psychogenic nonepileptic seizures. *Neurology* 2002; 58: 493-5.
12. Reuber M, Pukrop R, Bauer J, *et al.* Outcome in psychogenic nonepileptic seizures: 1 to 10-year follow-up in 164 patients. *Ann Neurol* 2003; 53: 305-11.
13. McKenzie P, Oto M, Russell A, *et al.* Early outcomes and predictors in 260 patients with psychogenic nonepileptic attacks. *Neurology* 2010; 74: 64-9.
14. Kotagal P, Costa M, Wyllie E, *et al.* Paroxysmal nonepileptic events in children and adolescents. *Pediatrics* 2002; 110: e46.
15. Behrouz R, Heriaud L, Benbadis SR. Late-onset psychogenic nonepileptic seizures. *Epilepsy Behav* 2006; 8: 649-50.
16. Al Marzooqi SM, Baker GA, Reilly J, *et al.* The perceived health status of people with psychologically derived non-epileptic attack disorder and epilepsy: a comparative study. *Seizure* 2004; 13: 71-5.
17. Testa SM, Schefft BK, Szaflarski JP, *et al.* Mood, personality, and health-related quality of life in epileptic and psychogenic seizure disorders. *Epilepsia* 2007; 48: 973-82.

18. Jones SG, O'Brien TJ, Adams SJ, *et al*. Clinical characteristics and outcome in patients with psychogenic nonepileptic seizures. *Psychosom Med* 2010; 72: 487-97.

19. Prigatano GP, Kirlin KA. Self-appraisal and objective assessment of cognitive and affective functioning in persons with epileptic and nonepileptic seizures. *Epilepsy Behav* 2009; 14: 387-92.

20. Lawton G, Mayor RJ, Howlett S, *et al*. Psychogenic nonepileptic seizures and health-related quality of life: the relationship with psychological distress and other physical symptoms. *Epilepsy Behav* 2009; 14: 167-71.

21. Rusch MD, Morris GL, Allen L, *et al*. Psychological treatment of nonepileptic events. *Epilepsy Behav* 2001; 2: 277-83.

22. Abubakr A, Kablinger A, Caldito G. Psychogenic seizures: clinical features and psychological analysis. *Epilepsy Behav* 2003; 4: 241-5.

23. Salmon P, Al-Marzooqi SM, Baker G, *et al*. Childhood family dysfunction and associated abuse in patients with nonepileptic seizures: towards a causal model. *Psychosom Med* 2003; 65: 695-700.

24. D'Alessio L, Giagante B, Oddo S, *et al*. Psychiatric disorders in patients with psychogenic non-epileptic seizures, with and without comorbid epilepsy. *Seizure* 2006; 15: 333-9.

25. LaFrance Jr WC, Miller IW, Ryan CE, *et al*. Cognitive behavioral therapy for psychogenic nonepileptic seizures. *Epilepsy Behav* 2009; 14: 591-6.

26. Szaflarski JP, Szaflarski M, Hughes C, *et al*. Psychopathology and quality of life: psychogenic non-epileptic seizures versus epilepsy. *Medical Science Monitor* 2003; 9: 113-8.

27. Mazza M, Marca GD, Martini A, *et al*. Non-epileptic seizures (NES) are predicted by depressive and dissociative symptoms. *Epilepsy Res* 2009; 84: 91-6.

28. Reuber M, House AO, Pukrop R, *et al*. Somatization, dissociation and general psychopathology in patients with psychogenic non-epileptic seizures. *Epilepsy Res* 2003; 57: 159-67.

29. Marchetti RL, Kurcgant D, Neto JG, *et al*. Psychiatric diagnoses of patients with psychogenic non-epileptic seizures. *Seizure* 2008; 17: 247-53.

30. Bodde NM, Bartelet DC, Ploegmakers M, *et al*. MMPI-II personality profiles of patients with psychogenic nonepileptic seizures. *Epilepsy Behav* 2011; 20: 674-80.

31. Galimberti CA, Teresa Ratti M, Murelli R, *et al*. Patients with psychogenic nonepileptic seizures, alone or epilepsy-associated, share a psychological profile distinct from that of epilepsy patients. *J Neurol* 2003; 250: 338-46.

32. Harden CL, Jovine L, Burgut FT, *et al*. A comparison of personality disorder characteristics of patients with nonepileptic psychogenic pseudoseizures with those of patients with epilepsy. *Epilepsy Behav* 2009; 14: 481-3.

33. Reuber M, Mitchell AJ, Howlett S, *et al*. Measuring outcome in psychogenic nonepileptic seizures: how relevant is seizure remission? *Epilepsia* 2005; 46: 1788-95.

34. Arain AM, Hamadani AM, Islam S, *et al*. Predictors of early seizure remission after diagnosis of psychogenic nonepileptic seizures. *Epilepsy Behav* 2007; 11: 409-12.

35. Selwa LM, Geyer J, Nikakhtar N, *et al*. Nonepileptic seizure outcome varies by type of spell and duration of illness. *Epilepsia* 2000; 41: 1330-4.

36. LaFrance Jr WC, Rusch MD, Machan JT. What is 'treatment as usual' for nonepileptic seizures? *Epilepsy Behav* 2008; 12: 388-94.

37. Aboukasm A, Mahr G, Gahry BR, *et al*. Retrospective analysis of the effects of psychotherapeutic interventions on outcomes of psychogenic nonepileptic seizures. *Epilepsia* 1998; 39: 470-3.

38. LaFrance Jr WC, Barry JJ. Update on treatments of psychological nonepileptic seizures. *Epilepsy Behav* 2005; 7: 364-74.

39. Gaynor D, Cock H, Agrawal N. Psychological treatments for functional non-epileptic attacks: a systematic review. *Acta Neuropsychiatrica* 2009; 21: 158-68.

40. LaFrance Jr WC, Devinsky O. The treatment of nonepileptic seizures: historical perspectives and future directions. *Epilepsia* 2004; 45: 15-21.

41. Baker GA, Brooks JL, Goodfellow L, *et al*. Treatments for non-epileptic attack disorder. *Cochrane Database Syst Rev* 2007; 24: CD006370.

42. Zaroff CM, Myers L, Barr WB, *et al*. Group psychoeducation as treatment for psychological nonepileptic seizures. *Epilepsy Behav* 2004; 5: 587-92.

43. Hall-Patch L, Brown R, House A, *et al*. Acceptability and effectiveness of a strategy for the communication of the diagnosis of psychogenic nonepileptic seizures. *Epilepsia* 2010; 51: 70-8.

44. Ataoglu A, Ozcetin A, Icmeli C, *et al.* Paradoxical therapy in conversion reaction. *J Korean Med Sci* 2003; 18: 581-4.
45. Goldstein LH, Deale AC, Mitchell-O'Malley SJ, *et al.* An evaluation of cognitive behavioral therapy as a treatment for dissociative seizures: a pilot study. *Cogn Behav Neurol* 2004; 17: 41-9.
46. Goldstein LH, Chalder T, Chigwedere C, *et al.* Cognitive-behavioral therapy for psychogenic nonepileptic seizures: a pilot RCT. *Neurology* 2010; 74: 1986-94.
47. Moene FC, Spinhoven P, Hoogduin KAL, *et al.* A randomised controlled clinical trial on the additional effect of hypnosis in a comprehensive treatment programme for in-patients with conversion disorder of the motor type. *Psychother Psychosom* 2002; 71: 66-76.
48. Moene FC, Spinhoven P, Hoogduin KAL, *et al.* A randomized controlled clinical trial of a hypnosis-based treatment for patients with conversion disorder, motor type. *Int J Clin Exp Hypn* 2003; 51: 29-50.
49. Barry JJ, Wittenberg D, Bullock KD, *et al.* Group therapy for patients with psychogenic nonepileptic seizures: a pilot study. *Epilepsy Behav* 2008; 13: 624-9.
50. Pintor L, Bailles E, Matrai S, *et al.* Efficiency of venlafaxine in patients with psychogenic nonepileptic seizures and anxiety and/or depressive disorders. *J Neuropsychiatry Clin Neurosci* 2010; 22: 401-8.
51. Oto M, Espie CA, Duncan R. An exploratory randomized controlled trial of immediate versus delayed withdrawal of antiepileptic drugs in patients with psychogenic nonepileptic attacks (PNEAs). *Epilepsia* 2010; 51: 1994-9.
52. Shen W, Bowman ES, Markand ON. Presenting the diagnosis of pseudoseizure. *Neurology* 1990; 40: 756-9.
53. Berkhoff M, Briellmann RS, Radanov BP, *et al.* Developmental background and outcome in patients with nonepileptic versus epileptic seizures: a controlled study. *Epilepsia* 1998; 39: 463-9.
54. Farias ST, Thieman C, Alsaadi TM. Psychogenic nonepileptic seizures: acute change in event frequency after presentation of the diagnosis. *Epilepsy Behav* 2003; 4: 424-9.
55. Thompson NC, Osorio I, Hunter EE. Nonepileptic seizures: reframing the diagnosis. *Perspect Psychiatr Care* 2005; 41: 71-8.
56. Carton S, Thompson PJ, Duncan JS. Non-epileptic seizures: patients' understanding and reaction to the diagnosis and impact on outcome. *Seizure* 2003; 12: 287-94.
57. Shedler J. The efficacy of psychodynamic psychotherapy. *Am Psychol* 2010; 65: 98-109.
58. Gerber AJ, Kocsis JH, Milrod BL, *et al.* A quality-based review of randomized controlled trials of psychodynamic psychotherapy. *Am J Psychiatry* 2011; 168: 19-28.
59. Arch JJ, Craske MG. First-line treatment: a critical appraisal of cognitive behavioral therapy developments and alternatives. *Psychiatr Clin North Am* 2009; 32: 525-47.
60. McHugh RK, Smits JA, Otto MW. Empirically supported treatments for panic disorder. *Psychiatr Clin North Am* 2009; 32: 593-610.
61. Haby MM, Donnelly M, Corry J, *et al.* Cognitive behavioural therapy for depression, panic disorder and generalized anxiety disorder: a meta-regression of factors that may predict outcome. *Aust N Z J Psychiatry* 2006; 40: 9-19.
62. Mor N, Haran D. Cognitive-behavioral therapy for depression. *Isr J Psychiatry Relat Sci* 2009; 46: 269-73.
63. Keane TM, Marshall AD, Taft CT. Posttraumatic stress disorder: etiology, epidemiology, and treatment outcome. *Annu Rev Clin Psychol* 2006; 2: 161-97.
64. Bisson JI, Ehlers A, Matthews R, *et al.* Psychological treatments for chronic post-traumatic stress disorder. Systematic review and meta-analysis. *Br J Psychiatry* 2007; 190: 97-104.
65. Allen LA, Woolfolk RL, Escobar JI, *et al.* Cognitive-behavioral therapy for somatization disorder: a randomized controlled trial. *Arch Intern Med* 2006; 166: 1512-8.
66. Kroenke K. Efficacy of treatment for somatoform disorders: a review of randomized controlled trials. *Psychosom Med* 2007; 69: 881-8.
67. Thompson R, Isaac CL, Rowse G, *et al.* What is it like to receive a diagnosis of nonepileptic seizures? *Epilepsy Behav* 2009; 14: 508-15.
68. Ruddy R, House A. Psychosocial interventions for conversion disorder. *Cochrane Database Syst Rev* 2005; 19: CD005331.
69. Reiter JM, Andrews D, Janis C. Taking Control of Your Epilepsy: A Workbook for Patients and Professionals. Santa Rosa, CA, USA: Andrews/Reiter Epilepsy Research Program, 1987.
70. Noyes R, Jr., Happel RL, Muller BA, *et al.* Fluvoxamine for somatoform disorders: an open trial. *Gen Hosp Psychiatry* 1998; 20: 339-44.

71. Aragona M, Bancheri L, Perinelli D, *et al*. Randomized double-blind comparison of serotonergic (Citalopram) versus noradrenergic (Reboxetine) reuptake inhibitors in outpatients with somatoform, DSM-IV-TR pain disorder. *Eur J Pain* 2005; 9: 33-8.

72. Kroenke K, Messina N, 3rd, Benattia I, *et al*. Venlafaxine extended release in the short-term treatment of depressed and anxious primary care patients with multisomatoform disorder. *J Clin Psychiatry* 2006; 67: 72-80.

73. LaFrance Jr WC, Blum AS, Miller IW, *et al*. Methodological issues in conducting treatment trials for psychological nonepileptic seizures. *J Neuropsychiatry Clin Neurosci* 2007; 19: 391-8.

74. Voon V, Lang AE. Antidepressant treatment outcomes of psychogenic movement disorder. *J Clin Psychiatry* 2005; 66: 1529-34.

75. Hantke NC, Doherty MJ, Haltiner AM. Medication use profiles in patients with psychogenic nonepileptic seizures. *Epilepsy Behav* 2007; 10: 333-5.

76. Quigg M, Armstrong RF, Farace E, *et al*. Quality of life outcome is associated with cessation rather than reduction of psychogenic nonepileptic seizures. *Epilepsy Behav* 2002; 3: 455-9.

77. Johnson EK, Jones JE, Seidenberg M, *et al*. The relative impact of anxiety, depression, and clinical seizure features on health-related quality of life in epilepsy. *Epilepsia* 2004; 45: 544-50.

78. Loring DW, Meador KJ, Lee GP. Determinants of quality of life in epilepsy. *Epilepsy Behav* 2004; 5: 976-80.

79. Oto M, Espie C, Pelosi A, *et al*. The safety of antiepileptic drug withdrawal in patients with non-epileptic seizures. *J Neurol Neurosurg Psychiatry* 2005; 76: 1682-5.

80. Parra J, Iriarte J, Kanner AM, *et al*. De novo psychogenic nonepileptic seizures after epilepsy surgery. *Epilepsia* 1998; 39: 474-7.

81. Ney GC, Barr WB, Napolitano C, *et al*. New-onset psychogenic seizures after surgery for epilepsy. *Arch Neurol* 1998; 55: 726-30.

82. Davies KG, Blumer DP, Lobo S, *et al*. De novo nonepileptic seizures after cranial surgery for epilepsy: incidence and risk factors. *Epilepsy Behav* 2000; 1: 436-43.

83. Nedvizhenko AA. Epileptic and hysterical seizures arising after craniocerebral trauma. *Klinicheskaya Meditsina* 1981; 59: 88-9.

84. Westbrook LE, Devinsky O, Geocadin R. Nonepileptic seizures after head injury. *Epilepsia* 1998; 39: 978-82.

85. Reuber M, Fernandez G, Helmstaedter C, *et al*. Evidence of brain abnormality in patients with psychogenic nonepileptic seizures. *Epilepsy Behav* 2002; 3: 249-54.

86. Hudak AM, Trivedi K, Harper CR, *et al*. Evaluation of seizure-like episodes in survivors of moderate and severe traumatic brain injury. *J Head Trauma Rehabil* 2004; 19: 290-5.

87. Krahn LE, Rummans TA, Sharbrough FW, *et al*. Pseudoseizures after epilepsy surgery. *Psychosomatics* 1995; 36: 487-93.

88. Montenegro MA, Guerreiro MM, Scotoni AE, *et al*. De novo psychogenic seizures after epilepsy surgery: case report. *Arq Neuropsiquiatr* 2000; 58: 535-7.

89. Glosser G, Roberts D, Glosser DS. Nonepileptic seizures after resective epilepsy surgery. *Epilepsia* 1999; 40: 1750-4.

90. Henry TR, Drury I. Non-epileptic seizures in temporal lobectomy candidates with medically refractory seizures. *Neurology* 1997; 48: 1374-82.

91. Castro LHM. Epilepsy surgery in patients with coexisting psychogenic nonepileptic seizures: diagnosis and treatment. *Journal of Epilepsy and Clinical Neurophysiology* 2007; 13: 36-8.

92. Reuber M, Kurthen M, Fernandez G, *et al*. Epilepsy surgery in patients with additional psychogenic seizures. *Arch Neurol* 2002; 59: 82-6.

93. Kanner AM. Is the neurologist's role over once the diagnosis of psychogenic nonepileptic seizures is made? No! *Epilepsy Behav* 2008; 12: 1-2.

94. LaFrance Jr WC, Devinsky O. Treatment of nonepileptic seizures. *Epilepsy Behav* 2002; 3 (5 Suppl): 19-23.

95. Harden CL, Ferrando SJ. Delivering the diagnosis of psychogenic pseudoseizures: should the neurologist or the psychiatrist be responsible? *Epilepsy Behav* 2001; 2: 519-23.

Index